MANUAL OF NEPHROLOGY
Seventh Edition

MANUAL OF NEPHROLOGY

Seventh Edition

Edited by

Robert W. Schrier, MD

Professor of Medicine
Division of Renal Disease and Hypertension
University of Colorado
Health Sciences Center
Aurora, Colorado

Wolters Kluwer | Lippincott Williams & Wilkins
Health

Philadelphia · Baltimore · New York · London
Buenos Aires · Hong Kong · Sydney · Tokyo

3/11
$64.99
MATT

Acquisitions Editor: Lisa McAllister
Managing Editor: Ryan Shaw
Developmental Editor: Stacey Jensen
Project Manager: Jennifer Harper
Senior Manufacturing Manager: Benjamin Rivera
Marketing Manager: Kimberly S. Schonberger
Designer: Terry Mallon
Production Services: Laserwords Private Limited, Chennai, India

Sixth edition, © 2005 Lippincott Williams & Wilkins
Fifth edition, © 1999 Lippincott Williams & Wilkins
Fourth edition, © 1995 Little, Brown & Co.

Library of Congress Cataloging-in-Publication Data
Manual of nephrology/edited by Robert W. Schrier.—7th ed.
    p.; cm.
    Includes bibliographical references and index.
    ISBN 978-0-7817-9619-4
    1. Kidneys—Diseases—Handbooks, manuals, etc. 2. Nephrology—Handbooks, manuals, etc.
I. Schrier, Robert W.
    [DNLM: 1. Kidney Diseases—diagnosis—Handbooks. 2. Kidney Diseases—therapy—Handbooks.
3. Metabolic Diseases—diagnosis—Handbooks. 4. Metabolic Diseases—therapy—Handbooks.
WJ 39 M294 2009]
    RC903.M194 2009
    616.6′1—dc22
                                                        2008032469

To purchase additional copies of this book, call our customer service department at (800) 638-3030 or fax orders to (301) 223-2320. International customers should call (301) 223-2300.

Visit Lippincott Williams & Wilkins on the Internet: at LWW.com. Lippincott Williams & Wilkins customer service representatives are available from 8:30 am to 6 pm, EST.

10 9 8 7 6 5 4 3 2 1

CONTENTS

$\mathcal{T}$he seventh edition of the *Manual of Nephrology* continues to focus on the practical clinical aspects of the diagnosis and management of patients with electrolyte and acid-base disorders, urinary tract infections, kidney stones, glomerulonephritis and vasculitis, acute or chronic renal failure, hypertension, hypertension and renal disease in pregnancy, and drug dosing with renal impairment. Because of the growing number of patients with end-stage renal disease (ESRD), separate chapters are now included on treatment by chronic renal replacement therapy with dialysis and kidney transplantation. The *Manual of Nephrology* should continue to be of excellent clinical value for those caregivers encountering patients with the above disorders. This would include house officers, medical students, primary care physicians, nephrology fellows, nurse practitioners, and busy subspecialists outside of nephrology.

I am very appreciative of the outstanding contributions by the authors who have made every effort to update each chapter with recent advances in the diagnosis and management of the spectrum of hypertensive and kidney disorders. This includes adding several new authors who are outstanding clinician-educators. The *Manual of Nephrology* is again dedicated to Professor Hugh de Wardener who has made enormous contributions to the fields of hypertension and nephrology as a clinician, scientist, and educator for over 60 years.

Robert W. Schrier, MD

Sharon G. Adler, MD
Professor of Medicine
Division of Nephrology and Hypertension
University of California
UCLA School of Medicine
Los Angeles, California

George R. Aronoff, MD
Professor of Medicine and Pharmacology
Chief Division of Nephrology
University of Louisville School of Medicine
Louisville, Kentucky

Phyllis August, MD
Professor of Medicine and Obstetrics
and Gynecology
Weill Medical College of
Cornell University
New York, New York

Tomas Berl, MD
Professor of Medicine
Division of Renal Diseases
and Hypertension
University of Colorado Health
Sciences Center
Aurora, Colorado

Michael E. Brier, PhD
Professor of Medicine
Division of Nephrology
University of Louisville School of Medicine
Research Health Scientist
Department of Veterans Affairs
Louisville, Kentucky

Michel Chonchol, MD
Associate Professor of Medicine
Division of Renal Diseases
and Hypertension
University of Colorado Health
Sciences Center
Aurora, Colorado

Robert E. Cronin, MD
Professor of Medicine
VA Medical Center
Dallas, Texas

Charles L. Edelstein, MD
Professor of Medicine
Division of Renal Diseases
and Hypertension
University of Colorado Health
Sciences Center
Aurora, Colorado

David H. Ellison, MD
Professor of Medicine
Head, Division of Nephrology
and Hypertension
Oregon Health and Science University
Portland, Oregon

Kenneth Fairley, MD
Professorial Associate
Department of Medicine
University of Melbourne Hospital
Melbourne, Australia

Sarah Faubel, MD
Assistant Professor of Medicine
Division of Renal Diseases
and Hypertension
University of Colorado Health
Sciences Center
Aurora, Colorado

Eric Gibney, MD
Assistant Professor of Medicine
Division of Renal Diseases
Virginia Commonwealth University
Richmond, Virginia

Alkesh Jani, MD
Associate Professor of Medicine
Division of Renal Diseases
and Hypertension
University of Colorado Health
Sciences Center
Aurora, Colorado

William D. Kaehny, MD
Professor of Medicine
Division of Renal Diseases
and Hypertension
University of Colorado Health
Sciences Center
Aurora, Colorado

Catherine L. Kelleher, MD
Associate Professor of Medicine
Division of Renal Diseases
and Hypertension
University of Colorado Health
Sciences Center
Aurora, Colorado

Marilyn E. Levi, MD
Associate Professor of Medicine
Division of Infectious Diseases
University of Colorado Health
Sciences Center
Aurora, Colorado

Stuart L. Linas, MD
Professor of Medicine
Division of Renal Diseases
and Hypertension
University of Colorado Health
Sciences Center
Aurora, Colorado

Rebecca Moore, MD
Fellow
Division of Renal Diseases
and Hypertension
University of Colorado Health
Sciences Center
Aurora, Colorado

Charles R. Nolan, MD
Professor of Medicine
University of Texas Health Sciences Center
at San Antonio
San Antonio, Texas

Chirag Parikh, MD
Associate Professor of Medicine
Division of Nephrology
Yale School of Medicine
New Haven, Connecticut

Jeffrey G. Penfield, MD
Assistant Professor of Medicine
University of Texas Southwestern
Medical Center
Veterans Affairs North Texas Health
Care System
Dallas, Texas

Robert F. Reilly, MD
Professor of Medicine
Division of Nephrology
Yale University Medical School
New Haven, Connecticut

L. Barth Reller, MD
Professor of Medicine and Pathology
Departments of Medicine and Pathology
Duke University Medical Center
Durham, North Carolina

Robert W. Schrier, MD
Professor of Medicine
Division of Renal Diseases
and Hypertension
University of Colorado Health
Sciences Center
Aurora, Colorado

David M. Spiegel, MD
Professor of Medicine
Division of Renal Diseases
and Hypertension
University of Colorado Health
Sciences Center
Aurora, Colorado

Alexander Wiseman, MD
Associate Professor of Medicine
Division of Renal Diseases
and Hypertension
University of Colorado Health
Sciences Center
Aurora, Colorado

Joshua M. Thurman, MD
Assistant Professor of Medicine
Division of Renal Diseases
and Hypertension
University of Colorado Health
Sciences Center
Aurora, Colorado

Amir S. A. Naderi, MD
Fellow of Nephrology
Johns Hopkins University
School of Medicine
Baltimore, Maryland

THE EDEMATOUS PATIENT: CARDIAC FAILURE, CIRRHOSIS, AND NEPHROTIC SYNDROME

Robert W. Schrier and David H. Ellison

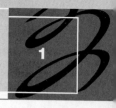

I. **BODY FLUID DISTRIBUTION.** Of the total fluids in the human body two-thirds reside inside the cell (i.e., intracellular fluid) and one-third resides outside cells [i.e., extracellular fluid (ECF)]. The patient with generalized edema has an excess of ECF. The ECF resides in two locations: in the vascular compartment (plasma fluid) and between the cells of the body, but outside of the vascular compartment (interstitial fluid). In the vascular compartment, approximately 85% of the fluid resides on the venous side of the circulation and 15% on the arterial side (Table 1-1). An excess of interstitial fluid constitutes edema. On applying digital pressure, the interstitial fluid can generally be moved from the area of pressure, leaving an indentation; this is described as *pitting* edema. This demonstrates that the excess interstitial fluid can move freely within its space between the body's cells. If digital pressure does not cause pitting in the edematous patient, then interstitial fluid cannot move freely. Such nonpitting edema can occur with lymphatic obstruction (i.e., lymphedema) or regional fibrosis of subcutaneous tissue, which may occur with chronic venous stasis.

Although generalized edema always signifies an excess of ECF, specifically in the interstitial compartment, the intravascular volume may be decreased, normal, or increased. For example, because two-thirds of ECF resides in the interstitial space and only one-third in the intravascular compartment, a rise in total ECF volume may occur as a consequence of excess interstitial fluid (i.e., generalized edema) although intravascular volume is decreased.

A. **Starling's law** states that the rate of fluid movement across a capillary wall is proportional to the hydraulic permeability of the capillary, the transcapillary hydrostatic pressure difference, and the transcapillary oncotic pressure difference. As shown in Figure 1-1, under normal conditions, fluid leaves the capillary at the arterial end because the transcapillary hydrostatic pressure difference favoring transudation exceeds the transcapillary oncotic pressure difference, which favors fluid resorption. In contrast, fluid returns to the capillary at the venous end because the transcapillary oncotic pressure difference exceeds the hydrostatic pressure difference. Because serum albumin is the major determinant of capillary oncotic pressure, which acts to maintain fluid in the capillary, hypoalbuminemia can lead to excess transudation of fluid from the vascular to interstitial compartment. Although hypoalbuminemia might be expected to lead commonly to edema, several factors act to buffer the effects of hypoalbuminemia on fluid transudation. First, an increase in transudation tends to dilute interstitial fluid, thereby reducing the interstitial protein concentration. Second, increases in interstitial fluid volume increase interstitial hydrostatic pressure. Third, the lymphatic flow into the jugular veins, which returns transudated fluid to the circulation, increases. In fact, in cirrhosis, where hepatic fibrosis causes high capillary hydrostatic pressures in association with hypoalbuminemia, the lymphatic flow can increase 20-fold to 20 L per day, attenuating the tendency to accumulate interstitial fluid. When these buffering factors are overwhelmed, interstitial fluid accumulation can lead to edema. Another factor that must be borne in mind as a cause of edema is an increase in the fluid permeability of the capillary wall (an increase in hydraulic conductivity). This increase is the cause of edema associated with hypersensitivity reactions and angioneurotic edema, and it may be a factor in edema associated with diabetes mellitus and idiopathic cyclic edema.

B. These comments refer to **generalized edema** (i.e., an increase in total body interstitial fluid), but it should be noted that such edema still may have a **predilection**

TABLE 1-1   Body Fluid Distribution

Compartment	Amount	Volume (L) in 70-kg man
Total body fluid	60% of body weight	42
Intracellular fluid (ICF)	40% of body weight	28
Extracellular fluid (ECF)	20% of body weight	14
Interstitial fluid	Two-thirds of ECF	9.4
Plasma fluid	One-third of ECF	4.6
Venous fluid	85% of plasma fluid	3.9
Arterial fluid	15% of plasma fluid	0.7

for specific areas of the body for various reasons. With cirrhosis, edema formation has a predilection for abdominal cavity because of portal hypertension as has already been mentioned. With the normal hours of upright posture, an accumulation of the edema fluid in the lower extremities should be expected, whereas excessive hours at bed rest in the supine position predispose to edema accumulation in the sacral and periorbital areas of the body. The physician must also be aware of the potential presence of localized edema, which must be differentiated from generalized edema.

C. Although generalized edema may have a predilection for certain body sites, it is nevertheless a **total-body phenomenon** of excessive interstitial fluid. Localized edema, on the other hand, is caused by local factors and therefore is not a total-body phenomenon. Venous obstruction, as can occur with thrombophlebitis, may cause localized edema of one lower extremity. Lymphatic obstruction (e.g., from malignancy) can also cause an excessive accumulation of interstitial fluid and, therefore, localized edema. The physical examination of a patient with ankle edema should, therefore, include a search for venous incompetence (e.g., varicose veins) and for evidence of lymphatic disease. It should be recognized, however, that deep venous disease may not be detectable on physical examination and therefore

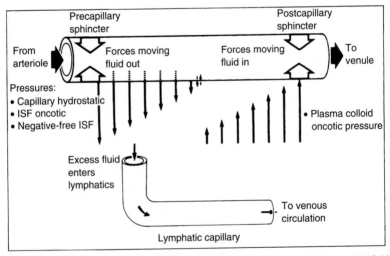

Figure 1-1. Effect of Starling forces on fluid movement across capillary wall. ISF, interstitial fluid.

may necessitate other diagnostic approaches (e.g., noninvasive ultrasonography). Therefore, if the venous disease is bilateral, the physician may mistakenly search for causes of generalized edema (e.g., cardiac failure and cirrhosis), when indeed the bilateral ankle edema is due to local factors. Pelvic lymphatic obstruction (e.g., malignancy) can also cause bilateral lower-extremity edema and thereby mimic generalized edema. Trauma, burns, inflammation, and cellulitis are other causes of localized edema.

II. **BODY FLUID VOLUME REGULATION.** The edematous patient has long presented a challenge in the understanding of body fluid volume regulation. In the healthy subject, if ECF is expanded by the administration of isotonic saline, the kidney will excrete the excessive amount of sodium and water, thereby returning ECF volume to normal. Such an important role of the kidney in volume regulation has been recognized for many years. What has not been understood, however, is why the kidneys continue to retain sodium and water in the edematous patient. It is understandable that when kidney disease is present and renal function is markedly impaired (i.e., acute or chronic renal failure), the kidney continues to retain sodium and water even to a degree causing hypertension and pulmonary edema. Much more perplexing are those circumstances in which the kidneys are known to be normal and yet continue to retain sodium and water in spite of the expansion of ECF and edema formation (e.g., cirrhosis, congestive heart failure). For example, if the kidneys from a cirrhotic patient are transplanted to a patient with end-stage renal disease but without liver disease, excessive renal sodium and water retention no longer occur. The conclusion has emerged, therefore, that neither total ECF nor its interstitial component, both of which are expanded in the patient with generalized edema, is the modulator of renal sodium and water excretion. Rather, as Peters suggested in the 1950s, some body fluid compartment other than total ECF or interstitial fluid volume must be the regulator of renal sodium and water excretion.

A. The term *effective blood volume* was coined to describe this undefined, enigmatic body fluid compartment that signals the kidney, through unknown pathways, to retain sodium and water in spite of an expansion of total ECF. That the kidney must be responding to cardiac output was suggested, providing an explanation for sodium and water retention in low-output cardiac failure. This idea, however, did not provide a universal explanation for generalized edema because many patients with decompensated cirrhosis, who were avidly retaining sodium and water, were found to have normal or elevated cardiac outputs.

B. **Total plasma or blood volume** was then considered as a possible candidate for the effective blood volume modulating renal sodium and water excretion. However, it was soon apparent that expanded plasma and blood volumes were frequently present in the renal sodium and water-retaining states, such as congestive heart failure and cirrhosis. The venous component of the plasma in the circulation has also been proposed as the modulator of renal sodium and water excretion and thereby of volume regulation, because a rise in the left atrial pressure is known to cause a water diuresis and natriuresis, mediated in part by a suppression of vasopressin and a decrease in neurally mediated renal vascular resistance. A rise in right and left atrial pressure also has been found to cause a rise in atrial natriuretic peptide. However, despite these effects on the low-pressure venous side of the circulation, renal sodium and water retention are hallmarks of congestive heart failure, a situation in which pressures in the atria and venous component of the circulation are routinely increased.

C. The **arterial portion of body fluids** (Table 1-1) is the remaining component that may be pivotal in the regulation of renal sodium and water excretion. More recently, the relationship between cardiac output and systemic arterial resistance [the effective arterial blood volume (EABV)] has been proposed as a predominant regulator of renal sodium and water reabsorption. This relationship establishes the "fullness" of the arterial vascular tree. In this context, a primary decrease in cardiac output or systemic arterial vasodilation, or a combination thereof, may cause arterial underfilling and thereby initiate and sustain a renal sodium and water-retaining state, which leads to generalized edema. The sodium- and water-retaining states that are initiated by a decline in cardiac output are shown

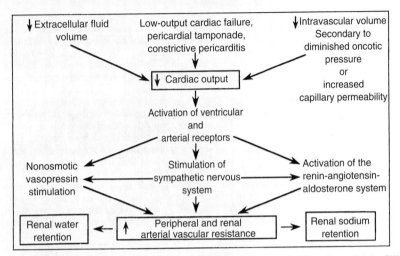

Figure 1-2. Decreased cardiac output as the initiator of arterial underfilling. (From Schrier RW. A unifying hypothesis of body fluid volume regulation. *J R Coll Physicians Lond* 1992;26:296. Reprinted with permission.)

in Figure 1-2 and include (a) ECF volume depletion (e.g., diarrhea, vomiting, hemorrhage); (b) low-output cardiac failure, pericardial tamponade, and constrictive pericarditis; (c) intravascular volume depletion secondary to protein loss and hypoalbuminemia (e.g., nephrotic syndrome, burns or other protein-losing dermopathies, protein-losing enteropathy), and (d) increased capillary permeability (capillary leak syndrome). The causes of increased renal sodium and water retention leading to generalized edema that are initiated by primary systemic arterial vasodilation are equally numerous and are shown in Figure 1-3. Severe anemia, beriberi,

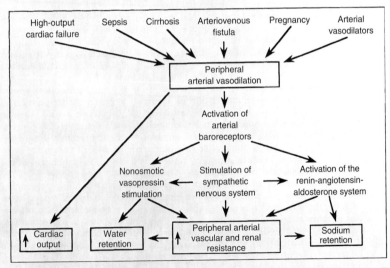

Figure 1-3. Systemic arterial vasodilation as the initiator of arterial underfilling. (From Schrier RW. A unifying hypothesis of body fluid volume regulation. *J R Coll Physicians Lond* 1992;26:296. Reprinted with permission.)

Paget's disease, and thyrotoxicosis are causes of high-output cardiac failure that may lead to sodium and water retention by the normal kidney. A wide-open large arteriovenous fistula, hepatic cirrhosis, sepsis, pregnancy, and vasodilating drugs (e.g., minoxidil or hydralazine) are other causes of systemic arterial vasodilation that decrease renal sodium and water excretion.

D. Two major **compensatory processes** protect against arterial underfilling, as defined by the interrelationship of cardiac output and systemic arterial vascular resistance. One compensatory process is very rapid and consists of a neurohumoral and systemic hemodynamic response. The other is slower and involves renal sodium and water retention. In the edematous patient, these compensatory responses have occurred to varying degrees depending on the time point when the patient is seen during the clinical course. Because of the occurrence of these compensatory processes, mean arterial pressure is a poor index of the integrity of the arterial circulation. Whether a primary fall in cardiac output or systemic arterial vasodilation is the initiator of arterial underfilling, the compensatory responses are quite similar. As depicted in Figures 1-2 and 1-3, the common neurohumoral response to a decreased EABV involves the stimulation of three vasoconstrictor pathways, namely the sympathetic nervous system, angiotensin, and vasopressin. In addition to direct effects, the sympathetic nervous system also increases angiotensin and vasopressin because increases in central sympathetic hypothalamic input and β-adrenergic stimulation through the renal nerves are important components of the increased nonosmotic vasopressin release and stimulation of renin secretion, respectively. With a primary fall in cardiac output or primary systemic arterial vasodilation, secondary increases in systemic arterial vascular resistance or cardiac output occur, respectively, to acutely maintain arterial pressure. This rapid compensation allows time for the slower renal sodium and water retention to occur and further attenuate arterial circulatory underfilling. With a decrease in ECF volume, such as occurs with acute gastrointestinal losses, sufficient sodium and water retention can occur to restore cardiac output to normal and therefore terminate renal sodium and water retention before edema forms. Such may not be the case with low-output cardiac failure because even these compensatory responses may not restore cardiac output totally to normal.

1. Therefore, the **neurohumoral** and **renal sodium- and water-retaining mechanisms** persist as important compensatory processes in maintaining EABV. However, neither the acute nor the chronic compensatory mechanisms are successful in restoring cardiac contractility, or reversing cardiac tamponade or constrictive pericardial tamponade. Compensatory renal sodium and water retention occurs with an expansion of the venous side of the circulation as arterial vascular filling improves but does not return to normal. The resultant rise in venous pressure enhances capillary hydrostatic pressure and thereby transudation of fluid into the interstitial fluid, with resultant edema formation. In hypoalbuminemia and the capillary leak syndrome, excessive transudation of fluid occurs across the capillary bed and also prevents the restoration of cardiac output; therefore, continuous renal sodium and water retention occurs and causes edema formation.

2. Systemic arterial vasodilation, the other major initiator of arterial underfilling, also generally cannot be totally reversed by the compensatory mechanisms and therefore may lead to edema formation. Systemic arterial vasodilation results in dilatation of precapillary arteriolar sphincters, thereby increasing capillary hydrostatic pressure and probably capillary surface area. A larger proportion of retained sodium and water therefore is transudated across the capillary bed into the interstitium in these edematous disorders (Fig. 1-3).

E. Another reason why low cardiac output or systemic arterial vasodilation may lead to edema formation is the inability of patients with these disorders, as compared with healthy subjects, to escape from the **sodium-retaining effect of aldosterone** (Fig. 1-4). In the healthy subject receiving large exogenous doses of aldosterone or another mineralocorticoid hormone, ECF expansion is associated with a rise in the glomerular filtration rate and a decrease in proximal tubular

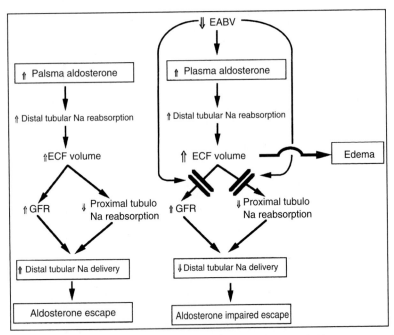

Figure 1-4. Aldosterone escape in a healthy subject (left side) and failure of aldosterone escape in patients with arterial underfilling (right side). (EABV, effective arterial blood volume; ECF, extracellular fluid; GFR, glomerular filtration rate.) (From Schrier RW. Body fluid regulation in health and disease: a unifying hypothesis. *Ann Intern Med* 1990;113:155–159. Adapted with permission.)

sodium and water reabsorption, which leads to an increase in sodium and water delivery to the distal nephron site of aldosterone action. This increase in distal sodium delivery is the major mediator of escape from the sodium-retaining effect of mineralocorticoids in healthy subjects, thereby avoiding edema formation. In contrast, in patients with cirrhosis or cardiac failure, the renal vasoconstriction that accompanies the compensatory neurohumoral response to arterial underfilling is associated with a decrease in distal sodium and water delivery to the distal nephron site of aldosterone action. This diminution in distal delivery, which occurs primarily because of a fall in the glomerular filtration rate and an increase in proximal tubular sodium reabsorption, results in a failure to escape from aldosterone and, therefore, causes edema formation. The importance of renal hemodynamics, particularly the glomerular filtration rate, in the aldosterone escape phenomena is emphasized by the observation that in pregnancy, a state of primary arterial vasodilation, aldosterone escape occurs despite arterial underfilling because of an associated 30% to 50% increase in the glomerular filtration rate. It still remains to be determined why pregnancy is associated with this large increase in the glomerular filtration rate, which occurs within 2 to 4 weeks of conception. The increase in the filtration rate cannot be due to plasma volume expansion, because this does not occur until several weeks after conception. The higher filtered load of sodium, and therefore distal sodium load in pregnancy, no doubt allows the escape from the sodium-retaining effect of aldosterone which is elevated in normal pregnancy. The occurrence of aldosterone escape in pregnancy attenuates edema formation when compared to other edematous disorders.

III. DIETARY AND DIURETIC TREATMENT OF EDEMA: GENERAL PRINCIPLES. The daily sodium intake in the United States is typically 4 to 6 g [1 g of sodium contains 43 mEq; 1 g of sodium chloride (NaCl) contains 17 mEq of sodium]. By not using added salt at meals, the daily sodium intake can be reduced to 4 g (172 mEq) whereas a typical "low-salt" diet contains 2 g (86 mEq). Diets that are lower in NaCl content can be prescribed, but many individuals find them unpalatable. If salt substitutes are used, it is important to remember that these contain potassium chloride; therefore potassium-sparing diuretics (i.e., spironolactone, eplerenone, triamterene, amiloride) should not be used with salt substitutes. Other drugs that increase serum potassium concentration must also be used with caution in the presence of salt substitute intake [i.e., converting enzyme inhibitors, angiotensin receptor blockers, β-blockers, and nonsteroidal anti-inflammatory drugs (NSAIDs)]. When prescribing dietary therapy for an edematous patient, it is important to emphasize that sodium chloride restriction is required, even if diuretic drugs are employed. The therapeutic potency of diuretic drugs varies inversely with dietary salt intake.

All commonly used **diuretic drugs** act by increasing urinary sodium excretion. They can be divided into five classes based on their predominant site of action along the nephron (Table 1-2). Osmotic diuretics (e.g., mannitol) and proximal diuretics (e.g., acetazolamide) are not employed as primary agents to treat edematous disorders. Loop diuretics (e.g., furosemide), distal convoluted tubule diuretics (DCT; e.g., hydrochlorothiazide), and collecting duct diuretics (e.g., spironolactone), however, all play important but distinct roles in treating edematous patients. The goal of the diuretic treatment of edema is to reduce ECF volume and to maintain the ECF volume at the reduced level. This requires an initial natriuresis, but, at steady state, urinary sodium chloride excretion returns close to baseline despite continued diuretic administration. Importantly, an increase in sodium and water excretion does *not* prove therapeutic efficacy if ECF volume does not decline. Conversely, a return to "basal"

 TABLE 1-2 **Physiologic Classification of Diuretic Drugs**

Osmotic diuretics
Proximal diuretics
   Carbonic anhydrase inhibitors
      Acetazolamide
Loop diuretics (maximal $FE_{Na} = 30\%$)
   Na-K-2Cl inhibitors
      Furosemide
      Bumetanide
      Torsemide
      Ethacrynic acid
DCT diuretics (maximal $FE_{Na} = 9\%$)
   NaCl inhibitors
      Chlorothiazide
      Hydrochlorothiazide
      Metolazone
      Chlorthalidone
      Indapamide[a]
      Many others
Collecting duct diuretics (maximal $FE_{Na} = 3\%$)
   Na channel blockers
      Amiloride
      Triameterene
   Aldosterone antagonists
      Spironolactone
      Eplerenone

DCT, distal convoluted tubule.
[a]Indapamide may have other actions as well.

levels of urinary sodium chloride excretion does not indicate diuretic resistance. The continued efficacy of a diuretic is documented by the rapid return to ECF volume expansion that occurs if the diuretic is discontinued.

A. When starting a loop diuretic as treatment for edema, it is important to establish a therapeutic goal, usually a target body weight. If a low dose does not lead to natriuresis, it can be doubled repeatedly until the maximum recommended dose is reached (Table 1-3). When a **diuretic drug is administered by mouth**, the magnitude of the natriuretic response is determined by the intrinsic potency of the drug, the dose, the bioavailability, the amount delivered to the kidney, the amount that enters the tubule fluid (most diuretics act from the luminal side), and the physiologic state of the individual. Except for proximal diuretics, the maximal natriuretic potency of a diuretic can be predicted from its site of action. In Table 1-2, it is shown that loop diuretics can maximally increase fractional sodium (Na) excretion to 30%, DCT diuretics can increase it to 9%, and sodium channel blockers can increase it to 3% of the filtered load. The intrinsic diuretic potency of a diuretic is defined by its dose–response curve, which is generally sigmoid. The steep sigmoid relation is the reason that loop diuretic drugs are often described as *threshold drugs*. When starting loop diuretic treatment, ensuring that each dose reaches the steep part of the dose–response curve before the dose frequency is adjusted is important. Because loop diuretics are rapid acting, many patients note an increase in urine output within several hours of taking the drug; this can be helpful in establishing that an adequate dose has been reached. Because loop diuretics are short acting, any increase in urine output more than 6 hours after a dose is unrelated to drug effects. Therefore, most loop diuretic drugs should be administered at least twice daily, when given by mouth.

B. The **bioavailability of diuretic drugs** varies widely among classes of drugs, among different drugs of the same class, and even within the same drug. The bioavailability of loop diuretics ranges from 10% to 100% (mean, 50% for furosemide; 80% to 100% for bumetanide and torsemide). Limited bioavailability can usually be overcome by appropriate dosing, but some drugs, such as furosemide, are variably absorbed by the same patient on different days, making precise titration difficult. Doubling the furosemide dose when changing from intravenous to oral therapy is customary, but the relation between intravenous and oral dose may vary. For example, the amount of sodium excreted during 24 hours is similar whether furosemide is administered to a healthy individual by mouth or by vein, despite its 50% bioavailability. This paradox results from the fact that oral furosemide absorption is slower than its clearance, leading to "absorption-limited" kinetics. Therefore, effective serum furosemide concentrations persist longer when the drug is given by mouth, because a reservoir in the gastrointestinal tract continues to supply furosemide to the body. This relation holds for a healthy individual. Predicting the precise relation between oral and intravenous doses, therefore, is difficult.

IV. DIURETIC RESISTANCE. Patients are considered to be **diuretic resistant** when an inadequate reduction in ECF volume is observed despite near-maximal doses of loop diuretics. Several causes of resistance can be determined by considering factors that affect diuretic efficacy, as discussed earlier.

A. Causes of diuretic resistance

    1. Excessive dietary NaCl intake is one cause of diuretic resistance. When NaCl intake is high, renal NaCl retention can occur between natriuretic periods, thereby maintaining the ECF volume expansion. Measuring the sodium excreted during 24 hours can be useful in diagnosing excessive intake. If the patient is at steady state (the weight is stable), then the urinary sodium excreted during 24 hours is equal to dietary NaCl intake. If sodium excretion exceeds 100 to 120 mM (approximately 2 to 3 g sodium per day), then dietary NaCl consumption is too high and dietary counseling should be undertaken.

    2. Impaired diuretic delivery to its active site in the kidney tubule is another cause of diuretic resistance. Most diuretics, including the loop diuretics, DCT diuretics, and amiloride, act from the luminal surface. Although diuretics are small molecules, most circulate while tightly bound to protein and reach tubule

TABLE 1-3 Ceiling Doses of Loop Diuretics

	Furosemide (mg)		Bumetanide (mg)		Torsemide (mg)	
	IV	PO	IV	PO	IV	PO
Renal insufficiency						
GFR 20–50 mL/min	80	80–160	2–3	2–3	50	50
GFR <20 mL/min	200	240	8–10	8–10	100	100
Severe acute renal failure	500	NA	12	NA	—	—
Nephrotic syndrome	120	240	3	3	50	50
Cirrhosis	40–80	80–160	1	1–2	10–20	10–20
Congestive heart failure	40–80	160–240	2–3	2–3	20–50	50

GFR, glomerular filtration rate; NA, not available.
Ceiling dose indicates the dose that produces the maximal increase in fractional sodium excretion. Larger doses may increase net daily natriuresis by increasing the *duration* of natriuresis without increasing the maximal rate.

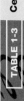

fluid primarily by tubular secretion. Loop and DCT diuretics are organic anions that circulate bound to albumin and reach tubule fluid primarily through the organic anion secretory pathway in the proximal tubule. Although experimental data suggest that diuretic resistance results when serum albumin concentrations are very low, because the volume of diuretic distribution increases, most studies suggest that this effect is only marginally significant clinically and is observed only when serum albumin concentration declines below 2 g per L. A variety of endogenous and exogenous substances that compete with diuretics for secretion into tubule fluid are more probable causes of diuretic resistance. Uremic anions, NSAIDS, probenecid, and penicillins all inhibit loop and DCT diuretic secretion into tubule fluid. Under some conditions, this may predispose to diuretic resistance, because the concentration of drug achieved in tubule fluid does not exceed the diuretic threshold. For example, chronic renal failure shifts the loop diuretic dose–response curve to the right, therefore requiring a higher dose to achieve maximal effect.

   3. **Diuretic binding to protein in tubule fluid** is another factor that may influence diuretic effectiveness. Diuretic drugs are normally bound to proteins in the plasma, but not once they are secreted into tubule fluid. This reflects the normally low protein concentrations in tubule fluid. In contrast, when serum proteins, such as albumin, are filtered in appreciable quantities, as in nephrotic syndrome, diuretic drugs interact with them and lose effectiveness. Despite experimental support, recent clinical studies have indicated that this phenomenon does not contribute significantly to diuretic resistance in nephrotic syndrome.

B. **Treatment of diuretic resistance.** Several strategies are available to achieve the effective control of ECF volume in patients who do not respond to full doses of effective loop diuretics.

   1. A diuretic of another class may be added to a regimen that includes a loop diuretic (Table 1-4). This strategy produces true synergy; the combination of agents is more effective than the *sum* of the responses to each agent alone. DCT diuretics are most commonly combined with loop diuretics. DCT diuretics inhibit the adaptive changes in the distal nephron that increase the reabsorptive capacity of the tubule and limit the potency of loop diuretics. Because DCT diuretics have longer half-lives than loop diuretics, they prevent or attenuate NaCl retention during the periods between doses of loop diuretics, thereby increasing their net effect. When two diuretics are combined, the DCT diuretic is generally administered some time before the loop diuretic (1 hour is reasonable) to ensure that NaCl transport in the distal nephron is blocked when it is flooded with solute. When intravenous therapy is indicated, chlorothiazide

TABLE 1-4   **Combination Diuretic Therapy (to Add to a Ceiling Dose of a Loop Diuretic)**

Distal convoluted tubule diuretics
   Metolazone 2.5–10 mg p.o. daily[a]
   Hydrochlorothiazide (or equivalent) 25–100 mg p.o. daily
   Chlorothiazide 500–1,000 mg i.v.
Proximal tubule diuretics
   Acetazolamide 250–375 mg daily or up to 500 mg i.v.
Collecting duct diuretics
   Spironolactone 100–200 mg daily
   Amiloride 5–10 mg daily

[a]Metolazone is generally best given for a limited period (3 to 5 d) or should be reduced in frequency to three times per week once extracellular fluid volume has declined to the target level. Only in patients who remain volume expanded should full doses be continued indefinitely, based on the target weight.

(500 to 1,000 mg) may be employed. Metolazone is the DCT diuretic most frequently combined with loop diuretics, because its half-life is relatively long (as formulated in zaroxylin) and because it has been reported to be effective even when renal failure is present. Other thiazide and thiazide-like diuretics, however, appear to be equally effective, even in severe renal failure. The dramatic effectiveness of combination diuretic therapy is accompanied by complications in a significant number of patients. Massive fluid and electrolyte losses (i.e., potassium and magnesium) have led to circulatory collapse during combination therapy, and patients must be followed up carefully. The lowest effective dose of DCT diuretic should be added to the loop diuretic regimen; patients can frequently be treated with combination therapy for only a few days and then must be placed back on a single-drug regimen. When continuous combination therapy is needed, low doses of DCT diuretic (2.5 mg metolazone or 25 mg hydrochlorothiazide) administered only two or three times per week may be sufficient.

2. For hospitalized patients who are resistant to diuretic therapy, the continuous infusion of loop diuretics is an alternative approach. **Continuous diuretic infusions** (Table 1-5) have several advantages over bolus diuretic administration. First, because they avoid peaks and troughs of diuretic concentration, continuous infusions prevent periods of positive NaCl balance (postdiuretic NaCl retention) from occurring. Second, continuous infusions are more efficient than bolus therapy (the amount of NaCl excreted per milligram of drug administered is greater). Third, some patients who are resistant to large doses of diuretics given by bolus respond to continuous infusion. Fourth, diuretic response can be titrated; in the intensive care unit, where obligate fluid administration must be balanced by fluid excretion, excellent control of NaCl and water excretion can be obtained. Finally, complications associated with high doses of loop diuretics, such as ototoxicity, appear to be less common when large doses are administered as a continuous infusion. Total daily furosemide doses exceeding 1 g have been tolerated well when administered over 24 hours. One approach is to administer a loading dose of 20 mg furosemide followed by a continuous infusion at 4 to 60 mg per hour. In patients with preserved renal function, therapy at the lower dosage range should be sufficient. When renal failure is present, higher doses may be used, but patients should be monitored carefully for side effects, such as ECF volume depletion and ototoxicity.

3. When therapy with diuretic drugs fails, **ultrafiltration** using hemodialysis equipment or a specialized ultrafiltration apparatus has been used. Although this approach is not recommended for routine use, in one controlled study, the response to volume removal through ultrafiltration was better sustained than after an equivalent volume removal through diuretics. In that study, loop diuretics induced a large rise in renin and angiotensin secretion, probably by stimulating the macula densa mechanism directly. This may explain the

TABLE 1-5	Continuous Infusion of Loop Diuretics			
		Infusion rate (mg/hr)		
Diuretic	Starting bolus (mg)	GFR <25 mL/min	GFR 25–75 mL/min	GFR >75 mL/min
Furosemide	40	20, then 40	10, then 20	10
Bumetanide	1	1, then 2	0.5, then 1	05
Torsemide	20	10, then 20	5, then 10	—
GFR, glomerular filtration rate.				

unique beneficial results sometimes observed following nonpharmacologic volume removal by ultrafiltration. Moreover, for the same volume of fluid removed by diuretics and ultrafiltration, more sodium is removed by ultrafiltration.

V. CONGESTIVE HEART FAILURE

A. Early **clinical symptoms** of cardiac failure occur before overt physical findings of pedal edema and pulmonary congestion. These symptoms relate to the compensatory renal sodium and water retention that accompanies arterial underfilling. The patient may present with a history of weight gain, weakness, dyspnea on exertion, decreased exercise tolerance, paroxysmal nocturnal dyspnea, and orthopnea. Nocturia may occur because cardiac output, and therefore renal perfusion, may be enhanced by the supine position. Patients with congestive heart failure may lose considerable weight during the first few days of hospitalization because of the supine position of bed rest, even without the administration of diuretics because of this nocturia. Although overt edema is not detectable early in the course of congestive heart failure, the patient may complain of swollen eyes on awakening and tight rings and shoes, particularly at the end of the day. With incipient edema, as much as 3 to 4 L of fluid can be retained before the occurrence of overt edema.

The period of incipient edema is then followed by more overt symptoms and physical findings: basilar pulmonary rales, ankle edema, distended neck veins at 30 degrees, tachycardia, and a gallop rhythm with a third heart sound. Although the chest x-ray may only show cephalization of pulmonary markings early in cardiac failure, increased hilar markings, Kerley's B lines, and pleural effusions occur later, generally accompanied by an enlarged heart size.

B. **Etiology.** Two mechanisms that reduce cardiac output are recognized to cause congestive heart failure: systolic dysfunction and diastolic dysfunction. Because specific, life-saving therapy is available for systolic dysfunction, it is essential to determine whether systolic dysfunction is present when a patient presents with the symptoms and signs of heart failure. Although physical examination, chest x-ray, and electrocardiogram are useful in this regard, additional diagnostic tests are usually indicated. An echocardiogram provides information about systolic (the ejection fraction) and diastolic function, and about valvular disease, which may require surgery. Occult hypothyroidism or hyperthyroidism and alcoholic cardiomyopathy may present as congestive heart failure; these entities are treatable. Uncontrolled hypertension may contribute to congestive heart failure, but disease of the coronary arteries is the most common cause. In one study, severe coronary artery disease was found in 9 of 38 patients undergoing cardiac transplantation for presumed idiopathic dilated cardiomyopathy, and in 3 of 4 patients with presumed alcoholic cardiomyopathy. These data suggest that cardiac catheterization may be indicated in virtually all patients who present with new-onset congestive heart failure. In patients with preexisting cardiac disease, a cardiac arrhythmia, pulmonary embolus, cessation of medicines, severe anemia or fever, dietary sodium indiscretion, and worsening of chronic obstructive lung disease with infection and resultant hypoxia are examples of potentially treatable precipitants of worsening of congestive heart failure. Drugs with a negative inotropic effect, such as verapamil, may worsen heart failure by decreasing cardiac output. A trial cessation of these drugs is the best means of determining their possible role in worsening congestive heart failure.

C. **Treatment.** When none of these specific primary or precipitating causes of congestive heart failure are detectable, then general principles of treatment must be considered.

Every patient with symptomatic systolic dysfunction or, if asymptomatic, an ejection fraction of less than 40% should be started on an **angiotensin-converting enzyme (ACE) inhibitor**, unless a specific contraindication exists. ACE inhibitors (and angiotensin receptor inhibitors) are unique agents that reduce blood pressure (reduce afterload), shift the renal function curve to the left (promote continued sodium losses), and block maladaptive neuroregulatory hormones (Fig. 1-5). These agents should be started at low doses (enalapril 2.5 mg b.i.d. or captopril 6.25 mg t.i.d.), but increased if tolerated to 10 b.i.d. of enalapril or 50 t.i.d. of captopril, unless side effects occur. If cough or angioedema limits ACE inhibitor use, then

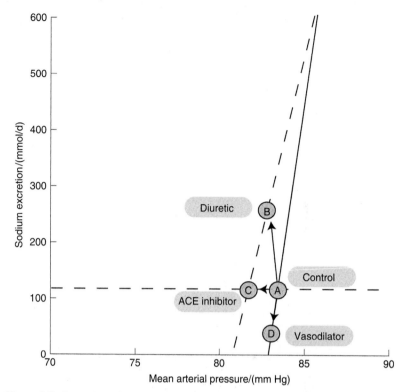

Figure 1-5. Comparison of diuretic, angiotensin-converting enzyme (ACE) inhibitor, and vasodilator effects on mean arterial pressure and natriuresis. The normal renal function curve is shown (*solid line*). Adding a vasodilator reduces mean arterial pressure but also reduces natriuresis because blood pressure declines. A diuretic moves the individual to a new renal function curve (*dashed line*), thereby increasing natriuresis, but has little effect on blood pressure. An ACE inhibitor moves the individual to a new renal function curve, maintaining natriuresis at a lower blood pressure.

an AT_1 angiotensin receptor blocker should be used (although angioedema may develop with AT_1 receptor blockers, the incidence is lower with this class of drugs). If neither class of drug can be employed safely, then therapy with hydralazine and isosorbide dihydrate or monohydrate should be used.

β-blockers have been shown to improve symptoms and mortality in patients with systolic dysfunction. Both selective β-blockers (metoprolol) and nonselective β-blockers with α blocking properties (carvedilol) are approved by the U.S. Food and Drug Administration (FDA) for the treatment of congestive heart failure. Because β-blockers can lead to symptomatic exacerbations of heart failure, these drugs are initiated in low doses only when patients are clinically stable and without expansion of the ECF volume.

The role of **digitalis glycosides** has been clarified by recent controlled studies. Digoxin significantly improves symptoms and reduces the incidence of hospitalization in patients with impaired left ventricular function, but it does not appear to prolong life. Therefore, the drug is indicated for symptomatic treatment when combined with ACE inhibitors and diuretics. In certain clinical states of heart failure, however, cardiac glycosides have been shown to be of little therapeutic value, for example, in association with thyrotoxicosis, chronic obstructive pulmonary disease, and cor pulmonale. Cardiac glycosides may actually worsen symptoms in patients with hypertrophic obstructive cardiomyopathy and subaortic stenosis, pericardial tamponade, and constrictive pericarditis. It should also be remembered that digoxin is excreted by the kidneys; therefore, the dosage interval should be increased in the patient with chronic renal disease (see Chapter 16). Also, the elderly patient should receive a decreased dose (e.g., 0.125 mg q.o.d.), even if the serum creatinine level is not increased. Although renal function deteriorates with age, serum creatinine levels may not rise in the elderly because of a concomitant loss of muscle mass. Although potentially useful acute therapy, phosphodiesterase inhibitors, such as milrinone, which also increase cardiac output, have been shown to increase mortality when used chronically. Therefore, the chronic use of these drugs should be avoided.

If symptomatic pulmonary congestion or peripheral edema is present, **diuretic therapy** is indicated (Fig. 1-5). A loop diuretic is usually employed as first-line therapy, although some patients may be managed using a thiazide. In patients with congestive heart failure, diuretic therapy must be instituted with full knowledge of the Starling-Frank curve of myocardial contractility (Fig. 1-6). The patient with congestive heart failure who responds to a diuretic will exhibit improved symptomatology as end-diastolic volume and pulmonary congestion decrease. However, because the Starling-Frank curve is usually either flat or upsloping even in failing hearts, an improvement in cardiac output may not occur. If, during the diuretic treatment of a patient with congestive heart failure, the serum creatinine and blood urea nitrogen levels begin to rise, it is likely that cardiac output has fallen. This situation is especially pronounced in patients who are receiving ACE

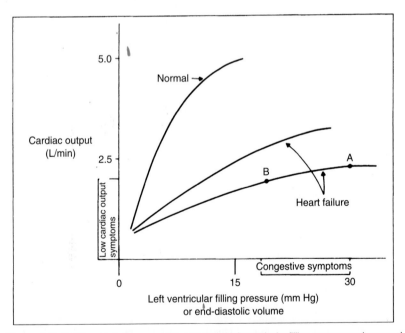

Figure 1-6. Relationship between cardiac output and left ventricular filling pressure under normal circumstances (*upper curve*) and low-output congestive heart failure (*lower curve*). Reduction of after-load [e.g., angiotensin-converting enzyme (ACE) inhibitor or a vasodilator] or improved contractility (inotropic agents) may shift the lower curve to the *middle curve*. Diuretic-induced preload reduction or other causes of volume depletion may decrease cardiac output (e.g., shift from point A to point B on the *lower curve*). (From Schrier RW, ed. *Renal and electrolyte disorders,* 4th ed. Boston: Little, Brown and Company, 1990. Reprinted with permission.)

inhibitor therapy. ACE inhibitors impair renal autoregulation and make patients prone to prerenal azotemia. When mild azotemia develops in a patient treated with diuretics and an ACE inhibitor, it is usually advisable to reduce the diuretic dose or liberalize dietary salt intake, provided that pulmonary congestion is not present simultaneously. This approach has been shown to permit the continued administration of ACE inhibitors in many patients. Some pedal edema may be preferable to a diuretic-induced decline in cardiac output as estimated by the occurrence or worsening of prerenal azotemia. Patients with congestive heart failure are especially sensitive to renal functional deterioration if NSAIDs are used together with diuretics and ACE inhibitors. Therefore, NSAIDS should be diligently avoided in this patient population.

Both congestive heart failure and treatment with loop diuretics stimulate the renin-angiotensin-aldosterone axis. Two large studies have provided evidence that **blocking mineralocorticoid (aldosterone) receptors** can improve mortality of such patients. In one trial, adding spironolactone (25 to 50 mg per day) to a regimen that included an ACE inhibitor and a diuretic (with or without digoxin) reduced all-cause mortality by 30% and reduced hospitalization for heart failure by 35%. This effect was felt to be independent of a negative sodium balance, but rather due to inhibition of cardiac fibrosis. Gynecomastia, which is a relatively common side effect of spironolactone owing to its estrogenic side effects, does not appear to occur with a newer more selective inhibitor mineralocorticoid receptor, eplerenone.

Hyperkalemia is of concern when aldosterone blockade is instituted. It is currently recommended that serum potassium be monitored 1 week after initiating therapy with an aldosterone blocker, after 1 month, and every 3 months thereafter. An increase in serum potassium greater than 5.5 mEq per L should prompt an evaluation of dietary potassium intake and for medications such as potassium supplements or NSAIDs that might be contributing to the hyperkalemia. If such factors are not detected, the dose of aldosterone blocker should be reduced 25 mg every other day. It is prudent to avoid the use of aldosterone blockers in patients with a creatinine clearance of less than 30 mL per minute and to be cautious in those with a creatinine clearance of between 30 and 50 mL per minute. These patients must be followed up very closely.

Complications of diuretic therapy are shown in Table 1-6. Although hyponatremia may be a complication of diuretic treatment, furosemide, when combined with ACE inhibitors, may ameliorate hyponatremia in some patients with congestive

TABLE 1-6	Complications of Diuretics

Contraction of the vascular volume
Orthostatic hypotension (from volume depletion)
Hypokalemia (loop and DCT diuretics)
Hyperkalemia (spironolactone, eplerenone, triamterene, and amiloride)
Gynecomastia (spironolactone)
Hyperuricemia
Hypercalcemia (thiazides)
Hypercholesterolemia
Hyponatremia (especially with DCT diuretics)
Metabolic alkalosis
Gastrointestinal upset
Hyperglycemia
Pancreatitis (DCT diuretics)
Allergic interstitial nephritis

DCT, distal convoluted tubule.

heart failure, possibly by improving cardiac output and diminishing urinary concentration. In patients with heart failure, hypokalemia and hypomagnesemia are frequent complications of diuretic treatment because of secondary hyperaldosteronism, which increases sodium delivery to the distal sites at which aldosterone stimulates potassium and hydrogen ion secretion. Severe renal magnesium wasting may also occur in the setting of secondary hyperaldosteronism and loop diuretic administration. Because both magnesium and potassium depletion cause similar deleterious effects on the heart, and potassium repletion is very difficult in the presence of magnesium depletion, supplemental replacement of both these cations is frequently necessary in patients with cardiac failure.

The treatment of patients with congestive heart failure and preserved systolic function is less clearly defined. Hypertension control is clearly paramount in these patients, because hypertension is a frequent cause of cardiac hypertrophy and diastolic dysfunction. Diuretics are usually necessary to improve symptoms of dyspnea and orthopnea. β-Blockers, ACE inhibitors, angiotensin receptor blockers, or nondihydropyridine calcium antagonists may be beneficial in some patients with diastolic dysfunction. Diastolic dysfunction is a very common cause of heart failure in elderly patients.

VI. HEPATIC CIRRHOSIS. The pathogenesis of renal sodium and water retention is similar in all varieties of cirrhosis, including alcoholic, viral, and biliary cirrhosis. Studies in both humans and animals indicate that renal sodium and water retention precedes the formation of ascites in cirrhosis. Therefore, the classic "underfill theory," which attributed the renal sodium and water retention of cirrhosis to ascites formation with resultant hypovolemia, seems untenable as a primary mechanism. Because plasma volume expansion secondary to renal sodium and water excretion occurs before ascites formation, the "overflow theory" of ascites formation was proposed. This postulated that an undefined process, triggered by the diseased liver (e.g., increased intrahepatic pressure), causes renal sodium and water retention that then overflows into the abdomen because of portal hypertension. This overflow theory, however, predicts that renal salt retention and ascites formation would be associated with decreased plasma levels of vasopressin, renin, aldosterone, and norepinephrine. Because these hormones rise progressively as cirrhosis advances from the states of compensation (no ascites) to decompensation (ascites) to hepatorenal syndrome, the overflow hypothesis also does not seem to explain the spectrum of renal sodium and water retention associated with advanced cirrhosis. More recently, the systemic arterial vasodilation theory has been proposed. This theory, summarized in Figure 1-7, is compatible with virtually all known observations in patients during the various stages of cirrhosis. According to this theory, cirrhosis causes systemic arterial vasodilation with activation of the neurohumoral axis. The cause of the primary arterial vasodilation in cirrhosis is not clear, but is known to present early, and occur primarily in the splanchnic circulation. Although several mediators, including substance P, vasoactive intestinal peptide, endotoxin, and glucagon have been proposed to play a role in splanchnic arterial vasodilation, recent information indicates that nitric oxide may be a crucial participant. The opening of existing splanchnic arteriovenous shunts may account for some early arterial vasodilation. Later, anatomically new portosystemic and arteriovenous shunting secondary to the portal hypertension may also occur.

A. Options for treating cirrhotic ascites and edema include dietary NaCl restriction, diuretic drugs, large-volume paracentesis, peritoneovenous shunting, portosystemic shunting [usually transjugular intrahepatic portosystemic shunting (TIPS)], and liver transplantation. Each of these approaches has a role in the treatment of cirrhotic ascites, but most patients can be treated successfully with NaCl dietary restriction, diuretics, and occasionally large-volume paracentesis.

The **initial therapy of cirrhotic ascites** is supportive, including dietary sodium restriction and cessation of alcohol. When these measures prove inadequate, diuretic treatment should begin with spironolactone. Spironolactone has several advantages. First, a controlled trial showed that spironolactone is more effective than furosemide alone in reducing ascites in cirrhotic patients. Second, spironolactone is a long-acting diuretic that can be given once per day in doses ranging from

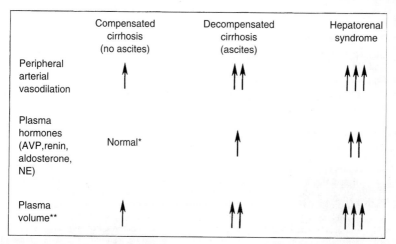

Figure 1-7. Systemic arterial vasodilation hypothesis. Stages of progression of cirrhosis. (AVP, arginine vasopressin; NE, norepinephrine.) *Given the positive sodium and water balance that has occurred, these plasma hormones would be suppressed in healthy subjects without liver disease. **The progressive renal sodium and water retention increases extracellular fluid, interstitial fluid, and plasma volume. However, the concomitant occurrence of hypoalbuminemia in decompensated cirrhosis and hepatorenal syndrome may attenuate the degree of volume expansion.

25 to 400 mg. Third, unlike most other diuretics, hypokalemia does not occur when spironolactone is administered. This is important because hypokalemia increases renal ammonia production and can precipitate encephalopathy. The most common side effect of spironolactone is painful gynecomastia. (Gynecomastia appears to be much less common with eplerenone, a newer, more selective antagonist, which may be substituted.) Although amiloride, another K-sparing diuretic, can be used as an alternative, spironolactone is more effective than amiloride in reducing ascites. In patients who do not respond to a low dose of spironolactone, it can be combined with furosemide, starting at 100 mg spironolactone and 40 mg furosemide (to a maximum of 400 mg spironolactone and 160 mg furosemide). This regimen has the advantages of once per day dosing and minimal hypokalemia. Diuretic resistance in cirrhosis has been defined as absence of response to 400 mg spironolactone and 160 mg furosemide.

B. The appropriate **rate of diuresis** depends on the presence or absence of systemic edema. Because mobilizing ascitic fluid into the vascular compartment is slow (approximately 500 mL per day), the rate of daily diuresis should be limited to 0.5 kg per day if systemic edema is absent. In the presence of systemic edema, most patients can tolerate up to 1.0 kg per day of fluid removal. Because ascites in the decompensated cirrhotic patient is associated with substantial complications including (a) spontaneous bacterial peritonitis (50% to 80% mortality), which does not occur in the absence of ascites; (b) impaired ambulation, decreased appetite, and back and abdominal pain; (c) an elevated diaphragm with decreased ventilation predisposing to hypoventilation, atelectasis, and pulmonary infections; and (d) negative cosmetic and psychological effects, the treatment of ascites with diuretics and sodium restriction is appropriate. This approach is successful in approximately 90% of patients, and complications are rare. Earlier studies demonstrating complications with diuretic therapy complications often utilized more aggressive diuretic regimens.

An alternate approach to diuretics is **large-volume paracentesis** in patients with advanced cirrhosis and ascites. Total paracentesis, occurring in increments over 3 days or, more commonly, at one setting has been shown to have few

Child-Pugh score >11
Serum bilirubin >5 mg/dL
Overt or chronic hepatic encephalopathy
Age older than 70
Serum creatinine >3 mg/dL
Cardiac dysfunction
Portal vein thrombosis

Figure 1-8. Contraindications to transjugular intrahepatic portosystemic shunt (TIPS).

complications; in some studies, paracentesis appears to have a lower incidence of complications than does diuretic treatment. Albumin 8 g for each liter of ascitic fluid removed should be infused to reduce hemodynamic compromise and the elaboration of vasoregulatory hormones. Patients often favor paracentesis because of the rapid improvement in symptoms and decreased hospitalizations; diuretics and salt restriction are still required between paracentesis. Portosystemic shunting is usually performed as TIPS. In two uncontrolled trials, TIPS led to an increase in urine output, a marked reduction in ascites, and a reduction in diuretic usage. Renal function also improved. Yet in a controlled trial, mortality increased in patients who received a TIPS as compared with controls, and TIPS can precipitate hepatic encephalopathy, especially in Child-Pugh class C patients. Contraindications are shown in Figure 1-8. A recent review of the literature confirmed that TIPS can effectively reduce or eliminate ascites, but carries a substantial complication rate. Therefore, it remains best reserved for truly refractory patients who will not receive a liver transplant. Similar considerations apply to peritoneovenous (LeVeen) shunting. In controlled trials, peritoneovenous shunting was shown to reduce ascites more effectively than paracentesis or diuretics, but this was associated with a high rate of complications (e.g., shunt clotting); and there was no survival advantage of the peritoneovenous shunt. Despite reports that the high complication rate can be reduced, most centers reserve this therapy for patients who are truly refractory to more conventional approaches and who are not candidates for liver transplantation.

The development of ascites in a patient with previously compensated cirrhosis may be an indication for liver transplantation if reversible hepatic insults or sodium-retaining drugs, for example, NSAIDs, have been excluded. In view of the morbidity and mortality associated with diuretic-resistant decompensated cirrhosis, the patient should be considered for placement on the liver transplantation list. Worsening of ascites in a previously stable individual is most often caused by progressive liver disease, but should also compel the search for hepatocellular carcinoma and portal vein thrombosis.

C. **Treatment aimed at the systemic arterial vasodilation** of cirrhosis has previously only been used in the acute setting of the patient with portal hypertension and bleeding esophageal varices. Portal venous hypertension is caused not only by the intrahepatic capillary fibrosis that increases resistance to flow but also by increased splanchnic flow. Therefore, the administration of vasopressin, which selectively constricts the splanchnic vasculature, has been shown to decrease portal venous pressure and thereby diminish esophageal variceal bleeding.

More chronic use of vasoconstrictors in association with albumin administration has emerged as a treatment for hepatorenal syndrome. This therapy has been shown to be effective in some patients with type 1 hepatorenal syndrome. The differences between type 1 and 2 hepatorenal syndromes are shown in Figure 1-9. The V_1 (vascular) vasopressin receptor agonist, terlipressin, has been approved for use with albumin in type 1 hepatorenal syndrome in Europe. However, because the V_2 antidiuretic receptor is already occupied in patients with advanced cirrhosis, vasopressin, a V_1 and V_2 agonist, can be used without worsening water retention. For chronic outpatient use, the α agonist, midodrine, has been used with albumin to

Type 1

   Rapidly progressive

   Serum creatinine double to >2.5 mg/dL or creatinine clearance <20 mL/min in <2 wk

   Prognosis 80% die in 2 wk

   Frequently precipitating events (e.g., spontaneous bacterial peritonitis)

Type 2

   Slower deterioration

   Serum creatinine >1.5 mg/dL or creatinine clearance <40 mL/min but decline is slow

   Most patients die within several weeks

   Most frequent cause of therapy resistant ascites

Figure 1-9. Two types of hepatorenal syndrome.

treat type 1 hepatorenal syndrome. The treatment approach with a vasoconstrictor and albumin has been shown to lower serum creatinine below 1.5 mg per dL over a 7- to 10-day period in 60% to 70% of patients with type 1 hepatorenal syndrome. No effect on mortality, however, has been demonstrated. Therefore, the therapeutic advantage of this approach is to allow time for reversibility of any acute hepatic insult or for liver transplantation.

Spontaneous bacterial peritonitis is probably the most frequent cause of type 1 hepatorenal syndrome, which frequently occurs on the background of type 2 hepatorenal syndrome. In a prospective, randomized study, the combination of albumin and cefotaxime has been shown to decrease the occurrence of renal failure and mortality as compared to cefotaxime alone in cirrhotic patients with spontaneous bacterial peritonitis (Fig. 1-10). A diagnostic peritoneal tap, therefore, should be undertaken in all cirrhotic patients with ascites in whom renal function is deteriorating independent of absence of fever, leukocytosis, or abdominal pain.

VII. NEPHROTIC SYNDROME. Another major cause of edema is nephrotic syndrome, the clinical hallmarks of which include proteinuria (greater than 3.5 g per day), hypoalbuminemia, hypercholesterolemia, and edema. The degree of the edema may range

Outcome variable	Cefotaxime ($n^\circ = 63$)	Cefotaxime plus albumin ($n^\circ = 63$)	p
Renal failure n° (%)	21 (33%)	6 (11%)	<0.002
Death in hospital n° (%)	18 (29%)	6 (10%)	<0.01
Death at 3 mo n° (%)	26 (41%)	14 (22%)	<0.03

Figure 1-10. Effects of albumin infusion on morbidity and mortality due to spontaneous bacterial peritonitis (SBP). (From Sort P, Navasa M, Arroyo V, et al. Effect of intravenous albumin on renal impairment and mortality in patients with cirrhosis and spontaneous bacterial peritonitis. *N Engl J Med* 1999;341:403–409. Reprinted with permission.)

from pedal edema to total body anasarca, including ascites and pleural effusions. The lower the plasma albumin concentration, the more likely the occurrence of anasarca; the degree of sodium intake is, however, also a determinant of the degree of edema. Nephrotic syndrome has many causes (see Chapter 8). Systemic causes of nephrotic syndrome include diabetes mellitus, lupus erythematosus, drugs (e.g., phenytoin, heavy metals, NSAIDs), carcinomas, and Hodgkin's disease, and primary renal diseases such as minimal-change nephropathy, membranous nephropathy, focal segmental glomerulosclerosis, and membranoproliferative glomerulonephritis.

A. The **pathogenesis** of ECF volume expansion in nephrotic syndrome appears to be more variable than the pathogenesis of edema in patients with congestive heart failure or cirrhotic ascites. Traditionally, ECF volume expansion in nephrotic syndrome was believed to depend on hypoalbuminemia and underfilling of the arterial circulation. Several observations, however, have raised questions about this hypothesis as always accounting for sodium retention in nephrotic patients. First, the interstitial oncotic pressure in healthy individuals is higher than previously appreciated. Transudation of fluid during ECF volume expansion reduces the interstitial oncotic pressure, thereby minimizing the change in transcapillary oncotic pressure. Second, patients recovering from minimal-change nephropathy frequently begin to excrete sodium before their serum albumin concentration rises. Third, the circulating concentrations of volume-regulatory hormones are not as high in many nephrotic patients as in patients with severe cirrhosis or congestive heart failure. These and other observations have **suggested a role for primary renal NaCl retention** (overflow hypothesis) in the pathogenesis of nephrotic edema.

B. Whereas "primary" renal NaCl retention may contribute to nephrotic edema in many patients, it is not often the only mechanism; some component of *underfill* often plays a role particularly in patients with serum albumin concentrations below 2.0 g per L. Evidence for its role includes the observation that "primary" renal NaCl retention alone may not lead to edema in the absence of a decrease in cardiac output or systemic arterial vasodilation. Chronic aldosterone infusion, for example, leads to hypertension and escape from renal sodium retention in the absence of edema formation. Furthermore, levels of vasoactive hormones, although below the levels commonly seen in cirrhosis and congestive heart failure, are often higher than would be expected on the basis of the level of ECF expansion. It appears, therefore, that nephrotic syndrome may reflect a combination of primary renal NaCl retention and/or relative arterial underfilling. A preponderance of one or the other mechanism may be observed in nephrotic syndrome from different causes. In general, a normal or near-normal glomerular filtration rate is associated with hypovolemic, vasoconstrictor nephrotic syndrome whereas a diminution in glomerular filtration rate, primary renal sodium retention, and evidence of volume expansion (e.g., decreased plasma renin activity) are characteristic of hypervolemic nephrotic syndrome.

C. **Treatment.** The initial focus of therapy must be aimed at those treatable, systemic causes of nephrotic syndrome such as systemic lupus erythematosus or drugs (e.g., phenytoin, NSAID). The treatment of the primary renal causes of nephrotic syndrome is described in Chapter 8.

   The treatment of edema in nephrotic patients involves **dietary sodium restriction and diuretics**. Because these patients may not be as underfilled as patients with cirrhosis or congestive heart failure, diuretic treatments are often tolerated well. In general, loop diuretics and mineralocorticoid antagonists are used as initial therapy. Some nephrotic patients may be relatively resistant to these drugs. Although low serum albumin concentrations may increase the volume of diuretic distribution, and filtered albumin may bind to diuretics in the tubule lumen, these factors do not appear to be the predominant causes of diuretic resistance. Rather, diuretic resistance may reflect a combination of reduced glomerular filtration rate and intense renal NaCl retention. When the glomerular filtration rate is reduced, endogenous organic anions impair diuretic secretion into the tubule lumen, the site where these drugs act to inhibit NaCl transport. Therefore, higher doses of loop diuretics are often required to achieve natriuresis.

The administration of albumin to patients with nephrotic syndrome can be costly and may cause pulmonary edema. One report, however, suggested that mixing albumin with a loop diuretic (6.25 g albumin per 40 mg furosemide) may induce diuresis in severely hypoalbuminemic patients. Recently, a double-blind, controlled study of nine nephrotic patients compared the effects of (a) 60 mg intravenous furosemide, (b) 60 mg intravenous furosemide plus 200 mL of a 20% solution of albumin, or (c) a sham infusion plus 200 mL of albumin. Coadministration of furosemide and albumin was significantly more effective than either albumin or furosemide alone. The authors noted that although adding albumin did increase natriuresis, the benefit was relatively small.

Suggested Readings

Abraham WT, Schrier RW. Cardiac failure and the kidney, Chapter 83. In: Schrier RW, ed. *Diseases of the kidney and urinary tract*, 8th ed. Philadelphia: Lippincott Williams & Wilkins, 2007:2159–2178.

Ellison DH. Diuretic therapy and resistance in congestive heart failure. *Cardiology* 2001;96:132–143.

Ellison DH, Okusa MD, Schrier Robert W. Mechanisms of diuretic action, Chapter 81. In: Schrier RW, ed. *Diseases of the kidney and urinary tract*, 8th ed. Philadelphia: Lippincott Williams & Wilkins, 2007:2122–2150.

Fliser D, Zurbruggen I, Mutschler E, et al. Coadministration of albumin and furosemide in patients with the nephrotic syndrome. *Kidney Int* 1999;55:629–634.

Okusa MD, Ellison DH. Physiology and pathophysiology of diuretic action, Chapter 37. In: Alpern RJ, Hebert SC, eds. *The kidney: physiology and pathophysioliogy*, 4th ed. Amerstdam: Elsevier Science, 2008:1051–1094.

Schrier RW. Pathogenesis of sodium and water retention in high and low output cardiac failure, cirrhosis, nephrotic syndrome, and pregnancy. *N Engl J Med* 1988;319:1065–1072, 1127–1134.

Schrier RW. A unifying hypothesis of body fluid volume regulation. *J R Coll Physicians Lond* 1992;26:297.

Schrier RW. How to use diuretics in heart failure patients, Chapter 9. In: Abraham W, Krum H, eds. *Heart failure: a practical approach to treatment*. New York: McGraw-Hill, 2007:91–104.

Schrier RW, Abraham WT. Hormones and hemodynamics in heart failure. *N Engl J Med* 1999;341(8):577–585.

Schrier RW, Abraham WT. The nephrotic syndrome, Chapter 85. In: Schrier RW, ed. *Diseases of the kidney and urinary tract*, 8th ed. Philadelphia: Lippincott Williams & Wilkins, 2007:2206–2647.

Schrier RW, Arroyo V, Bernardi M, et al. Systemic arterial vasodilation hypothesis: a proposal for the initiation of renal sodium and water retention in cirrhosis. *Hepatology* 1998;8:1151.

Schrier RW, Fassett RG. A critique of the overfill hypothesis of sodium and water retention in the nephrotic syndrome. *Kidney Int* 1998;53:1111–1117.

Schrier RW, Gurevitch AK, Abraham WT. Renal sodium excretion, edematous disorders, and diuretic use. In: Schrier RW, ed. *Renal and electrolyte disorders*, 6th ed. Philadelphia: Lippincott Williams & Wilkins, 2002:64–114.

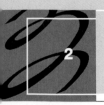

THE PATIENT WITH HYPONATREMIA OR HYPERNATREMIA

Robert W. Schrier and Tomas Berl

$\mathcal{C}$ontrol of serum sodium and osmolality. Under physiologic conditions, the concentration of sodium in plasma is kept in a very narrow range, between 138 and 142 mEq per L, despite great variations in water intake. Because sodium is the predominant cation in extracellular fluid (ECF), this reflects the equally narrow range in which the tonicity (osmolality) of body fluids is regulated, between 280 and 290 mOsm per kg. Therefore, calculated plasma osmolality can be expressed as follows:

$$P_{OSM} = 2[Na^+] + \frac{\text{blood urea nitrogen (mg/dL)}}{2.8} + \frac{\text{glucose (mg/dL)}}{18}$$

Serum sodium concentration and plasma osmolality are maintained in these normal ranges by the function of arginine vasopressin (AVP) and a very sensitive osmoreceptor that controls the secretion of this antidiuretic hormone. This hormone, in turn, is critical in determining water excretion by allowing urinary dilution in its absence and urinary concentration in its presence. Hyponatremic disorders supervene when water intake exceeds the patient's renal diluting capacity. Conversely, hypernatremia supervenes in settings associated with renal concentrating defects accompanied by inadequate water intake.

Hyponatremia. *Hyponatremia*, defined as a plasma sodium concentration of less than 135 mEq per L, is a frequent occurrence in the hospitalized patient. It has been suggested that approximately 10% to 15% of patients in hospitals have a low plasma sodium concentration at some time during their stay. Hyponatremia in the ambulatory outpatient is a much less frequent occurrence and is usually associated with a chronic disease state.

I. INTERPRETATION OF THE SERUM SODIUM. Under most clinical circumstances, a decrement in serum sodium reflects a hypo-osmolar state. However, recognizing the settings in which a normal or even low sodium level does not reflect a normal osmotic or a hypo-osmotic state is important. The addition to the ECF of osmotically active solutes that do not readily penetrate into cells, such as glucose, mannitol, or glycine, causes water to move from cells to ECF, thereby leading to cellular dehydration and a decrement in serum sodium concentration. This *translocational hyponatremia* does not reflect changes in total body water (TBW), but rather the movement of water from the intracellular to the extracellular compartment.

In hyperglycemia, for each 100 mg per dL rise in blood glucose, a 1.6 mEq per L fall in plasma sodium concentration occurs as water moves out of cells into the ECF. For example, in an untreated diabetic patient, as blood glucose rises from 200 to 1,200 mg per dL, the plasma sodium concentration is expected to fall from 140 to 124 mEq per L (1.6 mEq/L × 10 = 16 mEq) without a change in TBW and electrolytes. Conversely, treatment with insulin and lowering of the blood sugar from 1,200 to 200 mg per dL in this diabetic patient results in a comparable osmotic water movement from the ECF into cells and a return of plasma sodium concentration to 140 mEq per L without any change in TBW or electrolytes.

Hyponatremia can occur without a change in plasma osmolality; this is termed *pseudohyponatremia*. Pseudohyponatremia occurs when the solid phase of plasma, primarily lipids and proteins (usually 6% to 8%), is greatly increased, as in severe hypertriglyceridemia and paraproteinemic disorders. This falsely low reading is a consequence of the flame photometry methods that measure the concentration of Na^+ in whole plasma and not only in the liquid phase. It is estimated that a rise in plasma lipids by 4.6 g per L or in plasma proteins of 10 g per dL lowers serum sodium concentration by 1 mEq per L. This is not a problem when undiluted serum is analyzed with an ion-specific electrode that measures the concentration of sodium in serum water.

II. APPROACH TO THE HYPO-OSMOLAR HYPONATREMIC PATIENT. In the absence of pseudohyponatremia or an excess of osmotically active solute in the ECF, the most important initial step in the diagnosis of hyponatremia is an assessment of the ECF volume status.

Sodium is the primary cation in the ECF compartment. Therefore, sodium, with its accompanying anions, dictates ECF osmolality and fluid volume. Hence, ECF volume provides the best index of total body exchangeable sodium. A careful physical examination focused on the evaluation of ECF volume status therefore allows for the classification of the hyponatremic patient into one of three categories: (a) hyponatremia in the presence of an excess of total body sodium, (b) hyponatremia in the presence of a deficit of total body sodium, and (c) hyponatremia with a near-normal total body sodium. For example, the edematous patient is classified as having hyponatremia with an excess of total body sodium. The volume-depleted patient with flat neck veins, decreased skin turgor, dry mucous membranes, and orthostatic hypotension and tachycardia is classified as having hyponatremia with a deficit of total body sodium. The patient with neither edema nor evidence of ECF volume depletion is classified as having hyponatremia with near-normal total body sodium (Fig. 2-1).

A. In the **hypervolemic (edematous) hyponatremic patient**, both total body sodium and TBW are increased, water more so than sodium. These patients have cardiac failure, cirrhosis, nephrotic syndrome, or renal failure. When hyponatremia is secondary to cardiac and hepatic disease, the disease is advanced and readily evident on clinical examination. In the absence of the use of diuretics, the urinary sodium concentration in the hyponatremic edematous patient should be quite low (less than 10 mEq per L) because of avid tubular sodium reabsorption. The exception occurs in the presence of acute or chronic renal failure, in which, because of tubular dysfunction, the urinary sodium concentration is higher (greater than 20 mEq per L).

B. The diagnostic possibilities in the **hypovolemic hyponatremic patient** are entirely different. Again, a spot urinary sodium concentration is of value. If the volume-depleted hyponatremic patient has a low (less than 10 mEq per L) urine sodium concentration, the kidney is functioning normally by conserving sodium in response

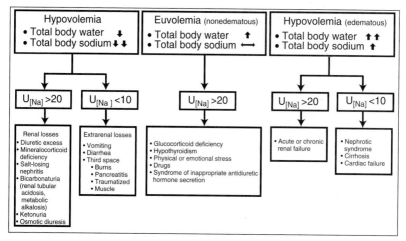

Figure 2-1. Diagnostic approach to hyponatremia. (↑, increased; ↑↑, greatly increased; ↓, decreased; ↓↓, greatly decreased; ↔, not increased or decreased; $U_{[Na]}$, urinary sodium concentration, in mEq per L.)

to ECF volume depletion. Conversely, if the urinary sodium concentration is greater than 20 mEq per L in a hypovolemic hyponatremic patient, the kidney is not responding appropriately to the ECF volume depletion, and renal losses of sodium and water must be considered as the likely cause of the hyponatremia.

1. In a hypovolemic hyponatremic patient with a **urinary sodium concentration of less than 10 mEq per L,** a gastrointestinal (or "third space") source of sodium and water losses must be sought. The source may be readily apparent if the patient presents with a history of vomiting, diarrhea, or both. In the absence of an obvious history of gastrointestinal fluid losses, several other diagnostic possibilities must be considered. Substantial ECF losses may occur into the abdominal cavity with peritonitis or pancreatitis, and into the bowel lumen with ileus or pseudomembranous colitis. The surreptitious cathartic abuser may present with evidence of ECF volume depletion and no history of gastrointestinal losses. The presence of hypokalemic metabolic acidosis and phenolphthalein in the urine may be a clue to this diagnosis. Loss of haustra on barium enema and melanosis coli on endoscopy are other clues to cathartic abuse. Burns or muscle damage may also lead to a state of hypovolemia and hyponatremia secondary to substantial fluid and electrolyte losses from skin or into muscle.

2. In a hypovolemic hyponatremic patient with a **urinary sodium level of greater than 20 mEq per L,** renal losses are occurring, and several different diagnostic possibilities must be considered.

   a. **Excessive use of diuretics** is foremost among these diagnoses. It occurs almost exclusively with thiazide diuretics, because these agents, unlike loop diuretics, alter only urinary diluting ability; urinary concentration remains unimpaired. A fall in plasma sodium concentration in a patient receiving diuretics may be the first clue that a diuretic dosage adjustment is needed. In some patients with diuretic abuse, ECF volume depletion is not readily apparent from clinical examination. An important clue, however, to the diagnosis of diuretic-induced hyponatremia is that virtually all these patients have an associated hypokalemic metabolic alkalosis if they are receiving potassium-losing diuretics. If, however, a potassium-sparing diuretic is involved (e.g., triamterene, amiloride, or spironolactone), neither hypokalemia nor metabolic alkalosis may be present. Cessation of use of the diuretic is the best means of confirming the diagnosis of diuretic-induced hyponatremia. However, it must be remembered that restoration of ECF volume also is necessary to correct the hyponatremia. In the hypokalemic patient, potassium replacement also may be necessary for complete correction of the plasma sodium concentration imbalance.

   Surreptitious diuretic abuse occurs among premenopausal women who use diuretics for weight loss or other cosmetic reasons (e.g., thick ankles or calves, "puffy" face). These patients may be difficult to distinguish from patients with surreptitious vomiting, because both may present with evidence of ECF volume depletion and hypokalemic metabolic alkalosis. The presence or absence of hyponatremia depends on the patient's water intake. The pivotal diagnostic test to distinguish between the hypovolemic hyponatremic patient with metabolic alkalosis who is a diuretic abuser and the patient who is a surreptitious vomiter is the urinary chloride concentration. Surreptitious vomiters have low (less than 10 mEq per L) concentrations and surreptitious diuretic abusers have high (greater than 20 mEq per L) concentrations.

   b. **Salt-losing nephritis.** Patients with medullary cystic disease, chronic interstitial nephritis, polycystic kidney disease, analgesic nephropathy, partial urinary tract obstruction, and, rarely, chronic glomerulonephritis may present with hypovolemic hyponatremia secondary to salt-losing nephritis. These patients generally have moderately advanced renal impairment with serum creatinine levels greater than 3 to 4 mg per dL. This diagnosis should virtually never be considered in patients with renal disease that is not associated with elevated serum creatinine. Patients with salt-losing nephritis may need supplemental sodium chloride (NaCl) intake to avoid ECF volume depletion, or they may become very susceptible to ECF volume depletion in association with either decreased intake or extrarenal (e.g., gastrointestinal) sodium and water losses. Because these patients may be pigmented secondary to uremic dermatitis and exhibit hyponatremia and volume depletion, their disease was initially described as mimicking Addison's disease.

c. **Mineralocorticoid deficiency.** The patient with Addison's disease (i.e., primary adrenal insufficiency) generally has associated hyperkalemia; prerenal azotemia generally does not increase serum creatinine to concentrations greater than 3 mg per dL. In patients with mineralocorticoid deficiency, ECF volume repletion may correct both the hyponatremia and the hyperkalemia. During periods of stress, the plasma cortisol level may be within the normal range. Therefore, if adrenal insufficiency is suspected, a 2-hour cosyntropin (Cortrosyn) stimulation test should be performed. In addition to a urinary sodium concentration of greater than 20 mEq per L, a urinary potassium concentration of less than 20 mEq per L may be another clue to mineralocorticoid deficiency. If fluid intake has been restricted, the patient with Addison's disease may not present with hyponatremia, and hyperkalemia may not be present if the ECF volume depletion is not severe. Therefore, a high index of suspicion is necessary to make the diagnosis of primary adrenal insufficiency. These patients may present with nonspecific symptoms such as weight loss, anorexia, abdominal pain, nausea, vomiting, diarrhea, and fever.

d. **Osmotic diuresis obligating anion and cation excretion** is another major diagnostic consideration in the hypovolemic hyponatremic patient with a urinary sodium concentration greater than 20 mEq per L.

   i. **Glucose, urea, or mannitol diuresis.** The uncontrolled diabetic patient may have substantial glucosuria, causing water and electrolyte losses and, thereby ECF volume depletion. The urea diuresis after the relief of a urinary tract obstruction is another example of an osmotic diuresis that can cause ECF volume depletion. A chronic mannitol infusion without electrolyte replacement can produce a similar situation.

   ii. **Bicarbonaturia.** Increased anion excretion also can obligate renal water and electrolyte losses. The most frequently encountered example of this is metabolic alkalosis with bicarbonaturia. The bicarbonate anion in the urine is accompanied by cations, including sodium and potassium, which maintain electrical neutrality. Bicarbonaturia may accompany the early development of metabolic alkalosis accompanying postoperative nasogastric suction or vomiting. Proximal renal tubular acidosis (e.g., in Fanconi's syndrome) is another condition in which bicarbonaturia causes renal electrolyte loss. In the absence of a urinary tract infection with urease-producing organisms, a urinary pH (measured by a pH meter) greater than 6.1 indicates the presence of bicarbonate in the urine.

   iii. **Ketonuria.** Ketoacid anions also can obligate renal electrolyte losses in spite of ECF volume depletion; this may contribute to urinary electrolyte losses in diabetic or alcoholic ketoacidosis or starvation.

C. **Euvolemic hyponatremia** is a commonly encountered form of hyponatremia in hospitalized patients. The urinary sodium concentration in euvolemic hyponatremia is generally greater than 20 mEq per L. However, if the patient is on a sodium-restricted diet or is volume depleted, the urinary sodium concentration may be less than 10 mEq per L. Refeeding with a normal salt intake or expansion of ECF volume with saline increases urinary sodium concentration to more than 20 mEq per L, but hyponatremia will persist in the patient with euvolemic hyponatremia. These patients show no signs of either an increase or decrease in total body sodium. Although the water retention leads to an excess in TBW, no edema is detected because two-thirds of the water is inside the cell. A limited number of diagnostic possibilities are available for hyponatremic patients who exhibit neither edema nor ECF volume depletion (i.e., euvolemic hyponatremic patients) (Fig. 2-1). Two endocrine disorders must be considered: hypothyroidism and secondary adrenal insufficiency associated with pituitary or hypothalamic disease.

1. The occurrence of hyponatremia with **hypothyroidism** generally suggests severe disease, including myxedema coma. In some patients, particularly the elderly, the diagnosis may not be readily apparent. Therefore, thyroid function must be assessed in the euvolemic hyponatremic patient.

2. **Glucocorticoid deficiency.** An intact renin-angiotensin-aldosterone system avoids ECF volume depletion in patients with secondary adrenal insufficiency, but it is clear that glucocorticoid deficiency alone can impair water excretion and cause hyponatremia. Although skull films and computed tomographic (CT) scans should always be obtained in the euvolemic hyponatremic patient when the cause of the hyponatremia is not obvious, normal skull films or CT scans do not exclude secondary adrenal insufficiency. A low plasma cortisol level associated with a low adrenocorticotropic hormone level supports the diagnosis of secondary adrenal insufficiency. In this setting, both secondary adrenal insufficiency and secondary hypothyroidism may contribute to the hyponatremia accompanying pituitary insufficiency.

3. **Emotional or physical stress** must be considered in the euvolemic hyponatremic patient before invoking the diagnosis of the syndrome of inappropriate antidiuretic hormone (SIADH). Acute pain or severe emotional stress (e.g., decompensated psychosis associated with continued water ingestion) may lead to acute and severe hyponatremia. It is likely that a combination of emotional stress and physical pain accounts for the frequently encountered secretion of vasopressin in the postoperative state, which in turn leads to hyponatremia in the face of hypotonic fluid administration.

4. A number of **pharmacologic agents** either stimulate the release of vasopressin or enhance its action. These include:
   a. Nicotine
   b. Chlorpropamide
   c. Tolbutamide
   d. Clofibrate
   e. Cyclophosphamide
   f. Morphine
   g. Barbiturates
   h. Vincristine
   i. Carbamazepine (Tegretol)
   j. Acetaminophen
   k. Nonsteroidal anti-inflammatory drugs (NSAIDs)
   l. Antipsychotics
   m. Antidepressants
   Therefore, determining whether the euvolemic hyponatremic patient is receiving such drugs is an important diagnostic step.

5. **SIADH** should be considered after exclusion of other diagnoses in the euvolemic hyponatremic patient. In general, the causes of SIADH include:
   a. **Carcinomas**, most frequently but not exclusively of the
      i. Lung
      ii. Duodenum
      iii. Pancreas
      iv. Head and neck
   b. **Pulmonary disorders**, including but not limited to
      i. Viral pneumonia
      ii. Bacterial pneumonia
      iii. Pulmonary abscess
      iv. Tuberculosis
      v. Aspergillosis
   c. **Central nervous system (CNS) disorders**
      i. Encephalitis (viral or bacterial)
      ii. Meningitis (viral, bacterial, or tubercular)
      iii. Acute psychosis
      iv. Stroke (cerebral thrombosis or hemorrhage)

      v. Acute intermittent porphyria
     vi. Brain tumor
    vii. Brain abscess
   viii. Subdural or subarachnoid hematoma or hemorrhage
     ix. Guillain-Barré syndrome
      x. Head trauma
  d. Acquired immunodeficiency syndrome

Therefore, SIADH occurs primarily in association with infections and with vascular and neoplastic processes in the CNS or lung.

III. SIGNS AND SYMPTOMS. The level of hyponatremia that may cause signs and symptoms varies with the rate of decline in the plasma sodium concentration and the age of the patient. In general, the young adult patient appears to tolerate a specific level of hyponatremia better than does the older patient. However, the acute (i.e., within a few hours) development of hyponatremia in a previously asymptomatic young patient may cause severe CNS signs and symptoms, such as depressed sensorium, seizures, and even death, when the plasma sodium concentration has reached only a level between 125 and 130 mEq per L. This is because the capacity of brain cells to extrude osmotically active particles, and thereby relieve the brain swelling that accompanies hyponatremia, requires a longer time to be invoked at the beginning of the condition. Conversely, this protective mechanism against brain swelling becomes very effective with the chronic development of hyponatremia over days or weeks, so that an elderly person may present without overt signs or symptoms even with a plasma sodium concentration below 110 mEq per L.

Gastrointestinal symptoms, including anorexia and nausea, may occur early with hyponatremia. The more severe later signs and symptoms relate to the CNS because the cell swelling that occurs with hyponatremia is tolerated worst within the rigid encasement of the skull. Severe hyponatremia of rapid onset may lead to brain edema and herniation and therefore requires rapid treatment. Cheyne-Stokes respiration may be a hallmark of severe acute hyponatremia. In addition to exposure, uremia, and hypothyroidism, hyponatremia also should be considered in the differential diagnosis of the hypothermic patient.

In summary, **symptoms** that may be associated with hyponatremia include:
A. Lethargy, apathy
B. Disorientation
C. Muscle cramps
D. Anorexia, nausea
E. Agitation
  Signs that may be associated with hyponatremia include:
F. Abnormal sensorium
G. Depressed deep tendon reflexes
H. Cheyne-Stokes respiration
 I. Hypothermia
 J. Pathologic reflexes
K. Pseudobulbar palsy
 L. Seizures

IV. THERAPY
  A. Factors affecting the approach to treatment. The presence or absence of symptoms and the duration of the hyponatremia are the primary guides to treatment strategy. Different time-dependent processes are involved in the adaptation to changes in tonicity, and the presence of cerebral symptoms reflects a failure of the adaptive response. In this regard, hyponatremia developing within 48 hours carries a greater risk of permanent neurologic sequelae from cerebral edema if the plasma sodium concentration is not corrected expeditiously. Conversely, patients with chronic hyponatremia are at risk of osmotic demyelination if the correction is excessive or too rapid.
  B. Cerebral adaptation to hypotonicity. Decreases in extracellular osmolality cause the movement of water into cells, increasing intracellular volume and causing tissue edema. Edema within the cranium raises intracranial pressure, leading to neurologic

syndromes. To prevent this complication, a volume-regulatory adaptation occurs. Early in the course of hyponatremia, within 1 to 3 hours, cerebral ECF volume decreases through the movement of fluid into the cerebrospinal fluid (CSF), which is then shunted into the systemic circulation. Thereafter, the brain adapts by losing cellular potassium and organic solutes, which tend to lower the intracellular osmolality without substantial gain of water. If hyponatremia persists, other organic osmolytes, such as phosphocreatine, myoinositol, and amino acids (e.g., glutamine and taurine) are lost. The loss of these solutes greatly decreases cerebral swelling. Patients in whom this adaptive response fails are prone to severe cerebral edema when they develop hyponatremia. Postoperative menstruant females, elderly women on a thiazide diuretic, psychiatric polydipsic patients, and hypoxemic patients are particularly prone to hyponatremia-related encephalopathy. Conversely, as noted earlier, patients who have had the adaptive response are at risk of osmotic demyelination syndrome if the hyponatremia is excessively or too rapidly corrected. For example, a rapid increase in plasma osmolality may cause excessive cerebral water loss in previously adapted brains. Alcoholic and malnourished subjects, burn victims, and patients with severe hypokalemia are at risk for this complication.

C. **Acute symptomatic hyponatremia**, developing in less than 48 hours, is almost inevitable in hospitalized patients receiving hypotonic fluids. Treatment should be prompt because the risk of acute cerebral edema exceeds the risk of osmotic demyelination. The aim should be to raise the serum Na^+ by 2 mmol per L per hour until symptoms resolve. Complete correction is unnecessary, although it is not unsafe. Hypertonic saline (3% NaCl) is infused at the rate of 1 to 2 mL per kg per hour, and a loop diuretic, such as furosemide, enhances solute-free water excretion and hastens the return to a normal serum Na^+. If severe neurologic symptoms (seizures, obtundation, or coma) are present, 3% NaCl may be infused at 4 to 6 mL per kg per hour. Even 29.2% NaCl (50 mL) has been used safely. Serum electrolytes should be carefully monitored.

D. **Chronic symptomatic hyponatremia.** If hyponatremia has been present for more than 48 hours or the duration is unknown, correction must be handled carefully. Whether it is the rate of correction of hyponatremia or the magnitude that predisposes to osmotic demyelination is unknown, but in practice dissociating the two is difficult, because a rapid correction rate usually means a greater correction over a given period of time.

The following guidelines are fundamental to successful therapy:

1. Because cerebral water is increased only by approximately 10% in severe chronic hyponatremia, promptly increase the serum Na^+ level by 10%, or by approximately 10 mEq per L.

2. After the initial correction, do not exceed a correction rate of 1.0 to 1.5 mEq per L per hour.

3. Do not increase the serum Na^+ by more than 12 mEq per L per 24 hours or 18 mEq per L per 48 hours.

It is important to take into account the rate of infusion and the electrolyte content of infused fluids and the rate of production and electrolyte content of the urine.

Once the desired increment in serum Na^+ concentration is obtained, the treatment should consist of water restriction.

E. The approach to the **chronic asymptomatic patient with hyponatremia** is different. Initial bedside evaluation includes searching for an underlying disorder. Hypothyroidism and adrenal insufficiency should be sought as possible etiologies, and hormones must be replaced if these deficiencies are found. A careful analysis of the patient's medications should be made and necessary adjustments undertaken.

For patients with SIADH, if the etiology is not identifiable or cannot be treated, the approach should be conservative because rapid changes in serum tonicity lead to a greater degree of cerebral water loss and possible osmotic demyelination. Various approaches can be considered.

1. **Fluid restriction** is an easy and usually successful option, if the patient complies. A calculation must be made of the fluid restriction that will maintain a specific serum Na^+. The daily osmolar load ingested divided by the minimal urinary

osmolality (a function of the severity of the diluting disorder) determines a patient's maximal urine volume. On a normal North American diet, the daily osmolar load is approximately 10 mOsm per kg of body weight; in a healthy person, the minimum urinary osmolality (given no circulating vasopressin) can be as low as 50 mOsm per kg. Therefore, the daily urine volume in a 70-kg man can be as high as 14 L (700 mOsm per 50 mOsm per L). If the patient has SIADH and the urinary osmolality cannot be lowered below 500 mOsm per kg, the same osmolar load of 700 mOsm per day allows for only 1.4 L of urine. Therefore, if the patient drinks more than 1.4 L per day, the serum Na^+ will fall. A measurement of urinary sodium (U_{Na}) and potassium concentration (U_K) can guide the degree of water restriction that is required. If $U_{Na} + U_K$ is greater than the serum sodium concentration, water restriction alone may not be sufficient to increase serum sodium concentration.

2. **Pharmacologic agents.** **Lithium** was the first drug used to antagonize the action of vasopressin in hyponatremic disorders. Lithium may be neurotoxic, and its effects are unpredictable. Therefore, **demeclocycline** has become the agent of choice. This drug inhibits the formation and action of cyclic adenosine monophosphate (AMP) in the renal collecting duct. The onset of action is 3 to 6 days after treatment is started. The dose must be decreased to the lowest level that keeps the serum sodium concentration within the desired range with unrestricted water intake; this dose is usually 300 to 900 mg daily. The drug should be given 1 to 2 hours after meals, and calcium-, aluminum-, and magnesium-containing antacids should be avoided. However, polyuria tends to make patients noncompliant. Skin photosensitivity may occur; in children, tooth or bone abnormalities may result. Nephrotoxicity also limits the drug's use, especially in patients with underlying liver disease or congestive heart failure, in whom the hepatic metabolism of demeclocycline may be impaired.

3. **Vasopressin antagonists.** The major therapeutic advance that has occurred in hyponatremic patients relates to the development of orally active, nonpeptide antagonists to the V_2 AVP receptor. AVP binds to the basolateral membrane of the principal cells of the renal collecting duct. Activation of this G-protein–linked V_2 receptor stimulates an adenylyl cyclase-cyclic AMP signaling pathway that upregulates the aquaporin-2 (AQP2) water channel expression and trafficking to the apical membrane (Fig. 2-2). The V_2 vasopressin antagonists bind more deeply in the principal cell transmembrane region than AVP. However, these V_2 antagonists do not activate the V_2 receptor, because of a lack of interaction with critical residues on the H1 helix of the receptor.

In Table 2-1, the nonpeptide AVP receptor antagonists which are in clinical trials are shown. The U.S. Food and Drug Administration (FDA) to date has only approved one of these antagonists for clinical use, namely conivaptan. Conivaptan is different from the other AVP receptor antagonists in that it antagonizes both the V_{1a} (vascular) and V_2 receptor. Moreover, it has only been approved to treat in-hospital hyponatremia by intravenous use for 4 days. The other three agents are selective V_2 receptor antagonists, which can be used chronically by oral administration. Conivaptan has been FDA approved to treat euvolemic hyponatremia, for example, SIADH and hypervolemic hyponatremia associated with cardiac failure. While the V_{1a} antagonist component may improve heart function by decreasing cardiac afterload, V_{1a} antagonist could theoretically increase splanchnic flow, thereby raising portal pressure in cirrhotic patients. Therefore, conivaptan is not approved to treat hyponatremia associated with cirrhosis. The other selective V_2 receptor antagonists, tolvaptan, lixivaptan, and satavaptan, have been shown to effectively increase solute-free water excretion and raise serum sodium concentrations in patients with cardiac failure, cirrhosis, and SIADH. Polyuria and thirst have been the major observed side effects of these agents. The major benefits of treating hyponatremia appear to relate to CNS function. Correction of hyponatremia with the V_2 receptor antagonists have been shown to improve mental function. Other studies have shown improved gait when raising severe sodium concentrations in "asymptomatic" hyponatremic

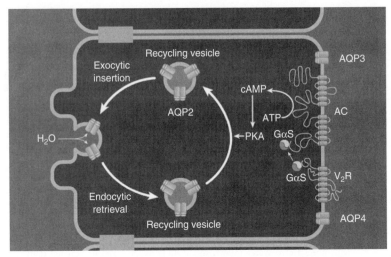

Figure 2-2. Signaling pathways for vasopressin-regulated water absorption. (AQP2, aquaporin-2; ATP, adenosine triphosphate; AC, adenylyl cyclase; PKA, protein kinase A; V_2R, vasopressin receptor.) (Used with permission of Bichet DG. Lithium, cyclic AMP signaling, A-kinase anchoring proteins, and aquaporin-2. *J Am Soc Nephrol* 2006;17:920–922.)

patients. Because falls and fractured hips, particularly in the elderly, are more common in hyponatremic patients, there are other clinical implications for using these V_2 receptor antagonists to treat hyponatremia. These relatively safe antagonists, therefore, have potential to more effectively correct acute and chronic hyponatremia as compared to severe fluid restriction, demeclocycline, urea, and so on. They, however, should not be used in hypovolemic hyponatremia, the treatment for which is ECF volume expansion.

4. **Increase in solute excretion.** Because urine flow can be significantly increased by obligating the excretion of solutes and thereby allowing a greater intake of water, measures to increase solute excretion have been used. A loop diuretic, when combined with high sodium intake (2 to 3 g additional NaCl), is effective. A single diuretic dose (40 mg furosemide) is usually sufficient. The dose should be doubled if the diuresis induced in the first 8 hours is less than 60% of

TABLE 2-1   Nonpeptide Arginine Vasopressin (AVP) Receptor Antagonists

	Tolvaptan	Lixivaptan	Satavaptan	Conivaptan
Receptor	V_2	V_2	V_2	V_{1a}/V_2
Route of administration	Oral	Oral	Oral	IV
Urine volume	↑	↑	↑	↑
Urine osmolality	↓	↓	↓	↓
Na^+ excretion/24 hr	↔	↔ Low dose ↑ High dose	↔	↔
Company	Otsuka	CardioKine	Sanofi-Aventis	Astrellas

(Used with permission of Lee CR, Watkins ML, Patterson JH, et al. Vasopressin: a new target for the treatment of hear failure. *Am Heart J* 2003;146:9–18.)

the total daily urine output. Administration of urea to increase the solute load increases urine flow by causing an osmotic diuresis. This permits a more liberal water intake without worsening the hyponatremia and without altering urinary concentration. The dose is usually 30 to 60 g of urea daily. The major limitations are gastrointestinal distress and unpalatability.

F. Hypovolemic and hypervolemic hyponatremia. Symptoms directly related to hyponatremia are unusual in hypovolemic hyponatremia because loss of both sodium and water limits osmotic shifts in the brain. Restoration of ECF volume with crystalloids or colloids interrupts the nonosmotic release of vasopressin. In patients with hypovolemic hyponatremia from diuretics, the drug must be discontinued and potassium repletion ensured. The treatment of hyponatremia in hypervolemic states is more difficult because it requires attention to the underlying disorder of heart failure or chronic liver disease. In congestive heart failure, both sodium and water restriction are critical. Refractory patients may be treated with a combination of an angiotensin-converting enzyme (ACE) inhibitor and a diuretic. The resultant increase in cardiac output with ACE inhibitors may increase solute-free water excretion and correct hyponatremia. Loop diuretics diminish the action of vasopressin on the collecting tubules, thereby increasing solute-free water excretion. Thiazide diuretics impair urinary dilution and may worsen hyponatremia. Water and salt restriction are also the mainstay of therapy in cirrhotic patients. For both disorders, orally active V_2-receptor antagonists are under investigation, and these aquaretics may be clinically available to treat hyponatremia in the near future.

Hypernatremia. *Hypernatremia*, defined as a plasma sodium concentration greater than 150 mEq per L, is less common than hyponatremia, probably not because of a more frequent occurrence of disorders of urinary dilution than of urinary concentration, but rather because of drinking behavior. Specifically, if an inability to dilute the urine is present, water intake of 1 to 2 L per day may cause hyponatremia. This amount of fluid intake may be ingested as routine behavior in spite of a hypo-osmolar stimulus to suppress thirst, which may explain the frequency of hyponatremia. Conversely, urinary-concentrating defects that cause renal water losses generally do not cause hypernatremia unless a disturbance in thirst is also present or the patient cannot drink or obtain adequate fluid to drink. The very young, the very old, and the very sick are, therefore, those populations that develop hypernatremia most frequently. In the absence of an inability to drink (e.g., with coma, nausea, and vomiting) or to obtain water (e.g., in infants or severely ill adults), the thirst mechanism is very effective in preventing hypernatremia. Whereas hyponatremia does not always reflect a hypotonic state (i.e., pseudohyponatremia or translocation hyponatremia), hypernatremia always denotes a hypertonic state.

I. APPROACH TO THE HYPERNATREMIC PATIENT. As is the case with hyponatremia, hypernatremic patients may have low, high, or normal total body sodium (Fig. 2-3). Such a classification allows the clinician to focus on the most likely diagnosis in each category.

A. Hypovolemic hypernatremic patient. The hypernatremic patient may have evidence of ECF volume depletion that has occurred secondary to either renal or extrarenal losses. These patients have sustained water losses that are greater than the sodium losses.

1. Extrarenal losses. If the losses have been from an extrarenal site (e.g., in diarrhea), then sodium and water conservation by the kidney should be readily apparent. In such patients, the urine sodium concentration is less than 10 mEq per L, and the urine is hypertonic. In fact, losses by hypotonic diarrhea are among the most common causes of hypernatremia in both children and adults, especially in those who are receiving recurring lactulose for underlying severe liver disease with encephalopathy.

2. Renal losses. In contrast, hypotonic electrolyte losses may occur in the urine during osmotic diuresis or use of loop diuretics. In these patients, evidence of renal sodium and water conservation is, of course, not present, because the urine is the source of the losses. Therefore, the urine is not hypertonic, and urine sodium concentration is generally greater than 20 mEq per L. In

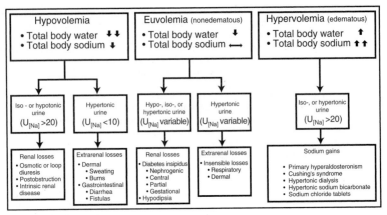

Figure 2-3. Diagnostic approach to hypernatremia. ($\uparrow$, increased; $\uparrow\uparrow$, greatly increased; $\downarrow$, decreased; $\downarrow\downarrow$, greatly decreased; $\leftrightarrow$, not increased or decreased; $U_{[Na]}$, urinary sodium concentration, in mEq per L.)

the hyperglycemic diabetic patient with good renal function and profound glucosuria, hypernatremia may be a presenting feature, because hypotonic renal losses may obscure any effect of hyperglycemia to shift water osmotically from cells to ECF. This is particularly true if the patient does not have access to water or is incapable of ingesting fluids (e.g., a comatose, ketoacidotic diabetic patient). In the setting of high-protein tube feedings, the high rate of urea excretion leads to significant renal water losses.

B. Hypervolemic hypernatremic patient. Patients with hypernatremia also may have evidence of ECF volume expansion. Generally, these patients have received excessive amounts of hypertonic NaCl or sodium bicarbonate. In such an acute setting, the incidence of ECF volume expansion is most likely to be associated with pulmonary congestion, elevated neck veins, or both, rather than with peripheral edema. This variety of hypervolemic hypernatremia is rather infrequent, but may occur with sodium bicarbonate administration during cardiac resuscitation or NaCl tablets taken during exercise in a high-temperature, high-humidity environment.

C. Euvolemic hypernatremia. Most patients with hypernatremia secondary to water loss appear euvolemic with normal total body sodium, because loss of water without sodium does not lead to overt volume contraction. Water loss in and of itself need not culminate in hypernatremia unless it is unaccompanied by water intake. Because such hypodipsia is uncommon, hypernatremia usually supervenes only in those who have no access to water or who have a neurologic deficit that does not allow them to seek it. Extrarenal water loss occurs from the skin and respiratory tract in febrile or other hypermetabolic states. Urine osmolality is very high, reflecting an intact osmoreceptor-vasopressin-renal response. Therefore, the defense against hyperosmolality requires both stimulation of thirst and the ability to respond by drinking water. The urine sodium concentration varies with sodium intake. The renal losses of water that lead to euvolemic hypernatremia are a consequence of a defect in vasopressin production or release (central diabetes insipidus), a failure of the collecting duct to respond to the hormone (nephrogenic diabetes insipidus), or excessive rapid degradation of vasopressin (gestational diabetes insipidus).

1. Approximately 50% of instances of **central diabetes insipidus** have no detectable underlying cause and therefore are classified as idiopathic. Trauma, surgical procedures in the area of the pituitary or hypothalamus, and brain neoplasms, either primary or secondary (e.g., from metastatic breast cancer), constitute most of the remaining causes of central diabetes insipidus. In addition, encephalitis, sarcoidosis, or eosinophilic granuloma may cause central diabetes insipidus. Central diabetes insipidus can be partial, with some preservation of vasopressin release. When the central diabetes insipidus is associated with hypothalamic lesions and hypodipsia, these patients present with hypernatremia and a urine osmolality above plasma. A congenital form of central diabetes insipidus has also been described.

2. **Nephrogenic diabetes insipidus.**   This disorder can be **congenital or acquired.** In 85% of congenital diabetes insipidus, the disorder is inherited as an x-linked mutation. The underlying defect resides in the vasopressin receptor that is localized to the x chromosome. The remaining 15% of cases of a rarer autosomal recessive form is related to a mutation in the vasopressin-dependent AQP2 water channel. A number of acquired causes have been described, many of them also associated with decreased AQP2 production:

   a. **Secondary to renal diseases.** Medullary or interstitial renal diseases are likely to be accompanied by vasopressin-resistant renal concentrating defects; the most frequent of these diseases are medullary cystic disease, chronic interstitial nephritis (e.g., analgesic nephropathy), polycystic kidney disease, and partial bilateral urinary tract obstruction. Far-advanced renal disease of any cause is uniformly associated with a renal concentrating defect. However, because of the very low glomerular filtration rate, the renal water loss (i.e., polyuria) is modest (2 to 4 L per day).

   b. **Secondary to hypercalcemia and hypokalemia.** Hypercalcemia secondary to any cause, including primary hyperparathyroidism, vitamin D intoxication, milk-alkali syndrome, hyperthyroidism, and tumor, may also cause acquired nephrogenic diabetes insipidus. Similarly, hypokalemia secondary to any cause, including primary aldosteronism, diarrhea, and chronic diuretic use, may cause nephrogenic diabetes insipidus. However, some of the polyuria accompanying hypercalcemia or hypokalemia may be due to stimulation of thirst and the resultant increase in water intake.

   c. **Drugs, dietary abnormalities, and other causes.** Various drugs impair the end-organ response to vasopressin and therefore cause a renal concentrating defect (see section I.C. 2.d.iii). Excess water intake as well as dietary sodium and protein restriction also have been shown to impair urinary concentration. Other unique causes of nephrogenic diabetes insipidus include multiple myeloma, amyloidosis, Sjögren's syndrome, and sarcoidosis.

   d. A **summary** of acquired causes of nephrogenic diabetes insipidus includes:

      i. **Chronic renal disease**
         - Polycystic kidney disease
         - Medullary cystic disease
         - Pyelonephritis
         - Urinary tract obstruction
         - Far-advanced renal failure
         - Analgesic nephropathy

      ii. **Electrolyte disorders**
         - Hypokalemia
         - Hypercalcemia

      iii. **Drugs**
         - Lithium
         - Demeclocycline
         - Acetohexamide
         - Tolazamide
         - Glyburide
         - Propoxyphene
         - Amphotericin
         - Methoxyflurane
         - Vinblastine
         - Colchicine

      iv. **Dietary abnormalities**
         - Excessive water intake

- Decreased sodium chloride intake
- Decreased protein intake

v. Miscellaneous
- Multiple myeloma
- Amyloidosis
- Sjögren's syndrome
- Sarcoidosis
- Sickle cell disease

3. **Diabetes insipidus secondary to vasopressinase.** Central diabetes insipidus and nephrogenic diabetes are not the only causes of polyuria during pregnancy. Vasopressinase is an enzyme, produced in the placenta, that causes *in vivo* degradation of AVP during pregnancy. Normally, an increase in vasopressin synthesis and release during pregnancy compensates for the increased degradation of the hormone. In rare cases, however, excessive vasopressinase has been incriminated in causing polyuria during pregnancy. Because vasopressinase cannot degrade deamino-8-D-arginine vasopressin, this is the treatment of choice for this pregnancy-related polyuria.

4. **Response to fluid deprivation and AVP in the diagnosis of polyuric disorder.** The various forms of diabetes insipidus must be differentiated from primary polydipsia in patients who present with polyuria. In Table 2-2, the procedure and interpretation of a water deprivation test are summarized. Patients with compulsive water drinking may present with polyuria and a blunted response to the fluid deprivation test; on cessation of fluid intake, hypernatremia does not develop in these patients and their renal concentration defect is primarily due to a resistance of the kidney to vasopressin. However, because patients with central or nephrogenic diabetes insipidus may present with polyuria and polydipsia in the absence of hypernatremia, awareness of the diagnosis of compulsive (psychogenic) water drinking is quite important. Menopausal women with previous psychiatric problems are particularly prone to compulsive water drinking. Psychoneurosis and psychosis are also frequently associated with increased water intake.

The differential diagnosis in the polyuric patient between compulsive water drinking and partial central diabetes insipidus is the most difficult. Fluid restriction with 3% to 5% loss of body weight will lead to a urine osmolality above plasma, albeit to a submaximal level in both circumstances. Administration of vasopressin will not increase urine osmolality further (less than 10%) in the patient with compulsive water drinking because the defect is at the level of

TABLE 2-2 Procedure and Interpretation of a Water Deprivation Test

Cause of polyuria	Urinary osmolality with water deprivation (mOsm/kg of water)	Increase in urinary osmolality after fluid deprivation with exogenous arginine vasopressin (AVP)
Normal	>800	Little or no increase
Complete central diabetes insipidus	<300	Substantially increased above plasma
Partial central diabetes insipidus	300–800	Increase of >10%
Nephrogenic diabetes insipidus	<300–500	Any increase <10%
Primary polydipsia	>500	Any increase <10%

the kidney, not inadequate endogenous vasopressin. In contrast, the patient with partial central diabetes insipidus will have a substantial increase in urinary osmolality (greater than 10%) with exogenous vasopressin because the defect is due to inadequate release of vasopressin.

Last, the patient with nephrogenic diabetes insipidus may occasionally have vasopressin-resistant hypotonic urine (e.g., hypercalcemic or hypokalemic nephropathy); therefore, the temporary absence of fluid intake because of an intercurrent illness can be associated with hypernatremia. In all hypernatremic patients who primarily have water losses without electrolyte losses, the urine sodium excretion concentration merely reflects sodium intake. During any solute-free water diuresis, the urinary sodium concentration declines so that sodium balance is maintained.

II. SIGNS AND SYMPTOMS. Polyuria and polydipsia may be prominent symptoms in the patient who subsequently develops hypernatremia in association with inadequate water intake.

  A. CNS dysfunction. Neurologic abnormalities constitute the most prominent manifestations of hypernatremic states. These neurologic manifestations appear to be due primarily to the cellular dehydration and shrinkage of brain cells that are associated with tearing of cerebral vessels. Capillary and venous congestion, subcortical and subarachnoid bleeding, and venous sinus thrombosis all have been described with hypernatremia.

  B. Prognosis of acute versus chronic hypernatremia. The signs and symptoms of hypernatremia are more severe in acute than in chronic hypernatremia. Indeed, 75% mortality has been reported in association with acute hypernatremia in adults with acute elevations of plasma sodium concentration above 160 mEq per L. These adults, however, frequently have severe primary diseases associated with their hypernatremia, and these primary diseases may largely account for the high mortality. A 45% mortality has been reported in children with acute hypernatremia, and as many as two-thirds of the surviving children may have neurologic sequelae.

  C. Idiogenic osmoles with chronic hypernatremia. The more benign course of chronic hypernatremia appears to be related to cellular mechanisms that protect against severe brain dehydration. The brain, however, requires some period of time, perhaps days, to adapt. In chronic hypernatremia, brain cells generate idiogenic osmoles, some of which appear to be amino acids; these idiogenic osmoles are osmotically active and restore brain water to near-control levels in spite of persistent hypernatremia. The presence of these idiogenic anions with chronic hypernatremia, although protective against brain dehydration and shrinkage, may predispose to brain edema if the hypernatremia is corrected too rapidly.

  D. Correlation of CNS dysfunction with degree of hyperosmolality. The earliest manifestations of hypernatremia are restlessness, increased irritability, and lethargy. These symptoms may be followed by muscular twitching, hyperreflexia, tremulousness, and ataxia. The level of hyperosmolality at which these signs and symptoms occur depends not only on the rapidity of the change in the plasma sodium concentration but also on the age of the patient; the very young and the very old exhibit the most severe manifestations. In general, however, these signs and symptoms may occur progressively with plasma osmolality in the range of 325 to 375 mOsm per kg of water. At plasma osmolalities above this level, tonic muscular spasticity, focal and grand mal seizures, and death may occur. The elderly patient with dementia or severe cerebrovascular disease may demonstrate these life-threatening signs and symptoms at a lower level of plasma hyperosmolality.

III. THERAPY. Hypernatremia is frequently a preventable electrolyte disorder if water losses are recognized and appropriately replaced. In most cases, hypernatremia can be treated by the judicious administration of water to patients with water-losing disorders who cannot obtain water. The treatment of hypernatremia depends on two important factors: ECF volume status and the rate of development of the hypernatremia.

  A. Correction of ECF volume depletion. When hypernatremia is associated with ECF volume depletion, the primary therapeutic goal is to administer isotonic saline until restoration of ECF volume is achieved, as assessed by normal neck veins and absence of orthostatic hypotension and tachycardia. Hypotonic (0.45%) NaCl or 5% glucose solutions can then be used to correct plasma osmolality.

B. **Correction of ECF volume expansion.** In contrast, if hypernatremia is associated with ECF volume expansion, diuretics (e.g., furosemide) with liberal fluid intake can be used to treat the hypernatremia. In the presence of advanced renal failure, the patient with hypernatremia and fluid overload may need to be dialyzed to treat the hypernatremia.

C. **Water-replacement method of calculation.** Last, the patient with euvolemic hypernatremia can be treated primarily with water replacement either orally or parenterally with 5% glucose in water. The method of calculation of the necessary water replacement for a 75-kg man with a plasma sodium of 154 mEq per L is as follows:

$$TBW = body\ weight \times 60\%\ or$$
$$TBW = 75 \times 0.6 = 45\ L$$

Then,

$$\frac{Actual\ plasma\ sodium}{Desired\ plasma\ sodium} \times TBW = \frac{154\ mEq/L}{140\ mEq/L} \times 45\ L = 49.5\ L$$

Therefore, the repletion of 4.5 L (49.5 − 45 L) positive water balance will correct the plasma sodium concentration. Ongoing water losses should not be overlooked.

D. **Rate of correction.** The recommended rate of correction of hypernatremia depends on the rate of development of the hypernatremia and the symptoms. More neurologic signs and symptoms are associated with acute hypernatremia; therefore, this biochemical abnormality should be corrected rapidly, over a few hours.

Conversely idiogenic osmoles appear to accumulate in brain cells during periods of chronic hypernatremia, a mechanism that protects against brain shrinkage. Therefore, the rapid correction of chronic hypernatremia can create an osmotic gradient between the ECF and intracellular compartments, with osmotic water movement into cells and subsequent brain edema. In general, therefore, chronic hypernatremia is best corrected gradually, at a rate not to exceed 2 mOsm per hour. One-half of the correction can be achieved in 24 hours and the other half in the next 24 hours or longer.

Suggested Readings

Berl T, Schrier RW. Disorders of water metabolism. In: Schrier RW, ed. *Renal and electrolyte disorders*, 6th ed. Philadelphia: Lippincott Williams & Wilkins, 2003:1–63.

Bichet D. Nephrogenic and central diabetes insipidus. In: Schrier RW, ed. *Diseases of the kidney and urinary tract*, 8th ed. Philadelphia: Lippincott Williams & Wilkins, 2007:2249–2269.

Cadnapaphornchai M, Kim Y-W, Gurevich A, et al. Urinary concentrating defect in hypothyroid rats: role of sodium, potassium, 2-chloride co-transporter and aquaporins. *J Am Soc Nephrol* 2003;14(3):566–574.

Chen YC, Cadnapaphornchai M, Summer S, et al. Molecular mechanism of impaired urinary concentrating ability in glucocorticoid deficient rats. *J Am Soc Nephrol* 2005;16:2864–2871.

Chen YC, Cadnapaphornchai M, Yang J, et al. Nonosmotic release of vasopressin and renal aquaporins in impaired urinary dilution in hypothyroidism. *Am J Physiol Renal Physiol* 2005;289:F672–F679.

Durr JA, Hoggard JG, Hunt JM, et al. Diabetes insipidus due to abnormally high circulating vasopressinase activity in a pregnancy. *N Engl J Med* 1987;316:1070–1074.

Schrier RW. Body water homeostasis: clinical disorders of urinary dilution and concentration. *J Am Soc Nephrol* 2006;17(7):1820–1832.

Schrier RW. Aquaporin-related disorders of water homeostasis. *Drug News Perspect* 2007;20(7):447–453.

Verbalis J. The syndrome of inappropriate anti-diuretic hormone secretion and other hypo-osmolar disorders. In: Schrier RW, ed. *Diseases of the kidney and urinary tract*, 8th ed. Philadelphia: Lippincott Williams & Wilkins, 2007:2214–2248.

Verbalis J, Goldsmith S, Greenberg A, et al. Hyponatremia treatment guidance consensus statement. *Am J Med* 2007;120(11 Suppl 1):S1–S12.

Wang W, Li C, Summer SN, et al. Molecular analysis of impaired urinary diluting capacity in glucocorticoid deficiency. *Am J Physiol Renal Physiol* 2006;290(5):F1135–F1142.

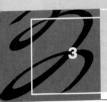

THE PATIENT WITH HYPOKALEMIA OR HYPERKALEMIA

Catherine L. Kelleher and Stuart L. Linas

 otassium is the most abundant cation in the human body. It regulates intracellular enzyme function and helps determine neuromuscular and cardiovascular tissue excitability. Ninety percent of total body potassium is located in intracellular fluid (ICF; primarily in muscle), 10% in the extracellular fluid (ECF), and less than 1% is in plasma. The ratio of extracellular potassium to intracellular potassium determines membrane potential. The acuity of changes in serum potassium concentration and membrane potential determines the severity of clinical symptoms and underlies the clinical findings caused by disorders of potassium metabolism.

I. OVERVIEW OF POTASSIUM PHYSIOLOGY. The typical Western diet contains 40 to 120 mEq of potassium a day. Tight control of the serum potassium between 3.5 and 5.5 mEq per day is primarily accomplished by the kidney where secretion varies between 40 and 120 mEq per day. Potassium losses in stool and sweat are small (5 to 10 mEq). In addition, the interplay of several hormonal systems as well as the internal acid–base environment contribute to the exchange of potassium between the ECF and ICF, which helps keep the serum potassium concentration tightly controlled. Although total body potassium declines with aging, and the rate of decline appears to be influenced by sex and race, the clinical significance of these observations is not clear.

A. Internal balance. After a meal, potassium is rapidly redistributed between the plasma and intracellular compartments. Several systems interact to regulate the transcellular movement of potassium.

    1. Insulin. A high serum potassium increases insulin levels. The binding of the insulin hormone to insulin receptors causes a hyperpolarization of cell membranes that facilitates potassium uptake in liver, fat, cardiac, and skeletal muscle. Insulin also activates Na-K-adenosine triphosphatase (ATPase) pumps and causes the cellular uptake of potassium.

    2. Catecholamines. Activation of the β_2 adrenoreceptor results in cellular potassium uptake in liver and muscle. This effect is transduced by cyclic adenosine monophosphate (cAMP) activation of Na-K-ATPase pumps, causing an influx of potassium in exchange for sodium. Therapeutic agents such as theophylline potentiate β_2 adrenoreceptor–mediated potassium uptake by inhibiting the degradation of cAMP.

    3. Aldosterone. Although this mineralocorticoid facilitates potassium uptake into muscle, clear proof of the clinical significance of this effect is lacking.

    4. Acid–base. Inorganic acidosis (e.g., hydrochloric acid) facilitates potassium movement from ICF to ECF. Protons enter cells, whereas impermeant inorganic ions do not. The resulting increases in ICF positive charge favor the outward movement of potassium. Because organic ions (lactate, ketoacids) are less restricted from entering cells, increases in serum potassium may not occur in organic acidosis.

    5. Tonicity. Hyperglycemia causes potassium-rich fluid to leave the cell, thereby increasing ECF potassium. Under most conditions, increases in insulin modulate and reverse the effect of increased extracellular tonicity. However, when insulin cannot be increased (e.g., type 1 diabetes mellitus) or hyperglycemia occurs rapidly (as with the administration of 50% glucose), hyperkalemia occurs. Rapid infusions of mannitol also may cause hyperkalemia.

B. External balance. Urinary potassium excretion is the result of a difference between the potassium secreted and potassium reabsorbed in the distal nephron. Potassium is freely filtered at the glomerulus. More than 50% of filtered potassium is reabsorbed in the proximal convoluted tubule through paracellular pathways. In the descending limb of Henle's loop, especially in deep nephrons, potassium concentration increases. In the medullary thick ascending limb of the loop of Henle, the Na–K–2Cl–cotransporter leads to the reabsorption of potassium. When the tubular fluid reaches the early distal convoluted tubule, only 10% to 15% of filtered potassium remains. Potassium is secreted by the principal cells of the cortical collecting and outer-medullary collecting duct. Potassium is reabsorbed in the collecting tubule, an effect mediated by intercalated cells. A fall in glomerular filtration rate (GFR) is not generally associated with decreased potassium excretion and hyperkalemia until the GFR is less than 20 mL per minute. The major factors regulating potassium excretion follow.

1. **Distal nephron flow rate and sodium delivery.** Under normal conditions, sodium delivered to the cortical collecting tubule is reabsorbed through amiloride-sensitive epithelial sodium channels (ENaCs) in the principal cells. The resulting negative potential in the tubular lumen results in increased potassium excretion through apical potassium channels [renal outer medullary potassium channel (ROMK)]. This system requires sodium delivery to the distal tubule. In addition, increases in tubular flow rate help maintain a low urinary potassium concentration, which favors the movement of potassium from cells into tubular fluid.

2. **Mineralocorticoids.** Aldosterone is the major mineralocorticoid; it increases potassium secretion into the tubular fluid by:
   a. Increasing the number and activity of apical amiloride sensitive ENaCs in the connecting tubule and cortical collecting duct in the distal tubule. This increases sodium reabsorption thereby creating a negative lumen and driving force for potassium excretion into the tubular lumen.
   b. Increasing basolateral Na-K-ATPase activity.

3. Increases or decreases in **dietary potassium** increase or decrease urinary potassium, respectively. Renal adaptation to high potassium intake is mediated by a potassium-induced increase in aldosterone secretion and by an increase in distal nephron Na-K-ATPase activity. In response to potassium restriction, mineralocorticoid activity decreases thereby causing a decline in potassium secretion.

4. Increases in relatively nonresorbable **anions** (e.g., bicarbonate, penicillins) trap secreted potassium in the tubular lumen and limit potassium reabsorption in the medullary collecting duct. The resulting renal potassium losses may lead to severe potassium depletion.

5. WNK kinases are a recently identified series of enzymes found to regulate potassium excretion. WNK4 decreases activity of the NaCl transporter in the distal tubules and decreases the number of potassium channels in the cortical collecting tubule. The net effect of WNK4 is to cause potassium retention.

II. HYPOKALEMIA

A. Diagnosis. The **initial approach** to hypokalemia is to determine whether it is spurious, secondary to a shift of potassium from the extracellular to intracellular compartments, or a result of a true decrease in total body potassium (Fig. 3-1).

Spurious hypokalemia occurs in the setting of extreme leukocytosis (*in vitro* white blood cells uptake potassium in the test tube) and is not associated with changes in either internal or external potassium balance.

Potassium shifts into cells may occur acutely in conditions associated with increases in endogenous insulin or catecholamines. For example, catecholamine release associated with shortness of breath (asthma, chronic obstructive pulmonary disease exacerbations, heart failure, chest pain syndromes including myocardial infarction or angina) or catecholamine release from a drug withdrawal syndrome (alcohol, narcotics, or barbiturates) shifts potassium into cells, thereby decreasing the serum potassium concentration. Hypokalemia may also be caused by insulin

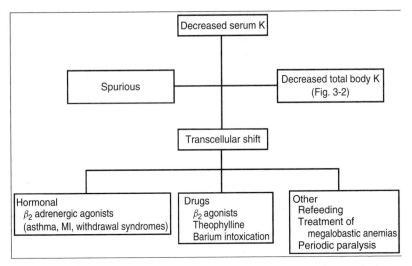

Figure 3-1. Diagnostic approach to hypokalemia. (K, potassium; MI, myocardial infarction.)

administration (correction of diabetic ketoacidosis, postresuscitation for hyperkalemia) or β_2-adrenoreceptor agonist (β_2 agonists, theophylline). Other common causes of decreases in serum potassium without decreases in total body potassium include hypokalemic periodic paralysis (familial and hyperthyroid types), treatment of megaloblastic anemias, and refeeding syndromes (probably insulin mediated). The refeeding syndrome, in which severely malnourished patients are begun on nasogastric feeding, is also seen in older adults in whom the clinical manifestations of malnutrition are less clinically apparent.

Decreases in total body potassium (Fig. 3-2) are caused by either inadequate potassium intake or by excessive renal or extrarenal potassium losses. The measurement of urinary potassium excretion (by 24-hour measurements or "spot" potassium concentrations) is used to distinguish renal versus extrarenal potassium loss. Urinary potassium concentrations less than 20 mEq per L suggest poor potassium intake or extrarenal potassium loss. Serum acid–base status is also helpful in evaluating the site of potassium loss. Metabolic acidosis may suggest gastrointestinal (GI) losses (diarrhea of any cause, e.g., infectious, toxic, laxative abuse). A normal serum pH is less helpful because hypokalemia can be secondary to both decreases in intake and GI losses. Metabolic alkalosis with urinary potassium of less than 20 mEq per L, although rare, is associated with laxative abuse, villous adenoma, or congenital chloride-losing diarrhea. Hypokalemia with a urinary potassium excretion of greater than 20 mEq per L suggests renal potassium wasting. The serum pH also is used to further evaluate etiologies. Metabolic acidosis suggests renal tubular acidosis (type 1 or type 2), diabetic ketoacidosis (osmotic diuresis), ureterosigmoidostomy, or carbonic anhydrase inhibitor use.

More commonly, renal potassium losses are associated with **metabolic alkalosis**. In this clinical setting, the urinary chloride concentration is helpful. A low urinary chloride concentration (less than 20 mEq per L) suggests potassium losses from upper GI losses, recent (but not current) diuretic use, or a posthypercapnic syndrome. Hypokalemia with a high urinary chloride concentration is further distinguished on the basis of the presence or absence of hypertension. In normotensive individuals, hypokalemia with metabolic alkalosis and a high urinary chloride occurs with diuretic use (loop or distal convoluted tubule–acting diuretics), Bartter's and Gitelman's syndrome, and with severe decreases in total body magnesium or potassium. Hypokalemia with renal potassium wasting, renal chloride wasting, and

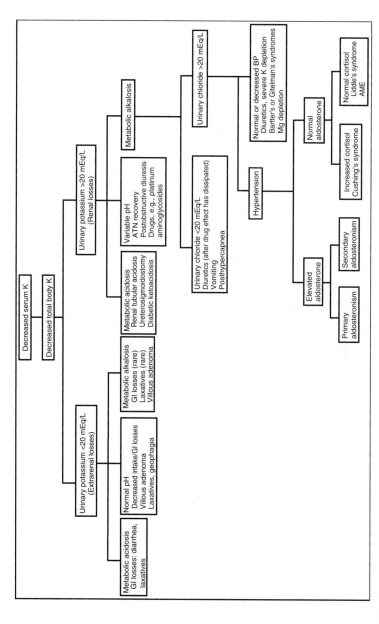

Figure 3-2. Diagnostic approach to hypokalemia. (AME, aseptic meningoencephalitis; ATN, acute tubular necroses; BP, blood pressure; GI, gastrointestinal; K, potassium.)

41

hypertension is further evaluated by urinary aldosterone concentrations. An elevated aldosterone level suggests either primary aldosteronism (adenoma, hyperplasia, glucocorticoid remedial) or secondary aldosteronism (renovascular or accelerated hypertension, diuretic use). Conversely, normal aldosterone levels with increases in serum cortisol suggest Cushing's syndrome or exogenous steroid use. Normal cortisol and aldosterone levels indicate Liddle's syndrome (caused by increases in the activity of the cortical collecting tubule sodium channel) or apparent mineralocorticoid excess syndrome [decreases in 11-β hydroxylsteroid dehydrogenase activity in kidney tissue (congenital, licorice ingestion) causing the mineralocorticoid receptor to respond to glucocorticoid]. Increases in urinary potassium excretion without a significant acid–base disorder are seen during the recovery phase of acute tubular necrosis, postobstructive diuresis, and magnesium depletion associated with drugs such as aminoglycosides and cisplatinum, or in myelomonocytic leukemia (secondary to lysozymuria).

Finally, hypokalemia is frequently associated with chronic alcoholism. The mechanism behind this electrolyte abnormality is not well defined but is probably multifactorial secondary to poor intake, diarrhea, alcohol withdrawal with respiratory alkalosis, and kaliuresis associated with hypomagnesemia.

Genetic disorders associated with hypokalemia

These disorders, mentioned earlier, are characterized by either excess mineralocorticoid production/activity or abnormal renal potassium excretion independent of mineralocorticoid activity. Disorders associated with increased aldosterone production include glucocorticoid-remediable aldosteronism and congenital adrenal hyperplasia.

Bartter's and Gitelman's syndromes are characterized by abnormalities in renal epithelial potassium metabolism. There are five variants of Bartter's syndrome. The phenotypes vary but all are associated with hypokalemia and normotension. Mutations have been identified in the butametanide-sensitive Na^+–K^+–$2Cl$–cotransporter gene (*NKCC2*), ROMK channel in the ascending loop of Henle, Barttin gene (β subunit for CIC-Ka and CIC-Kb chloride channels), CICKB, and calcium sensing receptor. Gitelman's syndrome is a hypokalemia tubulopathy associated with a mutation in the thiazide-sensitive NaCl cotransporter (TSC).

Liddle's syndrome is an autosomal recessive disorder caused by a gain-of-function mutation in the ENaC. As a result, extracellular volume is expanded with hypertension. However, as the ROMK channel is secondarily activated, potassium excretion is increased and hypokalemia results.

Although **cell-shift hypokalemia** and **decreases in total body potassium** do occur as isolated problems, they frequently occur **simultaneously**. Decreases in total body potassium potentiate the effects of drugs and hormones to shift potassium into cells. For example, small changes in potassium during insulin therapy may not cause hypokalemia if total body potassium is normal, but in the setting of total body potassium depletion (e.g., during the treatment of diabetic ketoacidosis or with diuretic use), cellular shifts of potassium during insulin therapy can result in profound hypokalemia.

B. The **manifestations** of hypokalemia are mainly cardiac and neuromuscular (Table 3-1). The most dramatic neuromuscular symptoms are paresis, paralysis, and respiratory failure. Potassium depletion causes supraventricular and ventricular arrhythmias, especially in patients on digitalis therapy. Although severe hypokalemia is more likely to cause complications, even minimal decreases in serum or total body potassium can be arrhythmogenic in patients with underlying heart disease or who are receiving digitalis therapy.

C. The **treatment** of hypokalemia depends on the underlying cause, the degree of potassium depletion, and the risk of potassium depletion to the patient. In general, hypokalemia secondary to cell shift is managed by treating underlying conditions. For example, hypokalemia in the setting of catecholamine increases, as in chest pain syndromes, is managed with appropriate treatments for the pain. However, when cell-shift hypokalemia is associated with life-threatening conditions such as paresis,

| TABLE 3-1 | Clinical Manifestations of Hypokalemia |

Cardiovascular
  Electrocardiographic abnormalities: U waves, QT prolongation, ST depression
    Predisposition to digitalis toxicity
    Atrial/ventricular arrhythmias
Neuromuscular
  Skeletal muscle
    Weakness
    Cramps
    Tetany
    Paralysis — flaccid
    Rhabdomyolysis
  Smooth muscle
    Constipation
    Ileus
    Urinary retention
Endocrine
  Carbohydrate intolerance
  Diabetes mellitus
  Decreased aldosterone
  Growth retardation
Renal/electrolyte
  Decreased renal blood flow, glomerular filtration rate
  Nephrogenic diabetes insipidus
  Increased ammoniagenesis (hepatic encephalopathy)
  Chloride wasting/metabolic alkalosis
  Cyst formation
  Interstitial nephritis
  Tubular vacuolization

paralysis, or hypokalemia in the setting of myocardial infarction, the administration of potassium is indicated. With potassium depletion, replacement therapy depends on the estimated degree of decreases in total body potassium. For example, decreases in total body potassium accompanied by a fall in serum potassium to 3.5 to 3.0 mEq per L are associated with a potassium deficit of 150 to 200 mEq. Decreases in serum potassium from 3 to 2 mEq per L are associated with 200- to 400-mEq additional decreases in total body potassium. Potassium can be administered intravenously, but in limited quantities (10 mEq per hour into a peripheral vein; 15 to 20 mEq per hour into a central vein). Larger potassium requirements can only be accomplished by oral therapy or with dialysis.

III. HYPERKALEMIA

A. The **approach** to hyperkalemia (Fig. 3-3) is to determine whether increases in serum potassium are spurious, caused by shifts of potassium from cellular to extracellular spaces, or represent a true increase in total body potassium.

Spurious hyperkalemia is caused by red blood cell hemolysis *in vitro*, ischemic blood draws, extreme thrombocytosis (greater than 1 million mL), or leukocytosis (greater than 50,000 mL). Spurious hyperkalemia is distinguished from true hyperkalemia by the absence of electrocardiographic (ECG) abnormalities. Hyperkalemia caused by **cell shifts** of potassium occurs acutely and results from decreased potassium transfer into cells (with decreases in insulin or β-adrenergic blocker therapy), increased potassium movement from cells to the extracellular space (with metabolic acidosis), hypertonicity (with hyperglycemia or the administration of mannitol), exercise, muscle breakdown (with rhabdomyolysis), or drug intoxications from digitalis or succinylcholine.

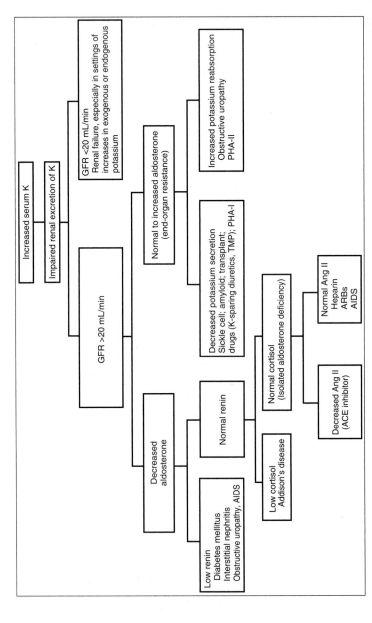

Figure 3-3. Diagnostic approach to hypokalemia. (ACE, angiotensin-converting enzyme; AIDS, acquired immunodeficiency syndrome; Ang, angiotensin; ARBs, adrenergic receptor binders; GFR, glomerular filtration rate; K, potassium; PHA, pseudohypoaldosteronism; TMP, trimethoprim-sulfa.)

Sustained hyperkalemia is caused by decreases in renal potassium excretion. This usually is not seen until the GFR is less than 20 mL per minute. However, it may be seen with less severe decreases in GFR when the kidney is challenged with a potassium load from potassium ingestion (e.g., diet, salt substitutes, or drugs, including potassium chloride and potassium citrate) and from increases in endogenous potassium production (e.g., GI bleed, resolving hematoma, rhabdomyolysis, catabolic states, tumor lysis). Hyperkalemia with less severe decreases in renal function is also associated with reductions in the distal nephron flow rate or low serum aldosterone levels as, for example, with hyporenin-hypoaldosteronism.

Last, hyperkalemia is also associated with less severe decreases in GFR when drugs that alter potassium physiology are administered. Hyperkalemia occurs in the setting of drugs that inhibit renin secretion (β-adrenergic blockers), renin activity (direct renin inhibition), angiotensin II generation (angiotensin-converting enzyme inhibitors), and the angiotensin receptor (AT_1). Hyperkalemia also occurs when drugs that block activation of the mineralocorticoid receptor (spironolactone, eplerenone) or inhibit the rate-limiting step in aldosterone synthesis (heparin) are administered. Drugs that directly inhibit ENaC such as amiloride, trimethoprim, and pentamidine cause hyperkalemia. The protease inhibitor, nafamostat, indirectly inhibits ENaC through inhibition of membrane-associated proteases. Nonsteroidal anti-inflammatory drugs (NSAIDs) may cause hyperkalemia. NSAIDs block prostaglandin production. As 70% of renin production is prostaglandin dependent, blocking the latter indirectly results in hyporeninemia. Cyclosporine, tacrolimus, and digoxin inhibit $Na^+–K^+–ATPase$, the enzyme responsible for potassium excretion in the collecting duct and this can cause hyperkalemia. Succinylcholine causes hyperkalemia by depolarizing skeletal muscle.

Clinical studies also suggest that older adults are at increased risk for hyperkalemia. Although no clear explanation exists for this observation, it may be related to an age-associated decline in aldosterone synthesis or possibly a decline in tubular sensitivity to its action. Commonly used medications causing hyperkalemia are shown in Table 3-2.

Hyperkalemia also occurs in the **setting of a relatively well-preserved GFR.** The causes of hyperkalemia in this setting are distinguished on the basis of plasma or urinary aldosterone levels. Decreases in aldosterone occur in the setting of normal, increased, or decreased plasma renin activity. Decreased plasma renin activity (hyporeninemic hypoaldosteronism) tends to occur in older adults and is associated with a number of renal diseases, including diabetes, interstitial nephritis (e.g., sickle cell anemia, analgesic use, heavy metal toxicity), obstructive uropathy, systemic lupus erythematosus, and amyloidosis. Decreases in plasma renin activity also are associated with acquired immunodeficiency syndrome (AIDS) nephropathy, transplantation, and medications including cyclosporine and NSAIDs. Hyper-reninemic hypoaldosteronism also occurs both with decreases in cortisol production (Addison's disease) and with normal cortisol production when medications such as angiotensin-converting enzyme inhibitors, angiotensin receptor blockers, and heparin are used. Finally, increases in serum potassium can be associated with normal to high levels of aldosterone and end-organ resistance to aldosterone. Aldosterone resistance is caused by drugs (such as potassium-sparing diuretics, trimethoprim, and pentamidine), interstitial renal diseases (systemic lupus erythematosus, sickle cell anemia), obstructive uropathy, or transplantation. It also occurs in an unusual hereditary disease called *pseudohypoaldosteronism type 1*, in which the etiology is either a decrease in aldosterone receptor number or decreased activity of the epithelial sodium channel in the distal convoluted tubule. Gordon's syndrome is associated with hyperkalemia in the setting of a normal GFR, decreased renal potassium excretion, and metabolic acidosis. Its mode of heritance is autosomal dominant. It is caused by a *WNK4* gene mutation causing a gain-of-function mutation in the thiazide-sensitive NaCl cotransporter (TSC) with an increase in ECF and as a result, suppression of plasma renin, decreased aldosterone, and hyperkalemia. Hyperkalemia in association with normal potassium secretion and increased potassium reabsorption occurs with obstructive uropathy.

| TABLE 3-2 | Commonly Used Medications Causing Hyperkalemia |

Medication	Mechanism
Digitalis overdose	Inhibition of the Na-K-ATPase pump
Angiotensin II inhibitors	Decreased aldosterone excretion
NSAIDs	Blocks prostaglandin stimulation of renin
Trimethoprim	A cationic agent that decreases the number of open sodium channels in the luminal membrane of cortical collecting ducts
Pentamidine	Same mechanism as trimethoprim—blocks distal potassium excretion
Spirolactone	Competes for aldosterone receptor in collecting tubule
Amiloride	Blocks sodium channel
Heparin	Decrease aldosterone
Salt substitutes	Contain potassium
Succinylcholine	Moves potassium from intracellular to extracellular fluid
Cyclosporine	Multifactorial, including hyporenin hypoaldosteronism and interference with aldosterone action in the potassium-secreting cells of the cortical collecting duct
Pentamidine	Blocks distal potassium secretion

ATPase, adenosine triphosphatase; NSAIDs, nonsteroidal anti-inflammatory drugs.

B. **Diagnosis.** The **urinary potassium excretion rate** or **transtubular potassium gradient (TTKG)** [(urine potassium/serum potassium)/(urine osmolarity/serum osmolarity)] is used to distinguish aldosterone deficiency/resistance from extrarenal causes of hyperkalemia (Table 3-2). This test measures the amount of potassium secreted by the distal tubule corrected by water absorption in the medullary collecting tubules. A normal value for the TTKG is 6 to 12. In the setting of hyperkalemia, a value greater than 10 suggests normal aldosterone levels and activity and points to an extrarenal cause of hyperkalemia. In contrast, renal causes of hyperkalemia (hypoaldosteronism) are associated with decreases in urinary potassium excretion (less than 20 mEq per day) and TTKG less than 5 to 7. In this setting, the administration of a mineralocorticoid (0.05 mg fludrocortisone) results in increases in urinary potassium excretion (greater than 40 mEq per day) and TTKG greater than 10 in patients with aldosterone deficiency. However, no increase in urinary potassium excretion or in TTKG suggests aldosterone resistance (e.g., sickle cell anemia).

C. The **clinical manifestations** of hyperkalemia are predominantly cardiac and neuromuscular. It is important to note that patients with hyperkalemia often present with vague GI complaints and nonspecific unwell feelings. ECG abnormalities associated with mild hyperkalemia include peaked T waves. With moderate hyperkalemia there is prolongation of the PR interval, decrease in amplitude of P waves, and widening of the QRS complex. With severe hyperkalemia, the P wave is absent, there is progressive widening of the QRS complex, and if left untreated, sine waves develop with asystole. Neuromuscular abnormalities include weakness, constipation, and paralysis.

D. The **treatment** of hyperkalemia (Fig. 3-4) depends on the presence or absence of ECG and neuromuscular abnormalities. In the absence of symptoms or ECG abnormalities, hyperkalemia is treated conservatively—for example, by decreasing dietary

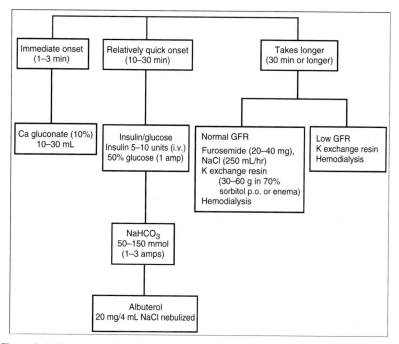

Figure 3-4. Treatment of hyperkalemia. (Ca, calcium; GFR, glomerular filtration rate; K, potassium.)

potassium or withdrawing offending drugs. In the presence of ECG abnormalities or symptoms, the goal of therapy is to stabilize cell membranes. First-line therapy includes calcium gluconate, 10 to 30 mL as a 10% solution (onset of action 1 or 2 minutes). Although the mechanism remains undefined, calcium "stabilizes" the cardiac membranes. Other therapies include sodium bicarbonate, 50 to 150 mEq (onset 15 to 30 minutes) and insulin 5 to 10 units intravenously (onset 5 to 10 minutes). Insulin increases the activity of the Na-K-ATPase pump in skeletal muscle and drives potassium into cells. Glucose, 25 g intravenously, is given simultaneously to prevent hypoglycemia. Blood sugars should be monitored for approximately 6 hours to identify and treat hypoglycemia from the insulin. Albuterol nebulizer, 20 mg in 4 mL normal saline (onset 15 to 30 minutes), also activates the Na-K-ATPase and drives potassium into cells. Potassium driven intracellularly generally begins to move extracellularly again after approximately 6 hours, increasing the serum potassium concentration. Therefore, therapy to remove potassium from the body should be started simultaneously. Reductions in total body potassium may be achieved through a potassium exchange resin. The primary potassium resin used is sodium polystyrene sulfonate. One gram of this medication binds approximately 1 mEq of potassium and releases 1 to 2 mEq of sodium back into the circulation. This medication may be given orally (onset 2 hours) or by enema with sorbitol to induce diarrhea (onset 30 to 60 minutes). Finally, if indicated, hemodialysis is initiated, removing 25 to 30 mEq of potassium per hour.

Suggested Readings

Allon M. Hyperkalemia in end stage renal disease: mechanisms and management. *J Am Soc Nephrol* 1995;6:1134–1142.

Ethier JH, Kanel KS, Magner PO, et al. The transtubular potassium concentration in patients with hypokalemia and hyperkalemia. *Am J Kidney Dis* 1990;15:309–315.

Gennari FJ. Hypokalemia. *N Engl J Med* 1998;339:451–458.

Halperin ML, Kamel SK. Electrolyte quintet: potassium. *Lancet* 1998;352:135–140.

Kahle KT, Ring AM, Lifton RP. Molecular physiology of the WNK kinases. *Annu Rev Physiol* 2008;70:329–355.

Kahle KT, Wilson FH, Lalioti M, et al. WNK kinases: molecular regulators of integrated epithelial cell transport. *Curr Opin Nephrol Hypertens* 2004;13:557–562.

Kamel KS, Halperin ML. Treatment of hypokalemia and hyperkalemia. In: Brad HR, Wilcox CS, eds. *Therapy in nephrology and hypertension*. Philadelphia: WB Saunders, 1999:270–278.

Kellerman PS, Linas SL. Disorders of potassium metabolism. In: Feehally J, Johnson R, eds. *Comprehensive clinical nephrology*. London: Mosby, 1999.

Landua D. Potassium-related inherited tubulopathies. *Cell Mol Life Sci* 2006;63:1962–1968.

Moonseong QH, Heshka S, Wang J, et al. Total body potassium differs by sex and age across the adult life span. *Am J Clin Nutr* 2003;78:72–77.

Musso C, Liakopoulos V, Miguel RD, et al. Algranati. Transtubular potassium concentration gradient: comparison between healthy old people and chronic renal failure patients. *Int Urol Nephrol* 2006;38:387–390.

Osorio FV, Linas SL. Disorders of potassium metabolism. In: Schrier RW, ed. *Atlas of diseases of the kidney*, Vol. 1, Sec. 1. Philadelphia: Blackwell Science, 1998.

Oster JR, Singer I, Fishman LM. Heparin-induced aldosterone suppression and hyperkalemia. *Am J Med* 1995;98:575–586.

Perazella M. Rastegar Asghar. Disorders of potassium and acid-base metabolism in association with renal disease. In: Schrier RW, ed. *Diseases of the kidney and urinary tract*, 7th ed. Philadelphia: Lippincott Williams & Wilkins, 2001:2577–2606.

Perazella MA, Mahnensmith RL. Hyperkalemia in the elderly. *J Gen Intern Med* 1997;10: 646–656.

Peterson L, Levi M. Disorders of potassium metabolism. In: Schrier RW, ed. *Renal and electrolyte disorders*, 6th ed. Philadelphia: Lippincott Williams & Wilkins, 2003:171–215.

Proctor G, Linas S. Type 2 pseudohypoaldosteronism: new insights into renal potassium, sodium, and chloride handling. *Am J Kidney Dis*, 2006;48(4):674–693.

Weiner ID, Linas SL, Wingo CS. Disorders of potassium metabolism. In: Johnson RJ, Feehally JF, ed. *Comprehensive clinical nephrology*, 2nd ed. St. Louis: Mosby, 2003; 109–121.

Weiner ID, Wingo CS. Hypokalemia: consequences, causes, and correction. *J Am Soc Nephrol* 1997;8:1179–1188.

Weiner ID, Wingo CS. Hyperkalemia: a potential silent killer. *J Am Soc Nephrol*, 1998;9: 1535–1543.

THE PATIENT WITH AN ACID–BASE DISORDER

William D. Kaehny

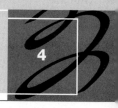

4

I. **Acid–base disorders** are the abdominal pains of the body fluids. They are important signs of disorders that have deranged physiology. Occasionally, acid–base disorders disrupt homeostasis sufficiently to move the arterial pH into a dangerous range (less than 7.10 or greater than 7.60). Depending on the overall status of the patient and the response of the cardiovascular system, the pH level may require direct attention. After the clinician detects the presence of an acid–base disorder from clinical and laboratory clues, he proceeds logically through a progression of steps to optimal management of the patient.

- A. **Step 1.** Measure pH. This identifies **acidemia or alkalemia**. The change in bicarbonate and partial pressure of CO_2 (Pco_2) indicates whether the primary process is metabolic or respiratory.
- B. **Step 2.** Check the compensatory or secondary response of the Pco_2 or HCO_3^- to see if the disorder is **simple** or **mixed**.
- C. **Step 3.** Calculate the serum **anion gap** (AG) to screen for an increase in organic anions such as lactate. Add any increase in AG (ΔAG) that is **potential HCO_3^-** to the serum total carbon dioxide content (tCO_2) to screen for a hidden metabolic alkalosis.
- D. **Step 4.** Determine the **cause** of the acid–base disorder from the clinical setting and laboratory tests.
- E. **Step 5. Treat** the underlying disorder, unless the pH is dangerous either acutely or chronically (such as acidosis affecting bone).

II. **WHEN TO SUSPECT ACID–BASE DISORDERS**

- A. **Clinical.** The underlying cause of the acid–base disorder is most frequently responsible for a patient's signs and symptoms. Certain clinical settings and findings should alert the clinician to the likelihood of an acid–base disorder. Coma, seizures, congestive heart failure, shock, vomiting, diarrhea, and renal failure generate changes in the Pco_2 or HCO_3^- levels. Marked changes in the pH occasionally may cause direct clinical manifestations. Severe alkalemia causes an irritability of heart and skeletal muscle. Severe acidemia causes a depression of heart pump function and vascular tone. Although central nervous system dysfunction appears frequently with acid–base disorders, changes in pH do not appear responsible. Rather, altered plasma osmolality and Pco_2 appear to be the causative agents.
- B. **Laboratory.** A thoughtful measurement of serum electrolytes in patients with abnormal losses or gains of body fluids is good practice. An abnormal serum tCO_2 is definite evidence of an acid–base disorder; an abnormal serum AG is very suggestive; an abnormal serum potassium is suspicious.
    1. **Serum tCO_2.** The HCO_3^- in blood can be estimated reasonably by measuring the tCO_2 in venous serum. The serum tCO_2 is 1 to 3 mmol per L greater than the arterial HCO_3^- because it is from venous blood, which has more HCO_3^-, and it includes dissolved CO_2 and trivial amounts of other substances. Normal sea level serum tCO_2 levels average 26 to 27 mmol per L. A value below 24 or above 30 likely marks a clinical acid–base disorder. An acid–base disorder of the mixed type may exist with a normal serum tCO_2.
    2. The **serum AG** is calculated from the venous serum sodium, chloride, and tCO_2:

$$AG = Na^+ - (Cl^- + tCO_2)$$

The units are mEq per L, because this calculation estimates the charge difference between the so-called unmeasured anions (serum total anions represented by Cl^-

and $HCO_3{}^-$) and unmeasured cations (total cations represented by Na^+). The average normal value is 9 ± 3 mEq per L, but may vary in different laboratories. Albumin contributes most to the AG. A fall in serum albumin of 1 g per dL from a normal of 4.4 decreases the AG by 2.5 mEq per L.

  a. Metabolic acidosis due to an organic acid such as lactic or acetoacetic acid is marked by an increased AG. An increase in the AG of 8 mEq per L to 17 or higher usually indicates the presence of organic acidosis, although at times the exact anion may not be identified. The anion of the organic acid replaces the $HCO_3{}^-$ lost in the buffering of the hydrogen ion (H^+) part of the acid and therefore increases the unmeasured anions. Importantly, a normal or slightly elevated AG does not rule out the presence of organic metabolic acidosis, such as diabetic ketoacidosis, because a patient with good renal perfusion and ample urine flow may excrete the ketoanions at a rate sufficient to keep the serum AG from rising markedly.

  b. Metabolic alkalosis. At times, a metabolic acidosis that increases the AG and lowers the $HCO_3{}^-$ may coincide with a process that generates a metabolic alkalosis. For example, vomiting that generates a high $HCO_3{}^-$ may be caused by diabetic ketoacidosis, which lowers the $HCO_3{}^-$. In this case, the serum tCO_2 (and arterial $HCO_3{}^-$) may be low or normal despite the elevating action of the metabolic alkalosis. The clue to the presence of such hidden metabolic alkalosis is derived in a Holmesian manner by adding the measured serum tCO_2 and the ΔAG (measured AG − 9). If this sum is greater than 30 mEq per L, a hidden metabolic alkalosis is likely present. The ΔAG is a marker of "lost" or potential $HCO_3{}^-$, that which was titrated by the H^+ of an organic acid. Pure metabolic alkalosis may directly increase the AG by up to 5 mEq per L due to effects on the albumin concentration and charge.

3. Serum potassium. Potassium metabolism is linked to acid–base metabolism at the levels of cell shifts, renal tubular functions, and gastrointestinal transport. Therefore, an abnormal serum potassium concentration alerts the clinician to the likelihood that an acid–base disorder is present also.

III. IDENTIFYING THE MAJOR ACID–BASE DISORDERS. When the clinician suspects that an acid–base disorder might be present and that patient management might be adjusted, a set of acid–base variables should be obtained: pH, Pco_2, and $HCO_3{}^-$.

  A. Chemistry and physiology of acid–base. Cellular, tissue, and organ systems apparently function best at an extracellular fluid (ECF) pH of approximately 7.40. Intracellular fluid (ICF) pH is heterogeneous within the cell, depending on organelles and metabolic activity, but averages approximately 7.00. ECF pH is a function of the state of available buffer molecules that respond to changes in pH by binding or releasing H^+ to keep pH close to 7.40. Therefore, buffers prevent extreme shifts in pH in the face of the gain or loss of acids or bases.

  Current clinical acid–base chemistry is based on the Bronsted-Lowry theory which designates acids as proton donors and bases as proton acceptors. The three key elements are the hydrogen ion activity (pH), carbonic acid (the acid), and bicarbonate (the base). The Pco_2 represents the acid in the modified Henderson-Hasselbalch equation. Base excess, used by some, is another concept derived from these elements in an attempt to explain whether alterations in these elements are due to metabolic or respiratory disorders.

  Another approach which appears useful in investigative, analytic settings uses the Stewart equations. These calculate the pH from three, so-called independent, variables: Pco_2, the strong ion difference, and total weak acid (mainly protein).

  1. Blood pH is the mathematical expression of the intensity of acidity or H^+ activity. H^+ concentration usually is expressed in nmol per L. H^+ concentration is 100 nmol per L at pH 7.00 and 40 nmol per L at pH 7.40. Within the pH range of 7.26 to 7.45, H^+ concentration is estimated accurately as (80 − the decimal of pH). For example, at pH 7.32, H^+ equals 80 minus 32 or 48 nmol per L. The pH is measured at body temperature with a glass, flow-through electrode.

2. The **partial pressure of carbon dioxide in blood, Pco_2**, represents the respiratory component in blood. The respiratory system determines the level at which the Pco_2 is set. Pco_2 substitutes for the buffer carbonic acid, H_2CO_3, in the acid–base equation. Pco_2 is measured in whole blood with a pH electrode that detects the change caused by the diffusion of CO_2 from the sample into a buffer solution.

3. **HCO$_3^-$** is the metabolic component of the acid–base equation, serving as the base of the H^+ binding partner in the buffer pair. HCO_3^- concentration is controlled by the buffering state, metabolic processes, and the kidneys. HCO_3^- concentration is calculated from the pH and Pco_2 using the Henderson-Hasselbalch equation. The fact that it is calculated makes it no less reliable a value than the serum tCO_2.

4. The **acid–base equation** allows the determination of the state of ECF acid–base balance, the presence of an acid–base disorder, the nature of the disorder, and the presence of a simple or mixed disorder:

$$pH = constant \times \left[HCO_3^-\right]/Pco_2$$

Therefore, the pH level depends on the ratio or mathematical relationship between the HCO_3^- and the Pco_2. An acid–base disorder is generated by an alteration from normal of either of these two factors. The resultant change in pH results in chemical shifts in the buffers, which mitigate the change in pH somewhat. A physiologic compensatory response occurs in the respiratory system for a metabolic disorder and in the kidneys for a respiratory disorder. A new steady state ensues, with the new pH set by the new values of the HCO_3^- concentration and Pco_2.

B. **Measurement of acid–base variables.** The determination of the acid–base state usually is based on an analysis of arterial blood, although arterialized venous blood analysis is equally valid. After warming the extremity, blood is drawn without air mixing from an artery or from a forearm vein without tourniquet. Although experimental studies show that ICF pH and mixed venous acid–base measurements correlate better with organ function, arterial blood measurements are more easily available and provide a readily interpretable view of the metabolic state of organs and their function. Keep in mind that tissue hypoperfusion, as in cardiopulmonary arrest or profound shock, makes tissue acidosis worse than that reflected by arterial blood acid–base values.

C. **Identification of a major acid–base disorder.** The basis of this approach is to determine the direction (up or down) in which the measured values differ from the arbitrary normal values for pH (7.40), Pco_2 (40 mm Hg), and HCO_3^- (24 mmol per L). First, determine if acidemia (pH down) or alkalemia (pH up) is present. Then determine if the primary generating change was in the HCO_3^- or in the Pco_2 (Table 4-1). The compensating factor should change in the same direction as the generating factor to yield a simple acid–base disorder.

1. **Example of a simple disorder.** Arterial blood analysis revealed the following values: pH 7.55, HCO_3^- 18 mmol per L, and Pco_2 21 mm Hg.

TABLE 4-1	Simple Acid–Base Disorders			
	Metabolic acidosis	**Metabolic alkalosis**	**Respiratory acidosis**	**Respiratory alkalosis**
Primary change	↓HCO$_3^-$	↑HCO$_3^-$	↑Pco_2	↓Pco_2
Compensation	↓Pco_2	↑Pco_2	↑HCO$_3^-$	↓HCO$_3^-$
Effect on pH	↓pH	↑pH	↓pH	↑pH

↓ decreased; ↑ increased.

    a. **Step 1.** The pH is up. Therefore, alkalemia is present and must be due to an increased HCO_3^- (as in metabolic alkalosis) or to a decreased Pco_2 (as in respiratory alkalosis).

    b. **Step 2.** The HCO_3^- is low and cannot be responsible for an increased pH.

    c. **Step 3.** Because the Pco_2 is low, it can account for the increased pH; this is respiratory alkalosis.

    d. **Step 4.** The HCO_3^- change is in same direction as that of the Pco_2; this is consistent with a compensation and a simple respiratory alkalosis.

  2. **Example of a mixed acid–base disorder.** Sampling of arterial blood yielded the following: pH 7.55, HCO_3^- 30 mmol per L, and Pco_2 35 mm Hg.

    a. **Step 1.** The pH is up. Therefore, alkalemia is present.

    b. **Step 2.** The HCO_3^- is increased and may be responsible for the increased pH.

    c. **Step 3.** The Pco_2 is low and it, too, can account for an increased pH.

    d. **Step 4.** The two acid–base determinants, that is, HCO_3^- and Pco_2, are changed from normal in opposite directions. Therefore, this is mixed metabolic and respiratory alkalosis. The metabolic alkalosis is dominant because the percent change in HCO_3^- is 6/24 or 25% whereas the percent change in Pco_2 is 5/40 or 12.5%.

IV. JUDGING WHETHER AN ACID–BASE DISORDER IS SIMPLE OR MIXED. When an underlying process generates an acid–base disorder by perturbing one member of the $HCO_3^- - Pco_2$ buffer pair (remember that Pco_2 represents H_2CO_3), the other partner is adjusted to compensate by the physiologic response of the body and changes in the same direction as the primary partner in order to reduce the magnitude of the change in pH. The time-honored term for this physiologic response is *compensation*. However, the physiologic response mechanisms may be activated by stimuli other than pH and actually may contribute to the maintenance of the abnormal pH. Therefore, some have termed these responses *maladaptive* because they are not always truly compensatory. For example, a low Pco_2 in response to metabolic acidosis actually causes the kidneys to reduce HCO_3^- reabsorption. Importantly, compensation does not restore the pH exactly to normal, because that would shut off the stimulus for the compensatory mechanism.

  A. Steps in judging whether an acid–base disorder is simple. After the major disorder is identified, determine whether the compensation for the primary event is appropriate.

    1. **Check directions of changes from normal of HCO_3^- and Pco_2.** The acid–base buffer pair change from normal in the same direction in all simple acid–base disorders. If they change in opposite directions, the disorder must be mixed.

    2. **Compare the magnitude of the compensation of the Pco_2 or HCO_3^- with the primary change in the HCO_3^- or Pco_2.** In metabolic disorders, the primary change occurs in the HCO_3^-, with the compensation occurring in the Pco_2. The opposite is true in the respiratory disorders. In Table 4-2 are contained guidelines or rules that can be used to judge whether compensation is appropriate. The respiratory disorders have two stages of compensation: acute, when only tissue buffering slightly changes the HCO_3^-, and chronic (after 24 hours), when the kidneys cause major changes in the HCO_3^- concentration. If the measured change in the compensating factor does not approximate the change predicted, a mixed disorder is likely. Two methods of predicting compensation appear in Table 4-2. One describes the expected changes in the buffer partner for a given change in the generating partner. For example, a fall in HCO_3^- of 10 mmol per L in metabolic acidosis is expected to result in hyperventilation that drops the Pco_2 by 10 to 15 mm Hg to 25 to 30 mm Hg. The other method relates the primary, generating factor change to a change in pH. For example, a fall in HCO_3^- of 10 mmol per L in metabolic acidosis is expected to decrease the pH by 0.1 to 7.30.

    3. **Check the AG for evidence of a hidden metabolic disorder.** An increase in the AG of more than 8 mEq per L to greater than 17 suggests the presence of metabolic acidosis due to an organic acid. Also if the ΔAG is added to the

TABLE 4-2	Appropriate Compensations in the Acid–Base Disorders	

	Change in P_{CO_2} per change in HCO_3^-	Change in pH per change in HCO_3^-
Metabolic acidosis	1.0–1.5 per 1	0.010 per 1
Metabolic alkalosis	0.25–1.00 per 1	0.015 per 1

	Change in HCO_3^- per change in P_{CO_2}	Change in pH per change in P_{CO_2}
Respiratory acidosis		
Acute	1 per 10	0.08 per 10
Chronic	4 per 10	0.03 per 10
Respiratory alkalosis		
Acute	1 per 10	0.08 per 10
Chronic	4 per 10	0.03 per 10

measured serum tCO_2, the theoretic maximum serum tCO_2 can be estimated. A value greater than 30 mmol per L suggests metabolic alkalosis.

B. Application of the rules

   1. The **primary event in metabolic acidosis** is a fall in HCO_3^-; the **compensation** is a fall in the P_{CO_2}, due to the stimulation of central nervous system receptors by the low pH. Hyperventilation increases the excretion of CO_2, and P_{CO_2} falls. For example, if the HCO_3^- falls from 24 mmol per L by 10 to 14 mmol per L, the P_{CO_2} should fall by 1.0 to 1.5 times as much, or 10 to 15 mm Hg, to a level of 25 to 30 mm Hg (40 − 10 = 30; 40 − 15 = 25).

   2. The **primary event in metabolic alkalosis** is a rise in HCO_3^-. The respiratory system responds to the rise in pH with hypoventilation, which reduces carbon dioxide excretion and results in a rise in P_{CO_2}. For example, if HCO_3^- rises by 16 mmol per L from 24 to 40 mmol per L, the P_{CO_2} should rise by 0.25 to 1.00 multiplied by the rise in HCO_3^- of 16, or by 4 to 16 mm Hg, to a level of 44 to 56 mm Hg (40 + 4 = 44; 40 +16 = 56). This response is tempered by the body's response to the concomitant hypoxemia resulting from hypoventilation.

   3. The **primary event in respiratory acidosis** is a rise in P_{CO_2}. During the acute phase (up to 24 hours), only buffering contributes measurably to the response. The HCO_3^- should increase, but not to as high as 30 mmol per L. In contrast, the kidneys respond to chronic elevations of P_{CO_2} by generating sufficient HCO_3^- to prevent the pH from falling to less than 7.20, even in the most severe cases of chronic respiratory acidosis.

   4. The **primary event in respiratory alkalosis** is a fall in P_{CO_2}. Initially, buffering occurs as a result of the release of H^+ from cells; later (hours) the kidneys dump HCO_3^- into the urine, with a resultant fall in blood HCO_3^-, as defined in Table 4-2.

C. Effects of respiratory responses to metabolic disorders. The kidneys respond to changes in P_{CO_2} regardless of the pH. A fall in P_{CO_2} causes renal HCO_3^- loss; a rise in P_{CO_2} causes renal HCO_3^- generation. Therefore, in chronic metabolic acidosis (lasting days), some of the reduction in bicarbonate actually is due to the compensatory fall in P_{CO_2} and not directly to the process causing the metabolic acidosis. Similarly, the increase in P_{CO_2} in chronic metabolic alkalosis contributes to the hyperbicarbonatemia.

D. Examples of mixed acid–base disorders. Four combinations of the "double" mixed acid–base disorders are possible. Two are important because they cause drastic changes in pH—metabolic and respiratory acidosis and metabolic and respiratory alkalosis. The other two disorders (metabolic acidosis with respiratory

| TABLE 4-3 | Example of a Mixed Acid–Base Disorder |

	Health	Emphysema	Emphysema and diarrhea
pH	7.40	7.32	7.10
P_{CO_2}	40	80	80
HCO_3^-	24	40	24

alkolosis and metabolic alkolosis with respiratory acidosis) tend to be associated with pH values close to normal and are not dangerous *per se*; however, they are important markers of underlying disease. Two other mixed disorders, so-called triple disorders, also have been described. The AG points to both metabolic acidosis and alkalosis developing simultaneously or sequentially in these disorders. The imposition of a respiratory disorder yields the infamous triple acid–base disorder.

1. **Metabolic acidosis and respiratory acidosis.** A patient with emphysema and carbon dioxide retention (chronic respiratory acidosis) develops diarrhea (metabolic acidosis). Note how the reduction in HCO_3^- to normal results in severe acidemia (Table 4-3).

2. **Metabolic alkalosis and respiratory acidosis.** The same emphysematous patient is given a diuretic for cor pulmonale. The bicarbonate level rises from 40 to 48 mmol per L, which, with the P_{CO_2} at 80 mm Hg, sets the pH at 7.40. Although this is a normal pH, some believe it is better for carbon dioxide-retaining patients to be mildly acidemic to keep ventilation stimulated.

3. **Triple acid–base disorder.** A more common mixture of disorders involves metabolic acidosis developing in a patient with metabolic alkalosis and super-imposed respiratory alkalosis. For example, a patient with metabolic alkalosis (HCO_3^- 32) from nasogastric suction becomes septic, which generates both lactic acidosis and pronounced hyperventilation, thereby causing independent respiratory alkalosis due to endotoxin (Table 4-4). Note that both the metabolic and respiratory alkaloses should cause only small increases in the AG. The lactic acidosis of septic shock results in a fall of from 32 to 24 mmol per L in the HCO_3^- with a reciprocal increase in AG. The AG of 33 is diagnostic of organic acidosis. The ΔAG of 26 (35 − 9) added to the serum tCO_2 of 9 yields 35 mmol

| TABLE 4-4 | Example of a Triple Mixed Acid–Base Disorder |

	Health	Nasogastric suction	Septic shock	Endotoxemia
ph	7.40	7.49	7.14	7.44
P_{CO_2}	40	44	24	12
HCO_3^-	24	32	8	8
Anion gap	9	11	33	35
Venous total carbon dioxide	26	35	9	9
Disorder		Metabolic alkalosis	Metabolic alkalosis Metabolic acidosis	Metabolic alkalosis Metabolic acidosis Respiratory alkalosis

per L, an estimate of the value before acidosis, indicative of metabolic alkalosis. The evidence for the presence of respiratory alkalosis is the high pH and low P_{CO_2} due to the hyperventilation caused by endotoxemia.

V. IDENTIFY THE UNDERLYING CAUSE OF AN ACID–BASE DISORDER. Usually, the cause of an acid–base disorder is obvious from the history, examination, and clinical course. However, on occasion, careful review of a thoughtful differential diagnosis is necessary to identify a remote causative disorder.

A. Causes of metabolic acidosis. The AG is used to divide the causes of metabolic acidosis into those with influx of organic acid into plasma (increased AG) and those with external losses of bicarbonate (normal AG; hyperchloremic). Some disorders belong to both groups at different stages (diabetic ketoacidosis) or are generated by mechanisms other than those described (renal failure). A list of causes is given in Table 4-5.

1. Metabolic acidosis with increased AG. Severe metabolic acidosis is caused by only three broad groups of disorders: ketoacidosis, lactic acidosis, and toxicities. In addition, renal failure may cause mild to moderate acidosis.

a. Ketoacidosis arises when glucose is not available to cells because of lack of insulin, cell dysfunction, or glucose depletion, and fatty acids are oxidized to yield energy, acetone (not an acid), and the two ketoacids (acetoacetic and β-hydroxybutyric). The H^+ produced are consumed (buffered) by HCO_3^-, producing carbonic acid, which dehydrates into water and carbon dioxide. The ketoanions accumulate in the serum in place of the HCO_3^-, further increasing the anion gap. The diagnostic test for ketoacidosis consists of

TABLE 4-5   Causes of Metabolic Acidosis

High anion gap type
  Ketoacidosis
    Diabetic
    Alcoholic
    Starvation
  Lactic acidosis
    Type A
    Type B
    D-Lactic acidosis
  Intoxications
    Ethylene glycol
    Methanol
    Salicylate
    Pyroglutamic acidosis from acetaminophen
  Advanced renal failure
Normal anion gap type
  Gastrointestinal HCO_3^- loss
    Diarrhea
    External fistulae
  Renal HCO_3^- loss
    Acetazolamide
    Proximal renal tubular acidosis (RTA)
    Distal RTA
    Hyperkalemic RTA
  Miscellaneous
    NH_4Cl ingestion
    Sulfur ingestion
    Toluene inhalation
    Pronounced dilution

testing the serum with a nitroprusside reagent, which only reacts with the acetoacetate. In diabetic ketoacidosis, the β-hydroxybutyrate–acetoacetate ratio averages 5:2 whereas in alcoholic ketoacidosis, it may reach as high as 20:1. In these cases, only urine, a concentrate of serum, may have a concentration of acetoacetate high enough to give a positive purple reaction with the reagent. **Diabetic ketoacidosis** occurs because of insulin deficiency. Hyperglycemia may be corrected by volume re-expansion but insulin is needed to stop ketogenesis. Volume expansion enhances the renal excretion of ketoanions, thereby correcting the increased AG. However, the kidneys take time to generate new HCO_3^- to replace that lost earlier in buffering H^+. Therefore, early in diabetic ketoacidosis, the AG usually is increased; during correction, the AG may return to normal despite a low HCO_3^-. Chloride replaces the ketoanions, and this stage is therefore called *hyperchloremic* or *normal anion gap metabolic acidosis*. **Alcoholic ketoacidosis** occurs because of volume depletion, which causes the α-adrenergic suppression of insulin release. The patient relates a story of severe vomiting following recently increased alcohol intake. Urine ketones are usually positive. Blood glucose ranges between 50 and 250 mg per dL. **Starvation** ketoacidosis occurs because of the use of fatty acids for energy maintenance. The degree of acidosis is mild, with arterial HCO_3^- not less than 18 mmol per L.

  b. Lactic acidosis arises when oxygen delivery to cells is inadequate for the demand (type A) or cell processes cannot use oxygen (type B). In this situation, glucose is metabolized through anaerobic glycolysis to pyruvate and then to the dead-end metabolite lactate. The H^+ produced from nicotinamide adenine dinucleotide (NADH) (one per lactate) are buffered by HCO_3^-, which is replaced in the blood by lactate. Therefore, the AG is increased. **Type A lactic acidosis** is caused by the primary inadequate delivery of oxygen to tissues. Shock is the most common mechanism. Hypovolemia, heart failure, and sepsis cause shock. Because carbon monoxide binds more avidly to hemoglobin than does oxygen, carbon monoxide poisoning can cause varying degrees of lactic acidosis. **Type B lactic acidosis** occurs when tissue oxygenation is normal but tissues cannot use the oxygen normally or need excessive amounts of oxygen. Causes of type B lactic acidosis include hepatic failure, malignancy, drugs, and seizures. Metformin is a biguanide hypoglycemic agent that rarely (8 per 100,000) causes lactic acidosis. Renal, liver, and heart failure are risk factors. Reverse transcriptase inhibitors for acquired immunodeficiency syndrome (AIDS) also cause lactic acidosis due to injury to cell mitochondria. Lactic acidosis has been seen in patients receiving large intravenous doses of lorazepam and diazepam due to the propylene glycol solvent. D-**lactic acidosis** is generated when colon bacteria metabolize malabsorbed sugars into both L- and D-lactate, which accumulates in the blood. The clinical manifestation is metabolic encephalopathy. At least two dozen inborn errors of metabolism result in pediatric lactic acidosis. The diagnosis is usually established by exclusion of ketoacidosis, toxicities, and advanced renal failure as causes for a high AG metabolic acidosis. L-Lactate can be measured by an automated assay, but measurement is often unnecessary.

  c. Four modern **toxicities** cause high AG metabolic acidosis: **ethylene glycol ingestion, methanol ingestion, salicylate intoxication, and pyroglutamic acidosis from acetaminophen.** Methanol and ethylene glycol are low molecular weight alcohols that readily enter cells. Metabolism generates H^+ that cause acidosis and formate (with methanol) or glycolate (with ethylene glycol) that causes a high AG. A clue to the presence of early stages of acidosis with elevated alcohol levels is an increased osmolal gap. This gap is the difference between the measured serum osmolality and the calculated osmolality (calc Sosm).

$$\text{Calc Sosm} = 2 \times [Na^+] + \text{glucose}/18 + [\text{urea nitrogen}]/2.8 + [\text{ethanol}]/4.6$$

If this difference between measured and calculated Sosm is greater than 25 mOsm per kg of serum, the presence of a toxic alcohol is likely. Needle-like or envelope-shaped calcium oxalate crystals in the urine suggest ethylene glycol ingestion. The combination of high AG metabolic acidosis and a high osmolal gap is an indication for specific analysis for methanol and ethylene glycol. The decision to measure levels of these alcohols, of course, must be tempered by the clinical setting. Salicylate intoxication is an important frequent unintentional chronic or intentional acute overdose that causes metabolic acidosis, respiratory alkalosis, or a mixed disorder. It should be suspected at the extremes of age. Another analgesic, acetaminophen, has been linked to pyroglutamic acidosis (5-oxoproline) in malnourished individuals, many with renal disease. Therapeutic doses taken chronically are involved. Most patients are women.

   d. Renal failure. Failure to excrete the daily acid load of 1 mmol per kg of body weight that is generated by metabolism results in metabolic acidosis. Bone buffers take up some hydrogen ions during chronic renal failure, and, therefore, the degree of acidosis is moderated until the end stages of kidney disease. Arterial bicarbonate usually remains above 15 mmol per L. In acute renal failure, venous tCO_2 or arterial HCO_3^- falls by approximately 0.5 mmol per L per day unless hypercatabolism increases daily acid production. The AG increases less than the HCO_3^- falls, resulting in hyperchloremic metabolic acidosis in early and middle stages of chronic renal failure. In advanced chronic renal failure, the serum AG rises approximately 0.5 mEq per L for each 1.0 mg per dL rise in serum creatinine. Retention of sulfate, phosphate, and organic anions causes the increase in AG.

2. Metabolic acidosis with normal AG (hyperchloremic) can be caused by three groups of disorders: gastrointestinal HCO_3^- loss, renal HCO_3^- loss or acid retention, and inorganic acid intake.

   a. Gastrointestinal bicarbonate loss. The gastrointestinal tract distal to the stomach has the capacity to absorb chloride and secrete bicarbonate. Therefore, diarrhea and external drainage of pancreatic, biliary, or small-bowel juices can cause external losses of bicarbonate-rich fluid. Relatively chloride-rich fluid remains behind. This generates hyperchloremic metabolic acidosis (normal AG). An interesting variety of this disorder occurs when normal urine, rich in sodium chloride (NaCl) from dietary sources, is drained into the gut through ureterosigmoidostomy or ileal loop conduit (both bladder replacement constructions). If contact time with mucosa is excessive, the gut reabsorbs the chloride in exchange for bicarbonate, resulting in hyperchloremic metabolic acidosis.

   b. Renal bicarbonate loss. The proximal renal tubule reabsorbs the bulk (85%) of filtered HCO_3^-. The carbonic anhydrase inhibitor **acetazolamide** blocks much of this reabsorption, resulting in urinary bicarbonate losses until arterial HCO_3^- falls to 16 to 18 mmol per L. The filtered load of HCO_3^- at this concentration can be completely reabsorbed by the distal nephron. Therefore, the urine becomes bicarbonate-free, with an acidic pH, in this new steady state. **Proximal renal tubular acidosis** (old type II RTA), a defect in proximal tubular HCO_3^- reabsorption, has identical features. Proximal RTA is unusual but may occur with Wilson's disease, multiple myeloma, transplant rejection, and in other disease states. **Distal RTA** (old type I) differs in that it is a defect of the collecting duct, in which the daily metabolic acid load is not excreted totally and a small HCO_3^- leak occurs every day. This leads to a mild-to-moderate normal AG, hyperchloremic metabolic acidosis, and hypercalciuria with calcium stones or nephrocalcinosis. Two varieties occur: **hypokalemic distal RTA and hyperkalemic distal RTA**. Hypokalemic distal RTA occurs when collecting duct potassium secretion is intact and in fact enhanced by the small amount of bicarbonaturia. Hyperkalemic distal RTA occurs due to two distinct mechanisms when collecting duct hydrogen ion and potassium secretion are impaired: hypoaldosteronism (old type IV RTA) or tubular defect. Hypokalemic distal RTA occurs with Sjögren's syndrome, amphotericin B toxicity, cirrhosis of the liver, medullary sponge kidney, and many other diseases. Chronic obstruction of the kidney, lupus erythematosus, and sickle cell disease can cause the tubular defect type of hyperkalemic distal RTA. Diabetes mellitus, mild chronic renal failure, and old age are associated with the hyporeninemic hypoaldosteronism type of hyperkalemic distal RTA.

Diagnosis of RTA is made by eliminating nonrenal causes for a normal AG metabolic acidosis (e.g., diarrhea). Proximal RTA is characterized by urinary wasting of more than 5% to 15% of the filtered load of HCO_3^- when serum levels are maintained close to normal. Hypokalemic distal RTA is characterized by the inability to decrease urine pH to less than 5.3 with oral furosemide and fludrocortisone. Hyperkalemic normal ion gap metabolic acidosis almost always is due to distal RTA. The tubular defect type is marked by an inability to acidify maximally (urine pH usually above 6.0), in contrast to the hypoaldosteronism type, in which the intensity of acidification is intact. In both types, renal ammonium excretion is reduced, and the urinary AG often is positive (see section **V.A.2.d**).

c. Inorganic acid intake. The ingestion of ammonium chloride to reduce appetite or acidify urine produces hyperchloremic metabolic acidosis. Inorganic sulfur, such as flowers of sulfur cathartic, is oxidized to form H_2SO_4. The hydrogen ions titrate the HCO_3^- down, and the sulfate is excreted rapidly with sodium. This leaves a low HCO_3^- with a normal AG. A similar process happens with toluene inhalation from paint or glue sniffing. Toluene is metabolized to hippuric acid, and the hippurate is excreted rapidly.

d. Diagnosis of distal RTA is made when urinary ammonium excretion is reduced during hyperchloremic, normal AG metabolic acidosis. A useful screening test for urinary ammonium is the **urinary anion gap** (UAG):

$$UAG = (Na^+ + K^+) - Cl^-$$

The UAG is an estimate of urinary ammonium that is elevated in gastrointestinal HCO_3^- loss but low in distal RTA. UAG is a negative value if urine ammonium is high (as in diarrhea; average, -20 mEq per L) whereas it is positive if urine ammonium is low (as in distal RTA; average, $+23$ mEq per L). Urinary sodium concentration must be ample.

B. Causes of metabolic alkalosis. Metabolic alkalosis is generated by three pathophysiological mechanisms: loss of volume, gain of volume due to mineralocorticoids, and miscellaneous factors. Metabolic alkalosis of the volume-depleted type is characterized by a low urine Cl^-, indicating the avidity of the kidney for solute, largely NaCl. During the generation phases of metabolic alkalosis, bicarbonaturia may occur and necessitate Na^+ and K^+ excretion. Therefore, urine Cl^- is a better marker than urine Na^+ of the stimulation of renal salt reabsorption by volume depletion. During the maintenance stage of metabolic alkalosis, bicarbonaturia is minimal, urine pH is acid, and urine Na^+ is low. Volume-depleted metabolic alkalosis is due to external losses of hydrogen ion or chloride. Volume-replete metabolic alkalosis is characterized by spot urine Cl^- concentrations of usually well over 20 mmol per L. The kidney is not avid for salt because of volume expansion (mild) and therefore excretes the daily Na^+ and Cl^- load without difficulty. This volume-regulated group of disorders is due to mineralocorticoid excess or occasionally to profound potassium depletion.

1. Metabolic alkaloses of the volume-depleted variety have in common the external loss of fluids rich in H^+ or Cl^-. The stomach, kidney, or skin may be the culprit (Table 4-6).

2. Metabolic alkaloses of the volume-replete variety are characterized by enhanced renal H^+ secretion despite normal or increased ECF volume. The stimulus for this sustained H^+ secretion is aldosterone (or a relative) or major cellular potassium depletion (Table 4-6). Gitelman's syndrome is an autosomal recessive disorder usually appearing in adults as hypokalemic, hypomagnesemic metabolic alkalosis. The distal convoluted tubule Na^+Cl^- cotransporter is

TABLE 4-6	Causes of Metabolic Alkalosis

Volume-depleted type
Gastric acid loss
Vomiting
Gastric suction
Renal chloride loss
Diuretics
Posthypercapnia
Cystic fibrosis
Volume-replete type
Mineralocorticoid excess
Hyperaldosteronism
Gitelman's syndrome
Bartter's syndrome
Cushing's syndrome
Licorice excess
Profound potassium depletion

defective. In contrast, Bartter's syndrome appears in childhood as hypokalemic metabolic alkalosis. In this syndrome, defects in loop of Henle Na^+Cl^- reabsorption lead to normotensive secondary hyperaldosteronism; loop diuretic abuse resembles these disorders.

C. Causes of respiratory acidosis. Two ventilatory abnormalities allow CO_2 retention and increased Pco_2: alveolar hypoventilation and severe ventilation–perfusion mismatch. Hypoxemia occurs in both settings. Disorders of respiratory drive, nerve conduction, thoracic cage, pleura, and lung parenchyma may cause hypercapnia (increased Pco_2). Renal compensation for chronic respiratory acidosis may produce very high HCO_3^- levels. If the Pco_2 is reduced by artificial ventilation, the high HCO_3^- may persist if not enough chloride is provided to replace it. This results in posthypercapnic metabolic alkalosis. Acetazolamide may be useful in this setting.

D. Causes of respiratory alkalosis. Disorders that drive ventilation independent of Pco_2 can cause hyperventilation and hypocapnia. Inflammatory and mass lesions of the brain, psychiatric disorders, and certain central-acting drugs and chemicals increase central respiratory drive and produce hypocapnia. Importantly, salicylates, endotoxin, and progesterone are among this group of drugs and chemicals. Disorders that cause hypoxemia are common causes of the hyperventilation that causes hypocapnia. Disorders that reduce lung or chest compliance such as mild pneumonia or pulmonary edema, vascular disorders such as emboli, and mixed disorders such as hepatic cirrhosis or cardiac failure can cause hypocapnia. Volume depletion is a primary stimulus to hyperventilation and hypocapnia.

VI. TREATING ACID–BASE DISORDERS. As discussed, acid–base disorders are markers of underlying diseases, and these diseases should be the targets of treatment.
  A. Step 1. Correct volume and electrolyte deficiencies.
  B. Step 2. Direct specific treatment at the underlying cause.
  C. Step 3. Manipulate the bicarbonate or Pco_2 only if the pH is adversely affecting organ function or if pH is less than 7.10 or greater than 7.60.
  D. Treatment of metabolic acidosis with alkali has not been shown to be efficacious in acute situations, including cardiopulmonary resuscitation, possibly because the HCO_3^- reaction with H^+ generates CO_2 at the tissue level and lowers cell pH. However, a mixture of carbonate and bicarbonate that produces less CO_2 also has not been shown to be of clinical benefit. At present, alkali therapy is recommended only for severe (pH less than 7.1) acute metabolic acidosis. In chronic distal RTA, alkali therapy reduces bone loss, hypercalciuria, and nephrocalcinosis. Oral alkali can be given as sodium bicarbonate tablets, 500 mg or 6 mmol, or as sodium or

potassium citrate solution, 1 mmol per mL. Usually 3 mmol per kg of body weight is the starting dose. Oral HCO_3^- is accompanied by a sodium or potassium load that must be watched for adverse effects.

1. Insulin is the specific **treatment for diabetic ketoacidosis.** HCO_3^- and phosphate administration are unnecessary, but potassium repletion is important. Volume and electrolyte repletion, plus glucose and thiamine, suffice to correct alcoholic ketoacidosis. Starvation requires only calories. Note that metabolism of ketoanions, as with all organic anions, produces HCO_3^-; metabolism corrects approximately half of the HCO_3^- deficit. If alkali is given unwisely, an overshoot metabolic alkalosis may result.

2. In the **treatment of lactic acidosis**, the restoration of tissue perfusion and oxygenation is desirable, but often difficult to attain. Attention to potassium and calcium levels is important.

3. **Treatment of intoxications.** Ethylene glycol and methanol poisoning require immediate fomepizole infusion to retard metabolism of the alcohol to toxic products. Hemodialysis is started if renal failure is present. An alternative approach is to infuse ethanol to maintain a blood level of 100 mg per dL to compete for alcohol dehydrogenase activity. The loading dose of ethanol is 0.6 to 1.0 g per kg of body weight followed by a maintenance infusion of 10 to 20 g per hour. Blood alcohol levels must be monitored frequently.

   Salicylate intoxication should be treated with urinary alkalinization by infusing a 5% glucose solution containing $NaHCO_3$, 150 mmol added per L, at 375 mL per hour, for 4 or more hours. Hemodialysis should be used to remove salicylate in patients with prominent renal failure, worsening mental status, recalcitrant acidosis, or general deterioration. Discontinuation of acetaminophen corrects pyroglutamic acidosis.

E. **Correction of metabolic alkalosis** very rarely, if ever, requires the administration of acid. If renal failure prohibits renal excretion of HCO_3^-, the patient usually requires dialysis for other reasons. A low bicarbonate dialysate can be used. If heart failure precludes the use of NaCl, then acetazolamide, 500 mg by mouth or intravenously, consistently reduces the serum tCO_2 by approximately 6 mmol per L. Acid infusion is fraught with the potential complications of hemolysis and vascular necrosis and is best avoided. Ammonium chloride can be given as a source of acid, but it causes gastric distress even when given intravenously and may cause ammonia intoxication.

   1. **Volume-depletion metabolic alkalosis is corrected** by providing ample chloride with sodium or potassium. Prevention, however, is preferable. Proton-pump inhibitors minimize gastric acid loss in patients with nasogastric suction. Use of the potassium-sparing diuretics spironolactone, triamterene, and amiloride reduces the frequency and severity of diuretic-induced alkalosis.

   2. **Treatment of volume-replete metabolic alkalosis.** If possible, the cause of increased mineralocorticoid production should be removed. For example, a functioning adrenal adenoma should be surgically excised. In the interim, the use of spironolactone in doses up to 400 mg per day with potassium chloride may be effective. Indomethacin may be beneficial in Bartter's syndrome.

F. **Respiratory acidosis *per se* does not require direct treatment.** Even at chronic P_{CO_2} levels above 100 mm Hg, the kidneys generate and maintain HCO_3^- levels sufficient to keep the pH above 7.20. However, adequate oxygenation is the critical issue in both acute and chronic respiratory acidosis.

G. **Definitive treatment of respiratory alkalosis** again requires the correction of the underlying condition causing hyperventilation. The provision of oxygen is essential for the hypoxemic patient.

H. **Treatment of mixed acid–base disorders**

   1. **Metabolic acidosis and respiratory acidosis.** The most rapid treatment is to provide assisted or controlled ventilation. The administration of base is not warranted. The correction of the cause of metabolic acidosis is a priority.

   2. In **metabolic alkalosis and respiratory acidosis**, the pH is often alkalemic. Acetazolamide given daily or every other day may be used to keep the pH near

7.35 to 7.40, which is a good level to avoid suppression or excessive stimulation of respiration.

3. **Metabolic alkalosis and respiratory alkalosis** in combination may produce severe alkalemia with dangerous arrhythmias. The most expedient treatment consists of intravenous morphine and a benzodiazepine, with immediate access to airway intubation and mechanical ventilation.

Suggested Readings

Batlle DC, Hizon M, Cohen E, et al. The use of the urinary anion gap in the diagnosis of hyperchloremic metabolic acidosis. *N Engl J Med* 1988;318:594–599.

Corey HE. Stewart and beyond: new models of acid-base balance. *Kidney Int* 2003;64: 777–787.

DuBose TD Jr. Hyperkalemic hyperchloremic metabolic acidosis: pathophysiologic insights. *Kidney Int* 1997;51:591–602.

Fenves AZ, Kirkpatrick HM III, Patel VV, et al. Increased anion gap metabolic acidosis as a result of 5-oxoproline (pyroglutamic acidosis): a role for acetaminophen. *Clin J Am Soc Nephrol* 2006;1:441–447.

Gabow PA, Kaehny WD, Fennessey PV, et al. Diagnostic importance of an increased serum anion gap. *N Engl J Med* 1980;303:854–858.

Galla JH. Metabolic alkalosis. *J Am Soc Nephrol* 2000;11:369–375.

Kraut JA, Kurtz I. Use of base in the treatment of severe acidemic states. *Am J Kidney Dis* 2001;38:703–727.

Kraut JA, Kurtz I. Toxic alcohol ingestions: clinical features, diagnosis, and management. *Clin J Am Soc Nephrol* 2008;3:208–225.

Kraut JA, Madias NE. Serum anion gap: its uses and limitations in clinical medicine. *Clin J Am Soc Nephrol* 2007;2:162–174.

Rastegar A. Use of the delta AG/delta HCO_3^- in the diagnosis of mixed acid-base disorders. *J Am Soc Nephrol* 2007;18:2429–2431.

Rodriguez-Soriano J. Renal tubular acidosis. The clinical entity. *J Am Soc Nephrol* 2002; 13:2160–2170.

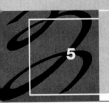

5

THE PATIENT WITH DISORDERS OF SERUM CALCIUM AND PHOSPHATE

Jeffrey G. Penfield and Robert F. Reilly

 DISORDERS OF SERUM CALCIUM

Most calcium in the body is in the form of hydroxyapatite in bone (99%). Although a small fraction of total body calcium is contained in the extracellular fluid (ECF), only the concentration of ionized calcium in the ECF is physiologically active and regulated. Approximately 60% of calcium in the ECF is ultrafilterable and exists either free in solution as ionized calcium (50%) or complexed to anions such as citrate, phosphate, sulfate, and bicarbonate (10%). The remaining 40% is bound to proteins (primarily albumin). Serum or plasma calcium concentration is measured as either total or ionized calcium. Total calcium concentration is measured with a colorimetric assay and includes ionized, complexed, and bound calcium. Ionized calcium concentration is measured with a calcium-specific electrode and represents physiologically regulated calcium. Conventional units of calcium are mg per dL or mEq per L and Standard International (SI) units are mmol per L. SI units (mmol per L) can be converted to mg per dL by multiplying by 4.

In Figure 5-1 are illustrated calcium fluxes between the ECF, intestine, kidney, and bone. Net intestinal calcium absorption amounts to approximately 200 mg of the normal dietary intake of 800 to 1,000 mg. In the steady state, this net intestinal absorption is matched by urinary excretion. As a result, 10,600 mg of the approximately 10,800 mg (98%) of calcium that is filtered daily is reabsorbed.

I. CALCIUM REGULATION. Plasma-ionized calcium is regulated through a complex and coordinated interplay of parathyroid hormone (PTH) and $1,25(OH)_2$ vitamin D_3 (calcitriol) in intestine, bone, and kidney. The parathyroid gland senses ECF-ionized calcium concentration through a calcium-sensing receptor. High concentrations of ECF calcium stimulate the receptor and activate second messenger pathways that, in turn, inhibit PTH release. Low ECF calcium concentration stimulates PTH secretion and production and increases parathyroid gland mass. The parathyroid gland responds quickly (within minutes) to alterations in ionized calcium concentration. An inverse sigmoid relationship exists between ECF calcium concentration and PTH secretion, with a nonsuppressible component present even at high plasma calcium concentration. The amount of hormone stored is enough to support basal secretion for 6 hours and stimulated secretion for 2 hours.

In bone, PTH in the presence of permissive amounts of calcitriol stimulates reabsorption by increasing osteoclast number and activity. In intestine, PTH enhances calcium and phosphate absorption indirectly by promoting the formation of calcitriol. In kidney, PTH augments distal tubular calcium reabsorption, stimulates calcitriol formation in the proximal tubule, and decreases proximal tubular phosphate and bicarbonate reabsorption.

Calcitriol is produced in proximal tubule through 1-α hydroxylation of $25(OH)$ vitamin D_3 (calcidiol). The calcitriol biosynthetic pathway is illustrated in Figure 5-2. Principal stimulators of 1-α hydroxylase are PTH and hypophosphatemia. The major function of calcitriol is to enhance calcium and phosphate availability for new bone formation and prevention of symptomatic hypocalcemia and hypophosphatemia. In intestine and kidney, calcitriol increases production of calcium-binding proteins (calbindins) that aid in transcellular calcium movement; this may be the rate-limiting step

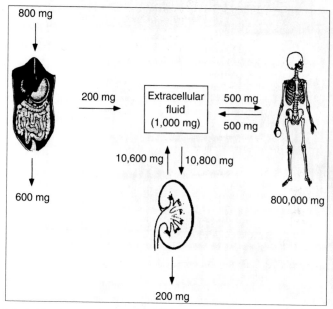

Figure 5-1. Calcium homeostasis.

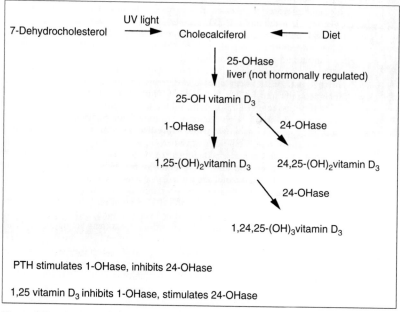

Figure 5-2. Vitamin D metabolism. (PTH, parathyroid hormone; UV, ultraviolet.)

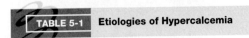

TABLE 5-1	Etiologies of Hypercalcemia

Hyperparathyroidism
Malignancy
Vitamin A and D intoxication
Milk-alkali syndrome
Thyrotoxicosis
Granulomatous disease
Immobilization
Paget's disease
Thiazide diuretic intake
Addison's disease
Pheochromocytoma
Lithium intake
Renal failure
Post renal transplant
Familial hypocalciuric hypercalcemia

in transepithelial calcium flux. In bone, calcitriol potentiates PTH actions, stimulates osteoclastic reabsorption, and induces differentiation of monocytes into osteoclasts.

In parathyroid gland, calcitriol binds to its receptor, leading to a decrease in PTH production. The *PTH* gene promoter contains regions that bind the calcitriol receptor. Binding results in a dramatic decrease in PTH expression. Calcitriol is the most potent suppressor of *PTH* gene transcription.

II. HYPERCALCEMIA

A. Etiology. Three basic pathophysiologic mechanisms contribute to hypercalcemia: increased calcium absorption from the gastrointestinal tract, decreased renal calcium excretion, and increased bone calcium resorption. The most common etiologies of hypercalcemia are listed in Table 5-1.

   1. Increased calcium absorption from the gastrointestinal tract plays a primary role in the hypercalcemia of the milk-alkali syndrome, vitamin D intoxication, and granulomatous disorders.

   a. Milk-alkali syndrome is the result of ingestion of excess calcium and alkali. In the past, peptic ulcer disease was treated with the Sippy regimen that included milk and sodium bicarbonate. This calcium and alkali source used to be the most common cause of the milk-alkali syndrome. The Sippy regimen was replaced with histamine antagonists and proton pump inhibitors so that milk and sodium bicarbonate are now rare causes of this syndrome. Currently, this syndrome most often occurs in elderly women consuming excess calcium carbonate or citrate for the treatment of osteoporosis. Alkalosis decreases renal calcium excretion and the resultant hypercalciuria, nephrocalcinosis, and subsequent renal insufficiency prevents correction of the alkalosis. Many of these patients are also receiving vitamin D supplements that increase intestinal calcium absorption. Diuretic use or vomiting can cause alkalosis. Patients present with the classic triad of hypercalcemia, metabolic alkalosis, and elevated serum creatinine concentration. Treatment is volume replacement with normal saline and avoidance of calcium and alkaline supplements. Bisphosphonates should be avoided because these agents prevent bone calcium release, which is not a contributing factor in this syndrome and can result in hypocalcemia. Treatment of hypercalcemia in these patients is often complicated by hypocalcemia resulting from sustained PTH suppression.

   b. Hypercalcemia in renal failure is uncommon, except in patients treated with calcium and vitamin D supplements. This disorder and the milk-alkali syndrome illustrate the important concept that hypercalcemia from excessive dietary calcium ingestion alone does not occur in the absence of renal impairment.

    c. **Vitamin D intoxication** also results in hypercalcemia. Calcium is absorbed primarily in the small intestine, and this process is stimulated by calcitriol.

    d. Hypercalcemia may also be secondary to **granulomatous disorders,** such as sarcoidosis. Activated macrophages produce calcitriol, which leads to increased intestinal absorption of dietary calcium. Hypercalciuria is seen more commonly than hypercalcemia. Lymphomas occasionally cause hypercalcemia through the same mechanism.

2. **Increased calcium resorption from bone** plays a primary role in hypercalcemia resulting from primary and secondary hyperparathyroidism, malignancy, hyperthyroidism, immobilization, Paget's disease, and vitamin A toxicity.

    a. **Primary hyperparathyroidism** is a common cause of hypercalcemia. Over the last several decades the incidence of primary hyperparathyroidism has been declining from 82.5 cases per 100,000 from 1974 to 1982 to 29.1 cases per 100,000 from 1983 to 1992 and most recently 21.6 cases per 100,000 from 1993 to 2001. The peak incidence in the 1970s may have been the result of a causative factor or the onset of automated serum calcium testing. A possible etiologic factor may have been the therapeutic use of head and neck radiation for a variety of conditions in the previous two decades. The underlying pathology is most often a solitary adenoma (80%). Among the remainder, 15% to 20% have diffuse hyperplasia, and approximately one-half of these have a familial syndrome [multiple endocrine neoplasia (MEN) type I, associated with pituitary adenomas and islet cell tumors, or MEN type II, associated with medullary carcinoma of the thyroid and pheochromocytoma]. Multiple adenomas are uncommon, and parathyroid carcinoma is rare (occurring in less than 1%). Hypercalcemia results from increased calcium reabsorption from bone, increased intestinal calcium absorption mediated by calcitriol, and increased distal tubular renal calcium reabsorption. In primary hyperparathyroidism, hypercalcemia is often mild, asymptomatic, and identified on routine blood chemistries in the outpatient setting. Patients most commonly present in the fifth and sixth decades. Women are affected two to three times more frequently than men, and two-thirds of all cases occur in postmenopausal women.

    b. **Tertiary hyperparathyroidism** leads to hypercalcemia after renal transplantation when plasma phosphorus concentration, vitamin D metabolism, and renal function improve, but PTH secretion remains high secondary to increased parathyroid mass. In most patients, PTH levels drop and hypercalcemia resolves during the first year following transplantation.

    c. **Malignancy** is also a common cause of hypercalcemia. Hypercalcemia of malignancy results from several pathophysiologic mechanisms: overproduction of PTH-related peptide (PTHrP), local bone reabsorption around sites of tumor infiltration (mediated through a variety of cytokines and osteolytic prostaglandins), and calcitriol production (e.g., with lymphomas). Patients with squamous cell lung cancer, breast cancer, multiple myeloma, and renal cell carcinoma are at highest risk. Hypercalcemia due to tumoral PTHrP production is often referred to as *humoral hypercalcemia of malignancy* (*HHM*). PTHrP has 70% amino acid identity to the first 13 amino acids of PTH and binds to the PTH receptor. It normally functions as a regulator of chondrocyte growth and differentiation in developing long bones, calcium mobilization from bones and into breast milk during lactation, transport of calcium across the placenta to the developing fetus, and regulation of uterine blood flow. HHM often presents with severe hypercalcemia (calcium concentration greater than 14 mg per dL) in a patient with either a known history of malignancy or evidence of malignancy at initial presentation. PTHrP is immunologically distinct from PTH and is not detected by standard PTH assays, but specific assays for PTHrP are commercially available. The normal range for PTHrP is less than 2.0 pmol per L. Assays that measure the

C-terminal fragment of PTHrP may show an increase when used in pregnant patients or patients with chronic kidney disease. Median survival from the onset of hypercalcemia with HHM is only 3 months. Squamous cell tumors, renal cell carcinomas, and most breast neoplasms produce PTHrP. The diagnoses of primary hyperparathyroidism and malignancy are not mutually exclusive. An increased incidence of primary hyperparathyroidism was reported in patients with malignancy.

Multiple myeloma is associated with hypercalcemia and localized osteolytic skeletal lesions. Approximately 30% of patients with myeloma experience hypercalcemia at some time during the course of their disease. Bone destruction occurs as a consequence of interleukin-6, interleukin-1, and tumor necrosis factor-beta release by malignant plasma cells. Bony lesions demonstrate a marked increase in osteoclastic resorption without manifestations of increased bone formation, in contrast to metastatic lesions of breast and prostate cancer, which generally show some increase in bone formation and radionuclide uptake at sites of increased osteoblastic activity.

d. Hyperthyroidism results in mild hypercalcemia in 10% to 20% of patients as a result of increased bone turnover. There is also an increased prevalence of hyperparathyroidism in patients with hyperthyroidism.

e. Paget's disease is an autosomal dominant disease of bone with focal areas of increased bone turnover, disorganized and structurally weak bone, and increased vascularity. Immobilization with Paget's disease can cause hypercalcemia, although this is more likely in children. In adults, hypercalciuria is more common than hypercalcemia.

f. Rare causes of hypercalcemia include lithium use (mild; interferes with the calcium-sensing receptor); thiazide diuretic use (occult primary hyperparathyroidism should be suspected); pheochromocytoma; primary adrenal insufficiency; and a rare genetic disorder, familial hypocalciuric hypercalcemia (FHH).

FHH is an autosomal dominant disorder caused by a heterozygous mutation in the calcium-sensing receptor. It presents with mild hypercalcemia early in life, hypocalciuria, and a normal or slightly increased PTH concentration in the absence of signs or symptoms of hypercalcemia. In patients with hypercalcemia, polyuria results from calcium-sensing receptor activation and decreased aquaporin 2 in the luminal membrane of the collecting duct. This functions to protect the kidney from stone formation by diluting hypercalciuric urine. In FHH, absence of the calcium-sensing receptor prevents both the associated polyuria and hypercalciuria (therefore kidney stones). As a result of the mutation, the calcium-sensing receptor is less sensitive to plasma calcium concentration, and a higher than normal calcium concentration is required to suppress PTH. One should be aware of FHH, because this condition is often misdiagnosed as primary hyperparathyroidism, and patients may be inappropriately subjected to neck exploration. FHH may account for a small percentage of patients who undergo surgery for primary hyperparathyroidism in whom no adenoma is found.

B. Signs and symptoms of hypercalcemia are related to the severity and rate of rise in plasma-ionized calcium concentration. Mild hypercalcemia is generally asymptomatic and often incidentally discovered on routine blood chemistries, as is the case in many patients with primary hyperparathyroidism. In contrast, severe hypercalcemia is often associated with neurologic and gastrointestinal symptoms. The patient may present with a wide range of central nervous system symptoms, from mild mental status changes to stupor and coma. Gastrointestinal symptoms include constipation, anorexia, nausea, and vomiting. Abdominal pain may result from hypercalcemia-induced peptic ulcer disease or pancreatitis. As discussed in Chapter 2, hypernatremia (see section I.C.2.b), hypercalcemia results in polyuria and secondary polydipsia that leads to ECF volume contraction, a reduction in the glomerular filtration rate (GFR), and an elevation in blood urea nitrogen (BUN) and creatinine concentrations. Hypercalcemia also potentiates the cardiac effects of digitalis toxicity.

C. Diagnosis. The most common causes of hypercalcemia are primary hyperparathyroidism and malignancy. These two disorders make up more than 90% of all cases. Initial evaluation includes a history and physical examination. Use of calcium supplements, antacids, vitamin preparations, and over-the-counter medications should be determined. A chest x-ray should be obtained to rule out pulmonary malignancies and granulomatous disorders.

1. **Initial laboratory examination** includes measurement of electrolytes, BUN, creatinine, and phosphorus; serum protein electrophoresis; and a 24-hour urine for calcium and creatinine. The presence of a high serum chloride concentration and a low serum phosphorus concentration in a ratio greater than 33:1 is suggestive of primary hyperparathyroidism resulting from PTH's effect of decreasing proximal tubular phosphate reabsorption. A low serum chloride concentration, a high serum bicarbonate concentration, and elevated BUN and creatinine concentrations are characteristic of milk-alkali syndrome. A monoclonal spike on either serum protein electrophoresis or urine electrophoresis is suggestive of multiple myeloma or light chain disease. A low serum phosphorus concentration is found in primary hyperparathyroidism and HHM. The 24-hour urinary calcium excretion is low in hypercalcemia caused by the milk-alkali syndrome, thiazide diuretic use, or FHH.

   As a general rule, primary hyperparathyroidism is the etiology in asymptomatic outpatients with a serum calcium concentration less than or equal to 11 mg per dL whereas malignancy is often the cause in symptomatic patients with an abrupt disease onset and serum calcium concentration greater than or equal to 14 mg per dL.

2. **Intact PTH concentration** is obtained after the initial evaluation is completed. The most common cause of an elevated PTH concentration is primary hyperparathyroidism, although an elevated PTH concentration may also be seen with lithium use and FHH. Occasionally, in primary hyperparathyroidism, PTH concentration will be inappropriately within the normal range compared to the serum calcium concentration. In all other conditions, PTH will be suppressed by hypercalcemia.

3. If no obvious malignancy is present and PTH concentration is not increased, the possibility of vitamin D intoxication or granulomatous disease should be evaluated further with an analysis of **calcidiol and calcitriol** concentration. An increased calcidiol concentration is seen with the ingestion of either vitamin D or calcidiol. An elevated calcitriol concentration is observed with calcitriol ingestion, granulomatous disease, lymphoma, and primary hyperparathyroidism.

4. As a final step, if calcitriol concentration is increased without an apparent cause, occult granulomatous disease can be evaluated with a **hydrocortisone suppression test**. After administration of 40 mg of hydrocortisone every 8 hours for 10 days, the hypercalcemia will resolve if it is the result of granulomatous disease.

D. Treatment of hypercalcemia varies depending on the severity of the serum calcium elevation. It is directed at increasing urinary calcium excretion, inhibiting bone resorption, and decreasing intestinal calcium absorption.

1. **Urinary calcium excretion is increased** by expanding the ECF volume and, subsequently, administering loop diuretics. Calcium reabsorption in proximal tubule is passive and parallels sodium reabsorption. ECF volume contraction, therefore, increases proximal sodium reabsorption and helps maintain hypercalcemia. Patients with hypercalcemia are often volume contracted. Hypercalcemia decreases sodium reabsorption in the thick ascending limb of the loop of Henle through activation of the calcium-sensing receptor, and it also antagonizes the effects of antidiuretic hormone. In the setting of a reduced GFR, higher doses of loop diuretics may be required. In the presence of little or no renal function and severe hypercalcemia, hemodialysis is indicated. If hypercalcemia is moderate, volume expansion and loop diuretics may be the only therapy required.

2. **An agent that inhibits bone resorption** is often required when hypercalcemia is moderate or severe. In the acute setting, calcitonin is often helpful because of its rapid onset of action (2 to 4 hours). Calcitonin inhibits osteoclastic bone reabsorption and increases renal calcium excretion. It reduces serum calcium concentration, however, by only 1 to 2 mg per dL, and tachyphylaxis often develops with repeated use. For these reasons, calcitonin should not be used as the sole agent to inhibit bone resorption.

   a. **Bisphosphonates** are the agents of choice for the management of hypercalcemia due to bone resorption. These analogs of inorganic pyrophosphate are selectively concentrated in bone, where they interfere with osteoclast attachment and function. Bisphosphonates have a slow onset (2 to 3 days) and a long duration of action (several weeks). Caution should be exercised in patients with milk-alkali syndrome. These patients do not have a defect in bone turnover and are susceptible to hypocalcemia with treatment.

   Etidronate was the first bisphosphonate approved for the treatment of hypercalcemia. The serum calcium concentration begins to fall on day 2 with etidronate and reaches a nadir on day 7. The hypocalcemic effect may be prolonged for several weeks. If serum calcium falls rapidly within the first 48 hours, the drug should be discontinued to avoid hypocalcemia. Etidronate can be given intravenously at a dosage of 7.5 mg per kg over 4 hours for 3 consecutive days. A single intravenous dose of 30 mg per kg as an infusion over 24 hours in 1 L of normal saline, however, may be more effective.

   Pamidronate is more potent than etidronate. It is given at a dose of either 60 or 90 mg intravenously over 4 hours. If serum calcium concentration is less than or equal to 13.5 mg per dL, 60 mg is given. If serum calcium concentration is greater than 13.5 mg per dL, 90 mg is administered. Serum calcium concentration gradually falls over the ensuing 2 to 4 days. A single dose is usually effective for 1 to 2 weeks. In most patients, serum calcium concentration normalizes after 7 days.

   Zolendronic acid is now the most commonly used bisphosphonate because it can be given intravenously which avoids esophageal damage from oral doses and it can be administered over a short interval (4 mg over 15 minutes). It is administered every 3 to 4 weeks and it may be longer lasting than pamidronate. The dose must be adjusted in patients with renal dysfunction as follows given the calculated GFR: greater than 60 mL per minute—4 mg; 50 to 60 mL per minute—3.5 mg; 40 to 49 mL per minute—3.3 mg; 30 to 39 mL per minute—3.0 mg; less than 30 mL per minute—no data available. The manufacturer recommends that the drug be discontinued if the serum creatinine concentration increases greater than or equal to 0.5 mg per dL above a normal baseline or greater than 1.0 mg per dL in those with a serum creatinine concentration greater than or equal to 1.4 mg per dL.

   Bisphosphonates are associated with significant toxicity including focal glomerular sclerosis with pamidronate and acute kidney injury with zolendronic acid. Most of these cases occurred in patients with preexisting chronic kidney disease or when recommended doses were exceeded. In addition, when bisphosphonates are used long term in patients with malignancy especially multiple myeloma and breast cancer they are associated with osteonecrosis of the jaw. Most of these patients have had recent tooth extraction or surgical tooth removal.

   b. **Plicamycin (Mithramycin)** can be used except in patients with severe hepatic, renal, and marrow disorders. Its effect begins in 12 hours and peaks at 48 hours. The dose can be repeated at 3- to 7-day intervals. Its side effect profile (nausea, hepatotoxicity, proteinuria, and thrombocytopenia) has led to decreased enthusiasm for its use.

   c. **Gallium nitrate** inhibits bone resorption by decreasing the acid secretion of osteoclasts and also enhancing hydroxyapatite crystallization of bone. It is an additional agent that can be employed to treat hypercalcemia of malignancy. It is administered as a continuous infusion at a dose of 100 to 200 mg per m^2

TABLE 5-2	Treatment of Hypercalcemia

Drug	Dosage
Normal saline	2–4 L/d initially
Furosemide	20–160 mg i.v. q8h after volume expansion
Salmon calcitonin	4 IU/kg s.c. q12 h
Etidronate disodium	7.5 mg/kg i.v. over 4 hr q.d. for 3–7 d, 30 mg/kg i.v. over 24 hr single dose
Pamidronate disodium	60–90 mg i.v. over 4 hr
Zolendronic acid	4 mg over 15 min. Dose adjusted for renal function
Plicamycin	25 μg/kg i.v. over 4 hr q.d. for 3–4 d
Corticosteroids	200–300 mg hydrocortisone i.v. q.d. for 3–5 d
Gallium nitrate	100–200 mg/m^2 for 5 d

for 5 consecutive days. Gallium nitrate should not be administered to patients with serum creatinine concentrations above 2.5 mg per dL, and it is probably best reserved for patients who have not responded to more conventional agents. A summary of treatment options is shown in Table 5-2.

3. **Measures to decrease intestinal calcium absorption** are often employed in outpatients with mild disease. Corticosteroids may be helpful in vitamin D intoxication, granulomatous disease, and certain neoplasms (lymphoma, myeloma). Alternatives to corticosteroids include ketoconazole and hydroxychloroquine. Oral phosphate can be administered, providing the patient does not have an elevated serum phosphorus concentration or renal failure. Oral phosphate, however, often causes diarrhea and only lowers the serum calcium concentration by approximately 1 mg per dL.

4. Whether to **surgically remove** a solitary parathyroid adenoma remains a difficult management issue. The following criteria for surgical intervention were suggested at a 1991 National Institutes of Health consensus conference: a total serum calcium concentration that is greater than 1 mg per dL above the upper limit of the normal range; evidence of overt bone disease; cortical bone mineral density that is more than 2 standard deviations (SDs) below the adjusted mean for age, sex, and race; reduction in renal function by more than 30%; a history of nephrolithiasis or nephrocalcinosis; urinary calcium excretion greater than 400 mg per day; and an episode of acute symptomatic hypercalcemia. It is estimated that approximately 50% of patients meet these criteria.

With the advent of minimally invasive parathyroid surgery, these criteria are likely to be liberalized. The adenoma is initially localized with sestamibi scanning. If a solitary hot spot is identified, the adenoma is resected under local anesthesia. PTH concentration is measured intraoperatively. Its concentration should fall within minutes (greater than 50% in 10 minutes) if the adenoma is successfully resected, given the short half-life of PTH (4 minutes). If PTH concentration remains elevated, then the patient is placed under general anesthesia and the opposite side of the neck explored. The combination of sestamibi scanning and intraoperative PTH concentration measurement results in the successful removal of solitary adenomas in the vast majority of cases.

III. HYPOCALCEMIA

A. **Etiology.** True hypocalcemia is the result of decreased calcium absorption from the gastrointestinal tract or decreased calcium resorption from bone. Given that 98% of total body calcium is contained within the skeleton, sustained hypocalcemia cannot occur without an abnormality of either PTH or calcitriol action in bone.

Total plasma calcium is composed of three components: ionized calcium (50%), complexed calcium (10%), and protein-bound calcium (40%). True hypocalcemia is present only when ionized calcium concentration is reduced. The reference range for ionized calcium concentration is 4.2 to 5.0 mg per dL (1.05 to 1.25 mmol per L).

Therefore, whenever a low total serum calcium concentration is observed, this value must be compared with the serum albumin concentration. For every decrease of 1 g per dL in serum albumin concentration from its normal concentration of 4 g per dL, a decrease of 0.8 mg per dL in total serum calcium concentration can be expected. Therefore, for each fall of 1 g per dL in serum albumin concentration, 0.8 mg per dL must be added to total serum calcium concentration. This correction factor was shown to be unreliable in patients with critical illness. Calcium binding to albumin is affected by ECF pH. Acidemia increases and alkalemia decreases ionized calcium concentration. Ionized calcium concentration increases approximately 0.2 mg per dL for each 0.1 decrease in pH. These correction factors are only general guidelines and should not be used as a substitute for the direct measurement of serum-ionized calcium concentration if clinical suspicion warrants.

True hypocalcemia is caused by decreased PTH secretion, end-organ resistance to PTH, or disorders of vitamin D metabolism. Occasionally, hypocalcemia occurs acutely as a result of either extravascular calcium deposition or intravascular calcium binding. The most common etiologies of true hypocalcemia are illustrated in Table 5-3.

1. **Hypoparathyroidism** is caused by a wide variety of acquired and inherited diseases that result from the impaired PTH synthesis and release or from peripheral tissue resistance to PTH.

   a. The most common cause of idiopathic hypoparathyroidism is **polyglandular autoimmune syndrome type I**, characterized by chronic mucocutaneous candidiasis and primary adrenal insufficiency. Occasionally, pernicious anemia, diabetes mellitus, vitiligo, and autoimmune thyroid disease also are associated. Mucocutaneous candidiasis often presents first in early childhood and is followed several years later by hypoparathyroidism. Adrenal insufficiency appears in adolescence. The combination of hypoparathyroidism, adrenal insufficiency, and mucocutaneous candidiasis is referred to as the *hypoparathyroidism, adrenal insufficiency, and mucocutaneous candidiasis*

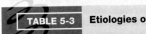

TABLE 5-3	Etiologies of Hypocalcemia

Hypoparathyroidism
   Idiopathic — HAM syndrome
   Familial
   Post surgery — hungry bone syndrome
   Infiltrative disorders
   Pseudohypoparathyroidism IA, IB, II
   Hypomagnesemia
Defects in vitamin D metabolism
   Nutritional
   Malabsorption
   Drugs
   Liver disease
   Renal disease
   Vitamin D–dependent rickets
Miscellaneous
   Tumor lysis syndrome
   Osteoblastic metastases
   Acute pancreatitis
   Toxic shock syndrome
   Sepsis

HAM, hypoparathyroidism, adrenal insufficiency, and mucocutaneous candidiasis.

(HAM) syndrome. Mutations in the autoimmune regulator *(AIRE)* gene, a transcription factor, were shown to cause the disease.

b. Familial hypocalcemia results from activating mutations in the calcium-sensing receptor that increase its sensitivity to calcium.

c. Parathyroid and radical neck surgery can result in a loss of glandular tissue. Surgical removal of parathyroid tissue in secondary or tertiary hyperparathyroidism is often complicated by severe hypocalcemia due to remineralization of bone, the so-called hungry bone syndrome.

d. Hypocalcemia also occurs after **thyroid surgery** (5% of cases); in approximately 0.5% of these patients hypocalcemia is permanent. Risk factors for the development of permanent hypocalcemia include removal of three or more parathyroid glands; postoperative PTH concentration less than or equal to 12 pg per mL; total serum calcium concentration less than or equal to 8 mg per dL after 1 week of oral calcium supplementation; and serum phosphorus concentration less than or equal to 4 mg per dL after 1 week of calcium supplementation.

e. Transient hypoparathyroidism may occur after the **removal of a parathyroid adenoma**.

f. Infiltrative disorders such as hemochromatosis, Wilson's disease, and infection with human immunodeficiency virus (HIV) can also decrease PTH secretion.

g. Severe hypomagnesemia is the most common cause of hypoparathyroidism. Magnesium deficiency results in end-organ resistance to PTH and a decrease in PTH secretion. Patients with hypocalcemia as a result of hypomagnesemia do not respond to calcium or vitamin D replacement until the magnesium deficit is replaced.

2. A variety of rare genetic disorders cause **end-organ resistance to PTH**, including pseudohypoparathyroidism types I and II. Patients with pseudohypoparathyroidism are classified on the basis of the response of nephrogenous cyclic adenosine monophosphate to PTH administration. A decreased response is indicative of type I and a normal response indicative of type II.

3. Defects in vitamin D metabolism also cause hypocalcemia. Etiologies include decreased intake of vitamin D, malabsorption, drugs, liver disease, kidney disease, and vitamin D–dependent rickets. Nutritional vitamin D deficiency is uncommon in the United States as a result of the supplementation of milk and other food products. It can occur, however, in poorly nourished patients with little sun exposure. Groups that were shown to be at high risk include the institutionalized elderly, postmenopausal women, and adolescents. Because vitamin D is fat soluble, vitamin D deficiency can be seen in gastrointestinal malabsorption from any cause. Anticonvulsants induce hypocalcemia through a variety of mechanisms including induction of the P-450 system with increased metabolism of vitamin D, inhibition of bone resorption, impaired calcium absorption from the gastrointestinal tract, and peripheral resistance to PTH action. This generally occurs in patients with additional predisposing factors, such as poor nutrition and decreased sun exposure. Phenobarbital enhances hepatic metabolism of vitamin D and calcidiol. Vitamin D deficiency can result from hepatocellular disease if disease is severe enough to impair 25-hydroxylation of vitamin D to calcidiol. Chronic kidney disease impairs 1-α hydroxylation of calcidiol to calcitriol. Vitamin D–dependent rickets is a result of either impaired hydroxylation of calcidiol to calcitriol (type I) or end-organ resistance to calcitriol (type II). Type I patients respond to physiologic calcitriol doses. Patients with type II disease have dramatically increased calcitriol concentrations, respond poorly to calcitriol therapy, and have mutations in the vitamin D receptor.

4. Less common causes of hypocalcemia include tumor lysis syndrome, osteoblastic metastases, acute pancreatitis, toxic shock syndrome, and sepsis. The acute addition or release of phosphate into the extracellular space may cause hypocalcemia through a variety of mechanisms. Calcium and phosphate may precipitate in tissues, although the exact tissue in which the deposition occurs has never been identified. In addition, phosphate infusion increases the rate of bone formation and inhibits PTH-induced bone resorption; both of these processes act to decrease serum calcium concentration.

B. As is the case for hypercalcemia, **signs and symptoms** of hypocalcemia depend not only on the degree of hypocalcemia but also on the rate of decline of serum calcium concentration. The threshold at which symptoms develop also depends on serum pH and whether concomitant hypomagnesemia, hypokalemia, or hyponatremia is present. Symptoms of neuromuscular excitability predominate. The patient may complain of circumoral and distal extremity paresthesias or of carpopedal spasm. Central nervous system manifestations include mental status changes, irritability, and seizures. On physical examination, hypotension, bradycardia, laryngeal spasm, and bronchospasm may be present. Chvostek's and Trousseau's signs should be checked. Chvostek's sign is a facial twitch elicited by tapping on the facial nerve just below the zygomatic arch with the mouth slightly open. A positive sign is occasionally observed in normal patients. Trousseau's sign is the development of wrist flexion, metacarpophalangeal joint flexion, hyperextended fingers, and thumb flexion after a sphygmomanometer cuff is inflated around the arm to 20 mm Hg above systolic pressure for 3 minutes.

C. Diagnosis. The differential diagnosis of true hypocalcemia is often straightforward, and a diagnostic algorithm is shown in Figure 5-3. The most common causes are magnesium deficiency, kidney failure, and complications of parathyroid surgery.

1. The first step in the evaluation of the patient with a decreased total serum calcium concentration is to **examine the serum albumin concentration** and, if necessary, measure ionized serum calcium concentration. If true hypocalcemia is documented, then blood analysis should be obtained for BUN, creatinine, magnesium, and phosphorus concentration, and a 24-hour urine sample should be collected to examine phosphorus and creatinine excretion.

Gadolinium-containing chelates used as contrast agents for magnetic resonance imaging may falsely lower serum calcium concentration. The effect persists for only 3 to 6 hours in those with normal renal function but can result in the spurious lowering of serum calcium concentration by up to 3 mg per dL or more. However, in patients with severe renal dysfunction serum calcium concentration may remain low for up to 4 days. This is an important entity to be aware of because in many reported cases patients were treated with intravenous calcium for the spuriously low serum calcium concentration.

2. The second step is to **evaluate serum magnesium concentration**. Hypomagnesemia is the most common cause of hypocalcemia in hospitalized patients. A high index of suspicion should be present in patients with a history of steatorrhea, diarrhea, or chronic alcoholism. These patients generally have severe hypomagnesemia, and hypocalcemia will not correct until magnesium losses are replaced. It frequently requires several days for serum calcium concentration to correct after magnesium deficiency is reversed.

3. Serum and urinary phosphorus concentrations are evaluated next. Hyperphosphatemia in the absence of kidney failure suggests a diagnosis of either hypoparathyroidism or pseudohypoparathyroidism. Measuring PTH concentration can differentiate these disorders. In primary hypoparathyroidism, PTH is low; in pseudohypoparathyroidism, PTH is increased. A decrease in serum phosphorus concentration indicates a defect in vitamin D metabolism. Hypocalcemia results in secondary hyperparathyroidism that, in turn, reduces proximal tubular phosphate reabsorption and results in phosphate wasting. Therefore, the fractional excretion (FE) of phosphate is expected to be high (more than 5%). In hypophosphatemia, the kidney has an extraordinary ability to conserve phosphate, and, in extrarenal disorders, the FE of phosphate is below 1%. If phosphaturia is noted, then calcidiol and calcitriol concentration should be measured. Calcidiol concentration is reduced with malabsorption, liver disease, and phenobarbital. Calcitriol concentration is reduced in kidney failure and increased in type II vitamin D–dependent rickets.

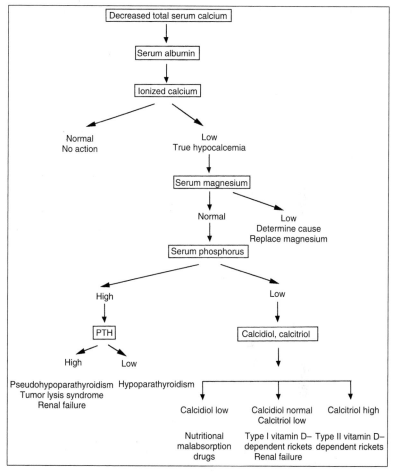

Figure 5-3. Evaluation of hypocalcemia. (PTH, parathyroid hormone.)

D. Management of hypocalcemia is dependent on both its severity and cause.
In an **emergency situation in which hypocalcemia is suspected and seizures, tetany, hypotension, or cardiac arrhythmias are present**, intravenous calcium should be administered (100 to 300 mg over 10 to 15 minutes) before results of the serum calcium concentration return from the clinical laboratory. Patients with symptomatic hypocalcemia or a total serum calcium concentration corrected for albumin of less than or equal to 7.5 mg per dL should be initially managed with parenteral calcium. Chronic, mild hypocalcemia, as seen in the outpatient setting, can be treated with oral calcium supplements, to which a vitamin D preparation may be added if necessary.

1. **Acute symptomatic hypocalcemia** is treated with intravenous calcium. In the absence of seizures, tetany, or cardiac arrhythmias, an infusion of 1.5 mg per kg of elemental calcium given over 4 to 6 hours raises the total serum calcium by 2 to 3 mg per dL. Calcium gluconate (10%) is supplied in 10-mL ampules and contains 94 mg of elemental calcium. The first ampule can be administered over several minutes, followed by a constant infusion begun at a rate of 0.5 to

TABLE 5-4	Oral Calcium Preparations	

Preparation	Formulation (mg)	Elemental calcium per tablet (mg)
Calcium carbonate	Tums 500	200
	Rolaids 550 mg	220	—
	Os-cal 1,250 mg	500	—
Calcium citrate	Citracal 950	200
Calcium lactate	650	85
Calcium gluconate	1,000	90

1.0 mg per kg per hour, with rate adjustments based on serial determinations of serum calcium concentration. Calcium gluceptate (10%) provides 90 mg of elemental calcium in a 5-mL ampule. Calcium chloride has higher bioavailability, and 272 mg of elemental calcium is contained in each 10-mL ampule. Treatment of hypocalcemia is ineffective in the presence of hypomagnesemia. In the setting of metabolic acidosis, hypocalcemia should be corrected before acidosis is reversed because excess protons in acidemia bind albumin in place of calcium resulting in an increase in ionized calcium concentration.

Patients with **hypoparathyroidism** are managed with calcium and vitamin D supplements. Serum calcium concentration should be maintained at the lower limit of normal. Oral elemental calcium, 1 to 3 g per day, is usually sufficient. A variety of oral calcium preparations are available, some of which are shown in Table 5-4. Calcium is best absorbed when taken between meals because an acid environment improves calcium absorption. Proton pump inhibitors are associated with decreased calcium absorption and osteoporosis. Calcium citrate is more soluble than calcium carbonate, especially in patients who require H_2 blockers or proton pump inhibitors. In the presence of severe hyperphosphatemia, calcium supplementation should be delayed, if possible, until the serum phosphorus concentration is reduced below 6 mg per dL using non calcium-containing phosphate binders. Severe hypocalcemia, however, may need to be treated despite hyperphosphatemia and clinical judgment must be used.

2. Calcitriol is the most potent of the **vitamin D preparations** and has the fastest onset and shortest duration of action, but is also the most expensive. A dose of 0.5 to 1.0 μg per day is usually required. As one moves back up the metabolic pathway to calcidiol, cholecalciferol, and ergocalciferol, cost decreases and duration of action increases. These agents, however, may be less efficacious in the presence of kidney or liver disease.

Patients with hypoparathyroidism have decreased distal tubular calcium reabsorption as a result of a lack of PTH. Therefore, the increase in filtered calcium load that results from calcium and vitamin D replacement can lead to hypercalciuria, nephrolithiasis, and nephrocalcinosis. If urinary calcium excretion exceeds 350 mg per day despite a serum calcium concentration in the low normal range, sodium intake should be restricted; if this is not effective, a thiazide diuretic should be added. The primary goal of treatment should be elimination of symptoms and not necessarily normalization of serum calcium concentration.

DISORDERS OF SERUM PHOSPHORUS

I. **OVERVIEW.** Approximately two-thirds of total plasma phosphorus is organic phosphorus (phospholipids) and one-third is inorganic. Clinical chemistry laboratories assay only the inorganic fraction. The reference range is 2.8 to 4.5 mg per dL (0.89 to 1.44 mmol per L) in adults. SI units (mmol per L) can be converted to conventional units (mg per dL) by multiplying by 3.1. Approximately 75% of inorganic phosphorus is free and circulates as either $HPO_4(-2)$ or $H_2PO_4(-1)$. The ratio of these two ions depends on ECF pH. At pH 7.4 80% is $HPO_4(-2)$ and 20% $H_2PO_4(-1)$. Of the remainder, 15% is protein bound, and 10% is complexed with either calcium or magnesium.

As is the case for calcium, most of the total body phosphorus is contained within the skeleton (50%). Approximately 14% is within skeletal muscle and viscera. Only a small fraction of the phosphorus pool is inorganic and available for synthesis of adenosine triphosphate (ATP). The average Western diet contains 800 to 1,400 mg of phosphorus per day, of which approximately 65% is absorbed in small intestine. Most of it is absorbed passively, but an active calcitriol-regulated component exists. PTH and calcitriol, through their effects in bone, intestine, and kidney, regulate phosphorus concentration. The major regulator of serum phosphorus concentration is renal phosphate excretion. In kidney, phosphate is reabsorbed primarily in proximal tubule (80%), where it is cotransported with sodium across the luminal membrane. The sodium-phosphate cotransporter is upregulated in response to phosphate depletion, and, under these circumstances, the kidney is capable of reducing the FE of phosphate to very low levels.

II. PHOSPHATE REGULATION. PTH acts directly in bone to increase phosphate entry into the ECF and indirectly in intestine by stimulating calcitriol production. Most dietary phosphate is reabsorbed in the small intestine, but a component of unregulated secretion is present in colon (100 to 200 mg per day). PTH reduces proximal tubular phosphate reabsorption in kidney. The net effect is to increase plasma calcium concentration while keeping serum phosphorus concentration constant. The major roles of calcitriol are to enhance calcium and phosphate availability for new bone formation and to defend the ECF from hypocalcemia and hypophosphatemia. PTH and hypophosphatemia stimulate calcitriol production in proximal tubule; although, the kidney is the primary regulator of serum phosphorus concentration. Hypophosphatemia causes insertion of sodium-phosphate cotransporters into the luminal membrane of the proximal tubule whereas PTH results in their removal. The ability of PTH to remove sodium-phosphate cotransporters from apical membrane is blunted in chronic phosphate depletion.

III. HYPERPHOSPHATEMIA

A. Etiology. Hyperphosphatemia can result from renal failure, an acute phosphate load from either exogenous or endogenous sources, or increased proximal tubular phosphate reabsorption. Etiologies are shown in Table 5-5.

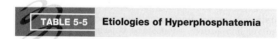

TABLE 5-5	Etiologies of Hyperphosphatemia

Decreased renal excretion
Acute renal failure
Chronic renal failure
Acute phosphate load
Tumor lysis syndrome
Rhabdomyolysis
Bowel infarction
Severe hemolysis
Vitamin D intoxication
Increased renal phosphate reabsorption
Hypoparathyroidism
Acromegaly
Thyrotoxicosis
Drugs — bisphosphonates
Tumoral calcinosis
Pseudohyperphosphatemia

1. **Renal failure** is the underlying cause in 90% or more of cases. As GFR begins to decline, the FE of phosphate increases. Once GFR falls below 30 mL per minute, however, phosphorus reabsorption is maximally suppressed, and the FE cannot increase further. As a result, renal excretion can no longer keep pace with dietary intake, and serum phosphorus concentration rises. A new steady state is eventually established, albeit at a higher serum phosphorus concentration.

2. **A sudden, massive phosphate load** may result in an increase in serum phosphorus concentration. Phosphate may be released from either the intracellular space, as is the case in tumor lysis syndrome or rhabdomyolysis, or it can be ingested and absorbed, as in vitamin D intoxication. Tumor lysis syndrome most commonly is seen with treatment of rapidly growing malignancies such as leukemias and lymphomas. It can occur after treatment of solid tumors such as small cell lung carcinoma, breast cancer, and neuroblastoma. Risk factors for tumor lysis syndrome in patients with solid tumors include pretreatment renal impairment, an increased lactate dehydrogenase level, and hyperuricemia. Increased lactate dehydrogenase levels and hyperuricemia are indicators of a large tumor burden.

3. **Primary increases in tubular phosphate reabsorption** are less common. They can occur in hypoparathyroidism; in acromegaly, as a result of direct stimulation of insulin-like growth factor (IGF) on phosphate transport; with bisphosphonates, through a direct effect on renal phosphate reabsorption; and in tumoral calcinosis. Tumoral calcinosis is an autosomal recessive disorder associated with hyperphosphatemia and soft tissue calcium deposition caused by mutations in three genes. The first is an inactivating mutation in GALNT3 that encodes a glycosyltransferase involved in O-linked glycosylation. It is thought that GALNT3 regulates fibroblast growth factor 23 (FGF23) glycosylation and that glycosylation is required for normal FGF23 function. The second mutation was identified in the *FGF23* gene itself. This mutation involves a serine residue that is thought to be involved in FGF23 glycosylation by GALNT3. The third mutation was described in the *Klotho* gene. Klotho binds to several FGF23 receptors and acts as a cofactor that is required for FGF23 signaling.

B. Many of the **signs and symptoms** of an acute rise in serum phosphorus concentration are secondary to concomitant hypocalcemia due to calcium deposition in soft tissues and a resultant fall in ECF-ionized calcium concentration. Hyperphosphatemia can also cause hypocalcemia by decreasing 1-α hydroxylase activity and calcitriol formation.

C. **Diagnosis.** Clinically unexplained, persistent hyperphosphatemia should raise the suspicion of pseudohyperphosphatemia, the most common cause of which is paraproteinemia. No consistent relationship of immunoglobulin type or subclass has been identified. This is a method-dependent artifact, and paraprotein interference may be a general problem in spectrophotometric assays. If paraproteinemia is absent, the cause is generally acute or chronic renal failure.

D. **Treatment** of hyperphosphatemia is aimed at reducing intestinal phosphate absorption. This is accomplished through the use of oral phosphate-binding drugs such as calcium carbonate, calcium acetate, sevelamer hydrochloride, lanthanum carbonate and aluminum hydroxide. These agents should be administered with meals. Aluminum hydroxide may be used in the short term, but chronic use in patients with kidney disease should be avoided because of the potential for aluminum toxicity. In patients with coexistent hypocalcemia, it is preferable to lower serum phosphorus below 6 mg per dL, if possible, before treating hypocalcemia to avoid the potential complication of metastatic calcification from calcium phosphate coprecipitation.

IV. HYPOPHOSPHATEMIA

A. **Etiology.** Hypophosphatemia may result from redistribution of phosphorus from the extracellular to the intracellular space, a decrease in intestinal phosphate absorption, a decrease in renal phosphate reabsorption, or extrarenal losses from the gastrointestinal tract or through dialysis. The differential diagnosis is presented in Table 5-6.

TABLE 5-6	Etiologies of Hypophosphatemia

Decreased dietary intake
  Alcoholism
  Phosphate-binding agents
Shift of phosphate into the intracellular fluid
  Respiratory alkalosis
  Refeeding
  Diabetic ketoacidosis
  Hungry bone syndrome
Increased renal excretion
  Hyperparathyroidism
  Vitamin D deficiency
  X-linked hypophosphatemic rickets
  Autosomal dominant hypophosphatemic rickets
  Fanconi's syndrome
  Drugs — acetazolamide
  Osmotic diuresis
  Oncogenic osteomalacia
  Post renal transplantation
Extrarenal losses
  Intestinal losses
  Dialysis
  Thermal injury

1. Respiratory alkalosis and the refeeding syndrome are the most common causes of a **phosphate shift from the ECF to the intracellular fluid (ICF)** in hospitalized patients. Respiratory alkalosis causes a rise in intracellular pH that stimulates phosphofructokinase, the rate-limiting step in glycolysis. This results in severe hypophosphatemia with serum phosphorus concentrations of less than 0.5 to 1.0 mg per dL. Intracellular shifts are also seen with the treatment of diabetic ketoacidosis and in "hungry bone syndrome," which occurs after parathyroidectomy for secondary hyperparathyroidism. In "hungry bone syndrome," serum calcium and phosphorus concentration fall dramatically in the postoperative period, although clinically, hypocalcemia is more of a management issue than hypophosphatemia.

2. **Decreased dietary intake** is an unusual cause of hypophosphatemia because oral intake almost always exceeds gastrointestinal losses, and the kidney is capable of reclaiming nearly all the filtered load of phosphate. In general, decreased intake must be combined with increased gastrointestinal losses (e.g., diarrhea) or the use of phosphate binders for hypophosphatemia to result.

3. **Increased urinary phosphate excretion** occurs in primary hyperparathyroidism, secondary hyperparathyroidism due to defects in vitamin D metabolism, Fanconi's syndrome, osmotic diuresis, acetazolamide use, oncogenic osteomalacia and other disorders of FGF23 homeostasis, imatinib use, after renal transplantation and with mutations in the sodium-phosphate cotransporter expressed in the proximal tubule. Oncogenic osteomalacia is a rare disorder associated with mesenchymal tumors. It is characterized by hypophosphatemia, phosphaturia, decreased calcitriol concentration, normal calcidiol concentration, and clinical and histologic evidence of osteomalacia. A considerable delay may occur between the presentation of the syndrome and discovery of the tumor. The tumor produces FGF23 that decreases the proximal tubular phosphate reabsorption and calcitriol production. Tumor removal results in resolution of phosphate wasting, osteomalacia, and normalization of FGF23 levels.

   FGF23 is produced by osteocytes, osteoclasts, and osteoblasts and is present in the circulation of healthy individuals, consistent with a physiologic role in regulating serum phosphorus. Animal studies have shown that FGF23 is phosphaturic. Dietary phosphorus changes within the physiologic range regulate serum concentrations of FGF23. When administered *in vivo*, it induces hypophosphatemia, suppresses $1,25(OH)_2$ vitamin D_3 concentration by inhibiting $1-\alpha$ hydroxylase activity, decreases type II sodium-phosphate cotransporters in proximal tubules, decreases PTH expression, and leads to osteomalacia. $1,25(OH)_2$ vitamin D_3 stimulates FGF23 production suggesting that it may play a counter-regulatory role in the maintenance of serum phosphorus concentration. $1,25(OH)_2$ vitamin D_3 induces phosphate mobilization from bone and an increase in serum phosphorus concentration. Two inherited renal phosphate wasting disorders, autosomal dominant hypophosphatemic rickets (ADHR) and X-linked hypophosphatemia (XLH), are the result of defects in FGF23 metabolism. Missense mutations in FGF23 cause ADHR.

ADHR is characterized by hypophosphatemia, renal phosphate wasting, short stature, and bony deformities. In ADHR, mutations at a proteolytic cleavage site prevent its cleavage and inactivation. *In vivo* studies showed that biologic activity is limited to full-length FGF23 (251 amino acids). The enzyme responsible for the cleavage of FGF23 has not been identified. One report suggested that PHEX, a cell surface metalloprotease, may cleave FGF23, but this has not been confirmed.

XLH is characterized by renal phosphate wasting, hypophosphatemia, growth retardation, defective cartilage and bone calcification, and resistance to phosphate and vitamin D repletion. Inactivating mutations of PHEX cause XLH. PHEX is a member of a family of zinc-dependent cell surface proteases that cleave small peptides such as endothelin. It is expressed predominantly in cartilage, bone, and teeth. Its physiologically relevant substrate is yet to be identified. Although it has been postulated that PHEX cleaves and inactivates FGF23, the large size of FGF23—251 amino acids—makes this less likely. Other intermediate small molecular weight substrates likely link PHEX function to FGF23.

Fibrous dysplasia of bone is the result of an activating mutation of GNAS1 that encodes the α subunit of the stimulatory G protein (G_s). FGF23 is expressed in the abnormal bone tissue and these patients may have renal phosphate wasting and hypophosphatemia. When fibrous dysplasia of bone is associated with precocious puberty and *café au lait* spots this triad is known as the *McCune-Albright syndrome*.

Hereditary hypophosphatemic rickets with hypercalciuria (HHRH) is inherited as an autosomal recessive disorder manifested by increased renal phosphate excretion, hypophosphatemia, and rickets. It is associated with increased $1,25(OH)_2$ vitamin D_3 concentration and hypercalciuria. Mutations were identified in SLC34A3, a proximal tubular sodium-phosphate cotransporter.

Post-transplant hypophosphatemia occurs in renal transplant recipients and is related to the use of immunosuppressant drugs, tertiary hyperparathyroidism, and an increased FGF23 levels. The effect of tertiary hyperparathyroidism usually resolves after the first year of transplantation, but may persist in some cases. Increasing the sensitivity of the calcium-sensing receptor with cinacalcet results in decreased calcium levels, increased phosphorus concentration, and decreased PTH levels in renal transplant recipients.

4. **Extrarenal losses** may occur through the intestines or through dialysis. Phosphorus is absorbed in the small bowel so high output ileostomies or cutaneous small bowel fistulas tend to result in hypophosphatemia more frequently than colostomies or diarrhea. Treatment with oral phosphate is difficult because it can exacerbate the diarrhea requiring admission for intravenous phosphate replacement.

Typically phosphorus is elevated in dialysis patients because dialysate removal is limited and oral phosphorus intake is often high. When oral intake is poor, phosphorus removal through dialysis can result in hypophosphatemia. This is particularly true with continuous dialysis modalities where removal is enhanced and most patients are not eating a regular diet.

Patients with significant thermal injuries will typically develop decreases in serum phosphorus concentrations several days after a burn related to phosphorus losses in the exudate.

B. Signs and symptoms. Hypophosphatemia results in a variety of clinical sequelae. The correction of moderate hypophosphatemia (serum phosphorus level 1.0 to 2.5 mg per dL) improves diaphragmatic function in patients with acute respiratory failure. In patients with severe hypophosphatemia (serum phosphorus level less than 1.0 mg per dL), failure to wean from mechanical ventilation until repletion of phosphate was demonstrated. *In vitro* hypophosphatemia causes a leftward shift in the oxygen dissociation curve. Neuromuscular symptoms include paresthesias, tremor, muscle weakness, and altered mental status; severe hypophosphatemia increases red cell fragility, which can lead to hemolysis and decreases chemotaxis, phagocytosis, and bacterial killing by white cells, with an increased susceptibility to infection as the possible result.

C. Diagnosis. FE of phosphate or 24-hour urinary phosphate excretion can be used to distinguish among the pathophysiologic mechanisms of hypophosphatemia. If the kidney is responding appropriately to decreased intestinal absorption or phosphate redistribution into cells, FE of phosphate is below 5%, and 24-hour urine phosphate excretion is less than 100 mg per day. When the kidney is the cause of hypophosphatemia, the FE of phosphate is greater than 5% and the 24-hour urine contains more than 100 mg per day of phosphate. In this case, a urinalysis for glycosuria, PTH concentration to rule out hyperparathyroidism, and the measurement of calcidiol and calcitriol concentrations are indicated.

D. Treatment is indicated for severe hypophosphatemia (less than or equal to 1 mg per dL) or symptoms. It is complicated by the fact that phosphate is largely an intracellular ion, and that serum phosphorus concentration is not a reliable indicator of total body phosphate stores. Hypophosphatemia is often associated with potassium and magnesium depletion. Phosphate repletion should be undertaken with extreme caution in the rare patient with renal insufficiency; the safest mode of therapy is oral, and hypophosphatemia usually can be corrected with 1,000 mg per day of phosphate. Alternative forms of oral phosphate replacement are listed in Table 5-7. Diarrhea is the most common complication.

Intravenous replacement carries the risk of hypocalcemia and hyperphosphatemia and is only warranted in patients with severe symptomatic hypophosphatemia. Sodium phosphate should be used unless the serum potassium is less than 4 mEq per L. Serum concentrations of phosphorus, calcium, magnesium, potassium, and urine output should be carefully monitored during intravenous replacement. Once serum phosphorus concentration has increased to more than 1 mg per dL, the patient should be switched to an oral preparation. The administration of doses larger than 0.32 mmol per kg over a 12-hour period is rarely warranted.

TABLE 5-7   Oral Phosphate Preparations

Preparation	Dosage	Contents
K-phos-neutral	2 tablets, b.i.d. or t.i.d.	250 mg phosphate, 12 mEq sodium, 2 mEq potassium per tablet
Fleets Phospho-Soda	5 mL b.i.d.	149 mg phosphate, 6 mEq sodium per mL
Neutra-Phos-K	1–2 capsules, b.i.d. or t.i.d.	250 mg phosphate, 14 mEq potassium per capsule
K-phos	2 tablets, t.i.d. or q.i.d.	114 mg phosphate, 3.68 mEq potassium per tablet

Suggested Readings

Amanzadeh J, Reilly RF. Hypophosphatemia: an evidence-based approach to its clinical consequences and management. *Nat Clin Pract Nephrol* 2006;2:136–148.

Beall DP, Henslee HB, Webb HR, et al. Milk-alkali syndrome: a historical review and description of the modern version of the syndrome. *Am J Med Sci* 2006;331:233–242.

Carmeliet G, Van Cromphaut S, Daci E, et al. Disorders of calcium homeostasis. *Best Pract Res Clin Endocrinol Metab* 2003;17:529–546.

Fiaschi-Taesch NM, Stewart AF. Minireview: parathyroid hormone-related protein as an intracrine factor—trafficking mechanisms and functional consequences. *Endocrinology* 2003;144:407–411.

Lumachi F, Brunello A, Roma A, et al. Medical treatment of malignancy-associated hypercalcemia. *Curr Med Chem* 2008;15:415–421.

Negri AL. Hereditary hypophosphatemias: new genes in the bone-kidney axis. *Nephrology* 2007;12:317–320.

Penfield JG, Reilly RF. What nephrologists need to know about gadolinium. *Nat Clin Pract Nephrol* 2007;3:654–668.

Quarles LD. FGF23, PHEX, and MEPE regulation of phosphate homeostasis and skeletal mineralization. *Am J Physiol Endocrinol Metab* 2003;285:E1–E9.

Razzaque MS, Lanske B. The emerging role of the fibroblast growth factor-23-klotho axis in renal regulation of phosphate homeostasis. *J Endocrinol* 2007;194:1–10.

Renkema KY, Alexander RT, Bindels RJ, et al. Calcium and phosphate homeostasis: concerted interplay of new regulators. *Ann Med* 2008;40:82–91.

Rodgers SE, Lew JI, Solorzano CC. Primary hyperparathyroidism. *Curr Opin Oncol* 2008;20:52–58.

Stalberg P, Delbridge L, van Heerden J, et al. Minimally invasive parathyroidectomy and thyroidectomy – current concepts. *Surgeon* 2007;5:301–308.

Tenenhouse HS, Murer H. Disorders of renal tubular phosphate transport. *J Am Soc Nephrol* 2003;14:240–248.

THE PATIENT WITH KIDNEY STONES

Amir S. A. Naderi and Robert F. Reilly

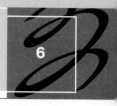

*N*ephrolithiasis is a common disorder in the United States, with an annual incidence of 7 to 21 per 10,000 patients. Kidney stones account for approximately 1 in every 100 hospital admissions, with men affected three to four times more frequently than women. It is estimated that, by the age of 70, as many as 20% of all white men and 7% of all white women will form a kidney stone. African Americans and Asians are affected less often. The peak incidence occurs between the ages of 20 and 30 years. In the United States, calcium-containing stones make up approximately 90% of all stones; they contain primarily calcium oxalate, either alone or in combination with calcium phosphate. The remaining 10% are composed of uric acid, struvite-carbonate, and cystine.

Kidney stones are a major cause of morbidity due to associated renal colic, urinary tract obstruction, urinary tract infection (UTI), and renal parenchymal damage. It was recently recognized that nephrolithiasis may be associated with end-stage renal disease (ESRD) and/or a declining glomerular filtration rate (GFR). According to United States Renal Data System reports between 1993 and 1997, stone disease was attributed as the cause of ESRD in 1.2% of patients. In Necker Hospital in France between 1989 and 2000 nephrolithiasis was felt to be the primary cause of ESRD in 3.2% of patients. Struvite stones accounted for 42.2% of these cases. In a case–control study of nephrolithiasis, there was a higher incidence of chronic kidney disease (CKD) noted in patients with kidney stones. This was only observed in those patients who did not report a history of hypertension. Finally, although the effect was small, an analysis of National Health and Nutrition Examination Survey III (NHANES III) data revealed an association between history of kidney stones and estimated GFR that was dependent on body mass index (BMI). Stone formers with a BMI greater than 27 kg per m^2 had a mean estimated GFR that was 3.4 mL per minute per 1.73 m^2 lower than similar nonstone formers.

A kidney stone can form only when urine is supersaturated with respect to a stone-forming salt. Interestingly, urine in many healthy subjects is often supersaturated with respect to calcium oxalate, calcium phosphate, or uric acid and crystalluria was described in as many as 15% to 20% of healthy subjects. However, urine of recurrent stone formers was noted to contain crystals in first morning voided specimens much more frequently than that of stone formers without subsequent recurrence suggesting that recurrence may depend on the degree and severity of crystalluria.

Several recent studies provided insight into the crystallization process. Calcium oxalate can crystallize as either calcium oxalate monohydrate (COM) or calcium oxalate dihydrate (COD). COM is the predominant species found in calcium oxalate stones and is the more thermodynamically stable of the two species. Macromolecular inhibitors block COM growth and favor COD formation. Using atomic force microscopy configured with nanoscale tips, which were modified by biologically relevant functional groups, it was shown that COD crystals do not adhere as well to organic compounds and to the surface of renal epithelia *in vitro*. This suggests that COD crystals in urine might protect against kidney stone formation given their reduced capacity to form stable aggregates and adhere to epithelial cells.

Urine is also often supersaturated with respect to brushite ($CaHPO_4 \cdot 2H_2O$), a calcium phosphate salt, especially after meals. Brushite can act as a nidus upon which calcium oxalate crystals can form. *In vitro* studies show that COM crystals once formed grow at the expense of brushite.

At least two other factors play a role in the pathogenesis of stone formation; heterogeneous nucleation and the presence of crystallization inhibitors in urine. The crystallization of a salt requires much less energy when a surface is present upon which it can precipitate (heterogeneous nucleation), as opposed to crystallization that occurs in the absence of such a surface (homogeneous nucleation). In addition, normal urine contains a variety of inorganic and organic substances that act as crystallization inhibitors. The most clinically important of these are citrate, magnesium, and pyrophosphate.

Sufficient energy must be generated for a crystal to form in solution. Once a crystal forms, it must either grow to sufficient size to occlude the tubular lumen or anchor itself to the urinary epithelium, which in turn provides a surface upon which it can grow. The typical transit time of a crystal through the nephron is on the order of 3 minutes, and this is too short a period for it to nucleate, grow, and occlude the tubular lumen.

A recent study of 19 stone formers shed additional light on how stones form in the kidney. In 15 patients with idiopathic hypercalciuria, the initial site of crystal formation, surprisingly, is in the basement membrane of the thin limb of the loop of Henle. The stone core is made up of calcium phosphate surrounded by calcium oxalate. The crystal deposit then migrates toward the renal pelvis where it acts as a base upon which a plaque forms, which is then bathed in urine supersaturated with stone-forming constituents. Why calcium phosphate precipitates at the basolateral surface of the thin limb of the loop of Henle remains a mystery. Four of 19 patients formed stones after intestinal bypass for obesity. In these patients, the mechanism for stone formation was different. Calcium phosphate crystals initially adhered to the inner medullary collecting duct. The calcium phosphate core then acts as a nidus for calcium oxalate precipitation that results in luminal occlusion and growth along the inner medullary collecting duct into the renal pelvis.

I. INITIAL PRESENTATION. A kidney stone most commonly presents with severe flank pain, sudden in onset, and is often associated with nausea and vomiting. The radiation of the pain may provide some clue as to where in the urinary tract the stone is lodged. Stones in the ureteropelvic junction cause flank pain that may radiate to the groin, whereas those lodged in the narrowest portion of the ureter, where it enters the bladder, are associated with signs of bladder irritation (dysuria, frequency, and urgency). Struvite-carbonate stones are, on occasion, incidentally discovered on abdominal radiograph. A careful abdominal examination and, in women, a pelvic examination are important to rule out other potential causes of abdominal pain.

A. Laboratory evaluation should include a complete blood cell count, serum chemistries, and urinalysis. The white blood cell count may be mildly elevated but is generally less than 15,000 per mm^3. A white blood cell count greater than 15,000 per mm^3 is suggestive of another intra-abdominal cause or an associated infection behind an obstructing calculus. An elevation of the serum blood urea nitrogen (BUN) and creatinine concentrations indicates prerenal azotemia, parenchymal renal disease, or obstruction of a solitary functioning kidney. A urinalysis should be performed routinely in any patient with abdominal pain. Microscopic hematuria is observed in approximately 90% of patients with nephrolithiasis.

B. Once the diagnosis is suspected based on the history, physical examination, and preliminary laboratory studies, **establishing a definitive diagnosis** is the focus of the next stage of the evaluation.

1. A **flat radiographic plate of the abdomen** is often obtained and is capable of identifying radiopaque stones (calcium oxalate, calcium phosphate, struvite-carbonate, and cystine) that are greater than or equal to 2 mm in size. It will miss radiolucent stones, the most common of which are composed of uric acid, and stones that overlie the bony pelvis. For these reasons, an abdominal flat plate is most valuable in ruling out other intra-abdominal processes.

2. An **ultrasonographic examination of the genitourinary tract** often identifies stones in the renal pelvis; however, most of the stones are lodged in the ureter, and the ultrasonographic examination often misses these.

3. The **intravenous pyelogram** (IVP) was formerly considered the gold standard for the diagnosis of nephrolithiasis and is still of considerable value in the acute setting. Although the stone itself may not be visualized on IVP, the site of obstruction is regularly identified. Structural or anatomic abnormalities that

may be present in the urinary tract and renal or ureteral complications can be recognized. Disadvantages of the IVP include the need for intravenous contrast and the prolonged waiting time often required to visualize the collecting system on the side of the obstruction.

4. **Spiral computed tomography** (CT), when available, is the test of choice in the patient with suspected nephrolithiasis. The advantages of spiral CT include higher sensitivity, faster scan times, and the lack of need for contrast.

C. **Management.** After the diagnosis is established, subsequent management is determined by: (a) the presence or absence of associated pyelonephritis, (b) whether parenteral narcotics are required for pain control, and (c) the likelihood of spontaneous stone passage. Obstructing calculi can be managed with observation alone if pain can be controlled with oral analgesics and spontaneous passage is likely. Extracorporeal shock wave lithotripsy may need to be employed for stones lodged in the upper ureter. Calculi in the lower ureter can be removed by cystoscopy and ureteroscopy. Hospital admission is necessary if there is evidence of renal parenchymal infection; when nausea, vomiting, or severe pain precludes oral analgesic use; or the stone is unlikely to pass spontaneously. The likelihood of spontaneous passage is determined by stone size and location in the ureter (Table 6-1). Small stones in the distal ureter will likely pass, whereas large stones in the upper ureter will likely require urologic consultation and intervention.

II. TYPES OF STONES

A. **Calcium-containing stones** make up 90% of all stones and are generally composed of a mixture of calcium oxalate and calcium phosphate. In mixed stones, calcium oxalate usually predominates, and pure calcium oxalate stones are more common than pure calcium phosphate stones. Calcium phosphate tends to precipitate in alkaline urine, as occurs with renal tubular acidosis (RTA), whereas the precipitation of calcium oxalate does not vary greatly with pH. Because urine is acidic in most patients, calcium oxalate stones are more common. The major risk factors for the formation of calcium-containing stones include hypercalciuria, hypocitraturia, hyperuricosuria, hyperoxaluria, low urine volume, and medullary sponge kidney. These risk factors can occur either alone or in combination. Their relative frequency is shown in Table 6-2.

1. **Hypercalciuria** is defined as urinary calcium excretion greater than 250 mg per 24 hours in women and greater than 300 mg per 24 hours in men. Hypercalciuria is present in approximately two-thirds of patients with calcium-containing stones and may result from an increased filtered load, decreased proximal reabsorption, or decreased distal reabsorption. Proximal calcium reabsorption parallels sodium. Any situation that decreases proximal sodium reabsorption such as extracellular fluid (ECF) volume expansion also decreases proximal calcium reabsorption. Distal tubular calcium reabsorption is stimulated by parathyroid hormone (PTH), thiazides, and amiloride, and inhibited by acidosis and phosphate depletion.

TABLE 6-1	Likelihood of Spontaneous Passage

	Likelihood of spontaneous passage (%)
Size	
>6 mm	25
4–6 mm	60
<4 mm	90
Location	
Upper ureter, >6 mm	1
Upper ureter, <4 mm	81
Lower ureter, <4 mm	93

TABLE 6-2	Risk Factors for Calcium-Containing Kidney Stones	
Risk factor	**Alone (%)**	**Combined (%)**
Hypercalciuria	60	80
Low urine volume	10	50
Hypocitraturia	10	50
Hyperuricosuria	10	40
Hyperoxaluria	2	15

Hypercalciuria may be idiopathic or secondary to primary hyperparathyroidism, RTA, sarcoidosis, immobilization, Paget's disease, hyperthyroidism, milk-alkali syndrome, and vitamin D intoxication. The idiopathic group makes up 90% of all hypercalciuria. This category of patients is characterized by increased $1,25(OH)_2$ vitamin D_3 concentration, suppressed PTH, and reduced bone mineral density. Three potential pathophysiologic mechanisms are postulated: increased intestinal calcium absorption, decreased renal calcium or phosphorus reabsorption, and enhanced bone demineralization. On the basis of a fast-and-calcium-load study, some authors advocate subdividing idiopathic hypercalciuria into absorptive hypercalciuria type I (due to primary intestinal calcium hyperabsorption with low-normal PTH), type II (dietary calcium-dependent hypercalciuria), type III (intestinal calcium hyperabsorption induced by elevated calcitriol levels secondary to renal phosphate leak), and renal leak hypercalciuria. The rationale for this approach is that the physiologic mechanism identified will help guide specific therapy.

Patients with absorptive hypercalciuria have exaggerated intestinal calcium reabsorption, which can be reduced by dietary calcium restriction. Some authors have expressed concern over the potential long-term effects of dietary calcium restriction. Patients with idiopathic hypercalciuria often have reduced bone mass and are in negative calcium balance, which may be further exacerbated by a low-calcium diet. In addition, a reciprocal relationship exists between free calcium and free oxalate in the intestinal lumen. Calcium acts to bind oxalate in the intestine and reduce absorption. If oral calcium intake is reduced, oxalate remains free in the intestinal lumen and its absorption increases. However, this may be reduced by concomitant oxalate restriction. Finally, as shown in Table 6-3, most randomized controlled trials demonstrating that a given pharmacologic intervention reduces the risk of calcium-containing stones did not subdivide patients based on results of a calcium load study. Whether patients with recurrent calcium oxalate stone formation should ingest a diet that is either liberal or restricted in calcium remains controversial and will be further discussed in the section on therapy.

In primary hyperparathyroidism, filtered calcium load is increased as a result of bone calcium release and increased intestinal calcium absorption mediated by $1,25(OH)_2$ vitamin D_3. An increase in filtered calcium load overcomes distal PTH action to increase tubular calcium reabsorption. In RTA, the decreased systemic pH results in increased calcium release from bone. In addition, acidosis directly inhibits distal nephron calcium reabsorption.

Macrophages in sarcoidosis produce $1,25(OH)_2$ vitamin D_3, which leads to the increased intestinal calcium absorption. Immobilization, Paget's disease, and hyperthyroidism cause hypercalciuria by releasing calcium from bone and increasing filtered calcium load.

2. **Hypocitraturia.** It is defined as less than 350 mg citrate excretion per day in men and less than 500 mg per day in women. Citrate combines with calcium in the tubular lumen to form a nondissociable but soluble complex. As a result,

TABLE 6-3 Randomized Trials in Calcium-Containing Nephrolithiasis

Author	Treatment	Dose	Condition	No. of patients; length of follow-up	Risk reduction (%)
Borghi	Water	—	First stone	199; 5 yr	55
Laerum	Hydrochlorothiazide	25 mg b.i.d.	Noncategorized, recurrent	50; 3 yr	54
Ettinger	Chlorthalidone	25–50 mg	Noncategorized, recurrent	54; 3 yr	48
Borghi	Indapamide	2.5 mg	Hypercalciuria, recurrent	75; 3 yr	95
Ettinger	Allopurinol	100 mg t.i.d.	Hyperuricosuria, recurrent	60; 3 yr	45
Barcelo	Potassium citrate	30–60 mEq	Hypocitraturia, recurrent	57; 3 yr	65
Ettinger	Potassium-magnesium-citrate	42/21/63 mEq	Noncategorized, recurrent	64; 3 yr	81
Ettinger	Potassium phosphate	1.4 g	Noncategorized, recurrent	71; 3 yr	None
Ettinger	Magnesium hydroxide	650–1,300 mg	Noncategorized, recurrent	52; 3 yr	None

b.i.d., twice daily; t.i.d., three times daily.

less free calcium is available to combine with oxalate. Citrate also prevents nucleation and aggregation of calcium oxalate. Chronic metabolic acidosis from any cause enhances proximal tubular citrate reabsorption and decreases urinary citrate concentration; this is the mechanism whereby chronic diarrhea, RTA, and increased dietary protein load result in hypocitraturia. Another important cause of hypocitraturia is hypokalemia, which increases expression of the sodium-citrate cotransporter present in the proximal tubular luminal membrane.

3. **Hyperuricosuria.** It is defined as uric acid excretion greater than 800 mg per day in men and greater than 750 mg per day in women. Uric acid and monosodium urate can act through several mechanisms to decrease calcium oxalate solubility in urine. They can act as a nidus upon which calcium salts can precipitate. Uric acid also binds naturally occurring macromolecular inhibitors and attenuates their activity. Finally, addition of increasing concentrations of sodium urate to normal human urine can induce calcium oxalate precipitation through a poorly understood physiologic phenomenon known as *salting out.*

4. **Hyperoxaluria.** It is defined as urinary oxalate excretion greater than 55 mg per day in men and greater than 45 mg per day in women. The etiologies of hyperoxaluria include enteric hyperoxaluria from inflammatory bowel disease, small bowel resection, jejunoileal bypass, Roux-en-Y gastric bypass, dietary excess (e.g., spinach, Swiss chard, rhubarb), and the rare genetic disorder primary hyperoxaluria. Urinary oxalate is derived from two major sources; 80% to 90% comes from endogenous production in liver and the remainder is obtained from dietary oxalate or ascorbic acid. In enteric hyperoxaluria, intestinal oxalate hyperabsorption occurs through two mechanisms. First, free fatty acids complex calcium and limit the amount of free calcium available to complex oxalate, thereby increasing the oxalate pool available for absorption. Second, bile salts and fatty acids increase colonic oxalate permeability. Additional risk factors for stone formation in these patients include intestinal fluid losses that decrease urine volume, and intestinal bicarbonate and potassium losses that result in hypocitraturia.

Recent studies suggest a correlation between decreased activity of the oxalate degrading bacteria *Oxalobacter formigenes* and the development of recurrent calcium oxalate–containing kidney stones. *O. formigenes* utilizes oxalate as its sole energy source and has the capacity to degrade 0.5 to 1.0 g of oxalate per day. In this process it converts oxalate to CO_2 and formate. It is unclear why intestinal colonization with *Oxalobacter* decreases with increasing age and in patients who form calcium oxalate stones. One possibility is that antibiotic therapy, especially recurrent courses of fluoroquinolones, act to eradicate the organism. Enteric colonization is much lower in nonstone formers exposed to a recent course of antibiotics when compared to unexposed subjects, 60% versus 17.1%, respectively, and 31% versus 10% in calcium oxalate stone formers. This may explain in part the increased frequency of calcium oxalate stone formation in disease states such as inflammatory bowel disease and cystic fibrosis, although patients with these disorders clearly have multiple other risk factors for stone formation.

Studies in colons of colonized rats showed that colonization with *Oxalobacter* results in net oxalate secretion across the colonic mucosa and a decrease in urinary oxalate excretion. Control rats showed net oxalate reabsorption. It was postulated that in addition to degrading luminal oxalate that *Oxalobacter* may also stimulate colonic oxalate secretion. Unidirectional flux data, however, seem to indicate that net oxalate secretion occurs as a result of decreased mucosal to serosal flux (reabsorption) rather than serosal to mucosal flux (secretion).

These exciting recent findings raise the potential for new future therapies in hyperoxaluric calcium oxalate stone formers. Patients could be tested for the absence of fecal *Oxalobacter* and those that lack the organism could undergo replacement with either the bacteria itself or the purified enzymes (formyl CoA transferase and oxalyl-coenzyme A decarboxylase) that metabolize oxalate.

Preliminary data published using Oxadrop (a 1:1:4:4 ratio of *Lactobacillus acidophilus, Lactobacillus brevis, Streptococcus thermophilus,* and

Bifidobacterium infantis) in patients with enteric hyperoxaluria showed that although urinary oxalate excretion was reduced, there were only small declines in urinary calcium oxalate supersaturation that were not statistically significant. Bacteria in Oxadrop do not contain the oxalate/formate exchanger found in *O. formigenes* and, therefore, may have lesser capacity to degrade oxalate. Further studies using bacterial preparations with increased oxalate derogatory capacity would be of interest.

5. **Low urinary volume.** This is perhaps the most intuitively obvious of risk factors for calcium-containing kidney stones. The lower the volume of solvent, the more likely that a given amount of salt will be supersaturating. This risk factor is particularly prominent in warm climates with low humidity.

6. **Medullary sponge kidney** should be suspected in women, or in men with no other risk factors for calcium-containing stones. Studies showed that as many as 3% to 12% of patients with calcium-containing stones have this disorder. It has a prevalence of approximately 1 in 5,000 and affects males and females equally. The anatomic abnormality is an irregular enlargement of medullary and inner papillary collecting ducts. The diagnosis is usually established in the fourth or fifth decade by an IVP that reveals radial, linear striations in papillae or cystic collections of contrast media in ectatic collecting ducts. Patients present with stones or recurrent UTI, often associated with distal RTA. Malformations of the terminal collecting duct result in urinary stasis that promotes crystal precipitation and attachment to the tubular epithelium.

In one report, nanobacteria were isolated from 30 of 30 calcium-containing stones. Nanobacteria are members of the *Proteobacterium* family, and grow in protein- and lipid-free environments. They are capable of nucleating carbonate apatite directly on their surfaces at physiologic pH. This finding awaits confirmation from other laboratories. A subsequent study failed to culture nanobacteria from 10 upper urinary tract stones.

Increasingly, obesity is being recognized as a risk factor for calcium oxalate and uric acid stone formation. As body size increases urinary oxalate and uric acid excretion also increase. In a prospective study of three large cohorts with 4,827 incident stones detected, body weight, BMI, waist circumference, and weight gain after age 21 were all associated with an increased risk of kidney stone formation. This effect was even more pronounced in women than men. In another study of 4,883 patients with nephrolithiasis who underwent stone evaluation in two different stone clinics, urinary pH was inversely related to body weight. A persistently low urinary pH is the most important risk factor for uric acid nephrolithiasis. This may in part explain the increasing incidence of stone formation observed over the last several decades in the United States. As the BMI of the population increases it would be expected that the incidence of stone formation will continue to rise well into the future.

B. **Uric acid stones** represent approximately 5% of all cases of nephrolithiasis in Western countries. The highest incidence was reported from Israel and the Middle East, where as many as 30% of all kidney stones consist solely of uric acid. This may be the result of the arid climate and reduced urinary volume. Uric acid is the major metabolic end product of purine metabolism in humans. Unlike most other mammals, humans do not express uricase, which degrades uric acid into the much more soluble allantoin. Uric acid stones are the most common radiolucent stone.

1. **Pathophysiology.** The principal determinant of uric acid crystallization is its relative insolubility at acidic pH. Uric acid is a weak organic acid with two dissociable protons. The first has a pK_a of 5.5, and the second a pK_a of 10. As a result, only the first proton is dissociated in urine. At pH less than 5.5, undissociated acid predominates, and it is more likely to crystallize (solubility 97 mg per L). As pH increases, uric acid dissociates into the more soluble sodium urate (solubility 1 g per L). Because of the great increase in solubility with increasing pH, uric acid stones are the only kidney stones that can be completely dissolved with medical therapy. The main determinants of uric acid solubility are pH, concentration, and other cations present in urine. A higher

sodium concentration decreases, whereas an increased potassium concentration increases, uric acid solubility. This may explain the complication of calcium-containing stone formation that can develop during sodium alkali therapy but not during treatment with potassium alkali. Sodium-containing alkalis also increase urinary calcium excretion secondary to ECF volume expansion.

2. **Signs and symptoms.** Patients with uric acid stones exhibit a lower mean urinary pH and ammonium ion excretion rate. As many as 75% demonstrate a mild defect in renal ammoniagenesis in response to an acid load. Urinary buffers other than ammonia are titrated more fully than in unaffected individuals, with a resultant urine pH approximating 4.5.

   Those with defects in ammoniagenesis, such as the elderly and patients with polycystic kidney disease, are at increased risk for uric acid lithiasis. Patients with type 2 diabetes mellitus are also at increased risk for uric acid stone formation, as they have a lower urine pH compared to healthy individuals. In one study, 33% of unselected uric acid stone formers had type 2 diabetes mellitus and 23% had impaired glucose tolerance. The low urine pH in patients with insulin resistance is due to impairment in urinary ammonium excretion. Insulin stimulates ammonia synthesis, as well as the activity of the Na^+/H^+ exchanger in the proximal tubule. Low insulin bioactivity leads to defective ammonia synthesis or transport into the lumen. In addition, insulin deficiency causes an increase in plasma free fatty acid concentration. Ammoniagenesis uses glutamine as substrate; the presence of an alternative non-nitrogen metabolic substrate such as free fatty acids or ketoanions inhibits ammoniagenesis. Uric acid stone formers also have a blunted urinary NH_4^+ response to acute acid load due to low NH_3 availability.

   Patients with type 2 diabetes mellitus also tend to have higher BMI and increasing weight is associated with lower urinary pH. In addition, type 2 diabetic patients also consume more dietary acid and this may contribute to their lower urinary pH. However, neither the increased acid consumption nor body weight alone completely explains the low urinary pH.

   The second most important risk factor is decreased urine volume. Hyperuricosuria is the least important risk factor and is seen in less than 25% of patients with recurrent uric acid stones.

3. A **definitive diagnosis** is established through stone analysis. The diagnosis is suggested by the presence of a radiolucent stone, although xanthine and 2,8-dihydroxyadenosine stones can also be radiolucent, or by the presence of uric acid crystals in unusually acidic urine.

C. **Struvite-carbonate stones** are also known as *infection stones* and are composed of a mixture of magnesium ammonium phosphate (struvite: $MgNH_4PO_4 \cdot 6H_2O$) and carbonate apatite [$Ca_{10}(PO_4)_6CO_3$]. Of all stones, 10% to 15% are estimated to be struvite-carbonate stones. This is likely an overestimate, however, given that these figures are based on reports from chemical stone analyses, and a greater proportion of stones chemically analyzed are obtained from surgical specimens. It is likely that struvite-carbonate stones make up no more than 5% of kidney stones. Their presence is also known as *stone cancer* because, before more recent therapeutic advances, they were the cause of numerous surgeries, renal failure, and death. Struvite-carbonate stones are the most common cause of staghorn calculi, although cystine, calcium oxalate, and urate stones may occasionally form staghorns. Struvite-carbonate becomes supersaturating in urine only in one circumstance: infection by urea-splitting organisms that secrete urease. The most common urease-producing bacteria include *Proteus, Morganella, Providencia, Pseudomonas,* and *Klebsiella. Escherichia coli* and *Citrobacter* do not produce urease.

1. **Risk factors.** Women with recurrent UTI and patients with spinal cord injury, other forms of neurogenic bladder, or ileal diversions of the ureter are most prone to form struvite-carbonate stones. Men with indwelling bladder catheters and complete spinal cord transection are at highest risk.

2. **Signs and symptoms.** Struvite stones may present in a variety of ways, including fever, hematuria, flank pain, recurrent UTI, and septicemia. They can

grow to a very large size and fill the renal pelvis as a staghorn calculus. The carbonate apatite component makes them radiopaque. Rarely, if ever, do they pass spontaneously, and 25% are discovered incidentally. If untreated, they result in loss of the affected kidney in 50% of cases.

3. **Pathophysiology.** For struvite-carbonate stones to form, urine must be alkaline, with a pH greater than 7.0 and supersaturated with ammonium hydroxide. Bacterial urease hydrolyzes urea to ammonia and carbon dioxide. The ammonia then hydrolyzes spontaneously to form ammonium hydroxide; the carbon dioxide hydrates to form carbonic acid and, subsequently, bicarbonate. At high pH, bicarbonate loses its proton to become carbonate. UTI with a urease-producing organism is the only situation in which urinary pH, ammonium, and carbonate are elevated simultaneously. The bacteria produce supersaturation in their own immediate environment. Crystals form around bacterial clusters, and bacteria permeate every crevice of a struvite-carbonate stone. The stone itself is an infected foreign body.

D. **Cystine stones.** Cystinuria is the result of an autosomal recessive defect in proximal tubular and jejunal reabsorption of the dibasic amino acids cysteine, ornithine, lysine, and arginine. Excessive amounts of these amino acids are excreted in urine, but clinical disease is due solely to the poor urinary cystine solubility. Cystine is a dimer of cysteine. Cystine stones make up less than 1% of all calculi in adults but may constitute as many as 5% to 8% of kidney stones in children. The prevalence of cystinuria is approximately 1 per 15,000 individuals in the United States. Pure cystine stones form only in homozygotes. A healthy adult excretes less than 19 mg of cystine per g of creatinine in 24 hours. Excretion of greater than 250 mg per g of creatinine is almost always indicative of homozygous cystinuria. Cystine stones are radiopaque due to the sulfhydryl moiety of cysteine.

1. **Pathophysiology.** Cystine solubility is approximately 250 mg per L, and this rises with increasing urinary pH. The pK_a of cysteine is 6.5; therefore, a gradual increase in solubility occurs as urinary pH rises from 6.5 to 7.5. Supersaturation occurs at cystine concentrations greater than 250 mg per L. If the cystine concentration can be maintained below 200 mg per L, cystine stones should not form. In patients with severe cystinuria (greater than 500 mg per day) as much as 4 L of urine is required at normal urinary pH to keep cystine concentration within the soluble range.

2. **Signs and symptoms.** Cystine stones begin to form in the first to fourth decades. Patients tend to have bilateral obstructive staghorn calculi with associated renal failure. Characteristic hexagonal crystals may be identified, particularly in first morning urine, which is usually acidic. Heterozygotes can form stones either with no cystine or with cystine as only a minor component, given that cystine can act as a nidus for crystallization of both calcium oxalate and calcium phosphate.

E. **Drug-related stones.** A variety of drugs can precipitate in urine, including sulfonamides, triamterene, acyclovir, and the antiretroviral agent indinavir. Microscopic hematuria occurs in up to 20% of patients on indinavir. Nephrolithiasis develops in 3%, and 5% experience either dysuria or flank pain that resolves when the drug is discontinued. Reports show that patients with flank pain may have abnormal CT scans with a decrease in contrast excretion in the medullary rays.

Topiramate is often used in the treatment of migraines and seizure disorders and is associated with an increased risk of kidney stone formation. It is an inhibitor of carbonic anhydrases II and IV, which are expressed in proximal and distal tubules. As a result, topiramate is associated with metabolic acidosis, hypercalciuria, and increased urinary pH, factors which result in urinary brushite supersaturation that can subsequently lead to calcium phosphate stone formation.

III. **EVALUATION OF THE PATIENT**

A. **Calcium-containing stones.** The first question to be addressed in the patient with calcium-containing stones is whether the stone disease is simple or complicated. Simple disease is defined as a single stone in the absence of an associated systemic disorder. Complicated calcium-containing stone disease is present if the patient has multiple stones, evidence of new stone formation, enlargement of old stones, or passage of gravel. This distinction is made based on the initial evaluation. A history should be obtained, looking for a family history of stone disease, skeletal disease, inflammatory bowel disease, and UTI. Environmental risk factors are evaluated, such as fluid intake, urine volume, immobilization, diet, medications, and vitamin ingestion. A physical examination is performed. Initial laboratory evaluation includes blood chemistries, urinalysis, and a flat radiographic plate of the abdomen to assess stone burden. Stone analysis should always be carried out if the patient has saved the stone. Stone analysis is inexpensive. It is also the only way to establish the diagnosis of a specific disorder and often helps to direct therapy. In addition, it was shown that in 15% of cases, analyses of 24-hour urines would not have predicted the chemical composition of the stone.

In the patient with complicated disease, two to three measurements of serum calcium concentration should be performed. If any serum calcium level is above 10 mg per dL, PTH concentration should be evaluated. Blood chemistries are examined. An IVP may be indicated to rule out structural abnormalities that predispose to stone formation. First morning void urine should be examined for cystine crystals. At least two 24-hour urine collections should be obtained on the patient's usual diet for calcium, citrate, uric acid, oxalate, sodium, phosphate, volume, pH, and creatinine. Further therapeutic intervention depends on results of these collections. Normal values for 24-hour urine collection are shown in Table 6-4. If a therapeutic intervention is undertaken, a 24-hour urine collection should be repeated in 6 to 8 weeks to verify its expected effect and then repeated yearly.

B. **Uric acid stones.** The etiologies of **uric acid stones** can be subdivided into three pathophysiologic groups based on risk factors. Low urine volume contributes to uric acid stones in gastrointestinal disorders such as Crohn's disease, ulcerative colitis, diarrhea, ileostomies, and dehydration. Acidic urinary pH plays an important role in primary gout and gastrointestinal disorders. Hyperuricosuria is divided into those with hyperuricemia (primary gout, enzyme disorders, myeloproliferative diseases, hemolytic anemia, and drugs) and those without hyperuricemia (dietary excess).

Primary gout is an inherited disorder most likely transmitted in an autosomal dominant manner with variable penetrance. It is associated with hyperuricemia, hyperuricosuria, and persistently acid urine. In affected patients, 10% to 20% have uric acid stones, and in 40% kidney stones precede the first articular gout attack. Because urine is always acidic, risk of uric acid lithiasis varies directly with serum and uric acid concentration.

Uric acid stones are typically round and smooth and are more likely to pass spontaneously than calcium-containing stones, which are often jagged. They are also radiolucent, as are xanthine, hypoxanthine, and 2,8-dihydroadenine stones. Xanthine, hypoxanthine, and 2,8-dihydroadenine stones should be suspected if a radiolucent stone fails to dissolve with alkali therapy.

C. **Struvite-carbonate stones.** Seventy-five percent of all staghorn calculi are composed of struvite-carbonate. Struvite-carbonate stones are large and less radiopaque than calcium-containing stones. As with any kidney stone, the definitive diagnosis is only established on chemical analysis, but a diagnosis of struvite-carbonate

TABLE 6-4	Normal Values for 24-Hour Urine Collection	
Substance	**Male (mg/24 hr)**	**Female (mg/24 hr)**
Calcium	<300	<250
Uric acid	<800	<750
Citrate	>350	>500
Oxalate	<55	<45

stones should be strongly suspected in any patient with an infected alkaline urine. In the presence of an infected acidic urine and a staghorn calculus, one should consider the possibility that the two are unrelated and that the calculus may be either calcium-containing or a uric acid stone. Stone analysis and culture should be carried out in all patients after either percutaneous nephrolithotomy or extracorporeal shock wave lithotripsy. Some patients, especially ambulatory men, have stones that contain a mixture of struvite-carbonate and calcium oxalate. These patients should always undergo complete metabolic evaluation, because virtually all have an underlying metabolic defect, and they are probably at higher risk for stone recurrence, even with complete stone removal.

Proteus mirabilis accounts for more than one-half of all urease-producing infections. Stone culture, when possible, is important, because urine culture is not always completely representative of the organisms present in the stone. If no organisms are cultured, then the possibility of infection with *Ureaplasma urealyticum*, which is often difficult to culture should be considered.

D. Cystine stones. The presence of characteristic hexagonal crystals in first morning void urine is diagnostic of cystinuria, although this is a very infrequent finding. The simplest and most rapid screening test for cystinuria is the sodium-nitroprusside test, which has a lower limit of detection of 75 mg per g of creatinine. The nitroprusside complex binds to sulfide groups and may yield a false-positive result in patients taking sulfur-containing drugs. Phosphotungstic acid has also been used as an alternative screening test. Patients with a positive screening test result should undergo 24-hour urine cystine quantitation. Cystine stones are usually less radiodense on radiography than calcium-containing or struvite-carbonate stones. They typically have a homogeneous structure without striation.

IV. TREATMENT

A. Calcium-containing stones. Treatment of calcium-containing stones is determined by whether the patient has simple or complicated disease. The American College of Physicians advises that the patient with a single, isolated stone and no associated systemic disease be managed with nonspecific forms of therapy alone, including increased fluid intake. This approach is appropriate in patients at low risk of recurrence. One may consider, however, performing more extensive studies in patients at high risk for recurrence (white males; 63% will form a second stone within 8 years) or in those who may experience substantial morbidity with a recurrence (patients who have undergone transplantation or patients with a solitary kidney).

The patient with complicated disease is managed with both nonspecific and specific treatment. Specific therapy varies depending on assessment of risk factors derived from analysis of 24-hour urines.

Although conventional upper limits of daily calciuria (95th percentiles) were defined as 250 mg per day for women and 300 mg per day for men, stone formers in the 70th percentiles (170 mg per day for women and 210 mg per day for men) may benefit from even lower calcium excretion rates. Data linking calcium excretion to stone risk are supportive of the idea that quantity of calciuria is a graded risk factor for development of calcium-containing kidney stones.

1. Nonspecific therapeutic options include manipulation of fluid intake and diet. Increasing fluid intake is the cheapest way to reduce urinary supersaturation with calcium oxalate and phosphate. In a prospective randomized trial of 199 first-time stone formers followed up for a 5-year period, risk of recurrent stone formation was reduced from 27% to 12% by raising urinary volume to more than 2 L per day with water ingestion. The average increase in urine volume in patients advised to increase fluid intake is approximately 300 mL per day.

Before 1993, most patients with calcium-containing stones were advised to restrict dietary calcium. Three large prospective cohort studies, however, in both men and women suggest that a low-calcium diet may actually increase the risk of forming calcium-containing stones. The postulated mechanism is that ingested calcium aids in complexing dietary oxalate, and a reduction in dietary calcium results in a reciprocal increase in intestinal oxalate absorption.

As a result, urinary supersaturation of calcium oxalate increases. Therefore, these authors recommend a liberal calcium intake in patients with calcium-containing stones. In these studies, however, ingestion of a high calcium diet was also associated with increased magnesium, potassium, and phosphate intake, which may have acted as confounding variables in reducing stone risk. A recent prospective, randomized controlled trial compared patients on a low-calcium diet to those on a normal calcium, low-sodium, low-protein diet. The relative risk for kidney stone formation was reduced by 51% in those on the normal calcium diet. As predicted, urinary oxalate increased in the low-calcium group, compatible with the reciprocal relationship hypothesis. However, there was no low-calcium, low-sodium, low-protein control group to directly assess the effects of decreasing dietary calcium intake alone. Observational studies showed an association between increased sodium intake and elevated risk of stone formation in women, whereas increased animal protein intake increases the risk of stone formation in men.

Pak et al. conducted a retrospective analysis of their stone registry to examine the potential effects of dietary restriction on urinary stone risk as assessed by 24-hour urine analysis. It should be stressed that this was an analysis of a surrogate rather than a hard endpoint (rate of new stone formation). Patients were subdivided into three groups: group 1 (urinary calcium excretion greater than 275 mg per day), group 2 (urinary calcium excretion 200 to 275 mg per day), and group 3 (urinary calcium less than 200 mg per day). Patients were than placed on a diet restricted in calcium, oxalate, and sodium. Urinary calcium excretion declined by 29% in group 1, 19% in group 2, and 10% in group 3. Relative supersaturation of calcium oxalate fell by 12% in group 1 and 6% in group 2, an effect that was statistically significant but less than the fall in urinary calcium. Calcium phosphate relative supersaturation fell in all three groups: 31% in group 1, 22% in group 2, and 17% in group 3. Urinary oxalate excretion did not increase.

These authors recommend that intake of oxalate, sodium, and meat products be limited in all patients with calcium-containing kidney stones. They also recommend that patients with urinary calcium excretion greater than 275 mg per day be treated with dietary calcium restriction (400 mg per day), thiazide diuretics, and potassium citrate. Patients with urinary calcium excretion between 200 and 275 mg per day are treated with mild calcium restriction (800 mg per day) and potassium citrate. Those with calcium excretion less than 200 mg per day are treated with a liberal calcium intake and potassium citrate.

Another study examined the effects of the Atkins diet on risk factors for calcium-containing stone disease. Net acid excretion increased by 56 mEq per day, urinary citrate decreased from an average of 763 mg per day to 449 mg per day, urinary pH fell from 6.09 to 5.67, and urinary calcium increased from 160 mg per day to 248 mg per day. Patients with a history of kidney stones should avoid this highly lithogenic diet.

On the basis of the studies discussed earlier the role of dietary calcium restriction in the prevention of calcium-containing stones remains controversial.

The question of whether supplemental calcium increases the risk of nephrolithiasis in women is controversial. One report suggested that any use of supplemental calcium raises the relative risk of stone disease approximately 20%. Risk in this study, however, did not increase with increasing dose. Although the relative risk of kidney stone formation is increased by supplemental calcium, one should bear in mind that women, in general, are at low risk for stone formation. In patients with a history of calcium-containing stones, urinary calcium excretion as well as calcium oxalate and phosphate saturation should be monitored closely. If saturation increases, consideration should be given to discontinuing the supplements.

2. **Specific forms of treatment** are directed by results of the 24-hour urine studies. Therapy is focused on agents shown to reduce relative risk of stone formation in

randomized placebo-controlled clinical trials with more than 1 year of follow-up (results shown in Table 6-3). This is important because of the "stone clinic effect." After patients present for evaluation of nephrolithiasis, the subsequent period is often associated with a reduced risk for new stone formation (the "stone clinic effect"). This is the result of at least two factors: (a) regression to the mean and (b) increased adherence to nonspecific forms of treatment. Trials with less than 12 to 24 months of follow-up should be viewed with skepticism if no effect is detected. At the start of treatment, patients at high risk for recurrence may have stones too small to be detected radiographically that grow and subsequently are identified as new stones. Because calcium-containing stones are often difficult to prevent from increasing in size once a nidus is established, this could minimize the treatment effect in high-risk patients. Agents that were shown to be effective in randomized placebo-controlled trials with a long duration of follow-up include thiazide diuretics, allopurinol, potassium citrate, and potassium magnesium citrate.

a. Hypercalciuria is managed initially with thiazide diuretics. Thiazides act directly to increase distal calcium reabsorption and indirectly to increase calcium reabsorption in the proximal tubule by inducing a state of mild volume contraction. Studies in transgenic mice in which distal nephron calcium transport pathways were knocked out argue that thiazides act primarily in the proximal tubule by inducing volume contraction. Volume contraction must be maintained and hypokalemia avoided for thiazide diuretics to remain maximally effective. Thiazides generally reduce urinary calcium by approximately 50%. The doses used in studies that show an effect are high (25 mg of hydrochlorothiazide twice a day or 50 mg of chlorthalidone once a day) with the exception of one study that used 2.5 mg of indapamide per day. If they are ineffective, noncompliance with the low-sodium diet is usually the reason. This can be monitored with a 24-hour urine for sodium. Amiloride acts independently of thiazides at a more distal site and can be added if required. Three randomized controlled trials in recurrent stone formers demonstrated a reduction in new stone formation risk with thiazide diuretics. Although all patients in these trials were calcium-containing stone formers, the minority were actually hypercalciuric. This suggests that thiazides may have additional effects beyond reducing urinary calcium or that the reduction of urinary calcium, even in the absence of hypercalciuria, may reduce the risk for recurrent kidney stone formation. Some have argued that the effect of thiazide diuretics may diminish with time, but this does not appear to be the case.

In patients who cannot tolerate thiazide diuretics, other potential therapies include sodium cellulose phosphate and orthophosphate. These are often poorly tolerated. Slow-release neutral phosphate appears to be better tolerated and may become the second-line agent of choice. Randomized controlled trials of potassium acid phosphate and magnesium hydroxide showed no benefit when compared to placebo.

b. Hypocitraturia is managed with potassium citrate or potassium-magnesium citrate. Each of these agents reduced the relative risk of stone formation in randomized controlled trials. Potassium-magnesium citrate may be especially beneficial in patients receiving thiazide diuretics, because potassium and magnesium losses induced by the diuretic are repleted. Patients with struvite-carbonate stones should not be given citrate, because it may increase deposition of magnesium ammonium phosphate and carbonate apatite. Citrate may also increase intestinal aluminum absorption in patients with renal failure. Currently, potassium-magnesium citrate is not clinically available. Citrate preparations are often difficult for patients to tolerate secondary to diarrhea. Slow-release preparations such as Urocit-K are well tolerated but are relatively expensive. In patients with urinary citrate levels less than 150 mg per 24 hours, 60 mEq of citrate should be administered daily in divided doses with meals. If urinary citrate is greater than 150 mg per 24 hours, the dose is 30 mEq per day.

    c. Hyperuricosuria is probably best managed with allopurinol. Whether alkalinization is of benefit is unclear, because heterogeneous nucleation and "salting out" can both be initiated by sodium urate. Citrate may reduce calcium oxalate precipitation in this setting, but this remains to be proved.

    d. Hyperoxaluria is managed with a low-oxalate diet. Enteric hyperoxaluria should be initially treated with a low-fat, low-oxalate diet. If this is unsuccessful, calcium carbonate, cholestyramine, or both can be added. As described earlier, modification of the digestive microflora by oral intake of the bacterial mixture Oxadrop is a promising new approach to decrease hyperoxaluria and potentially stone formation. However, larger randomized controlled trials are needed before use of this treatment can be widely recommended. It remains to be determined if enteral administration of the oxalate degrading bacterium *O. formigenes* is safe and effective in reducing urinary oxalate excretion.

    e. Urinary volume should be increased to at least 2 L per day. This is best accomplished by drinking water, which is the only liquid shown to reduce stone formation rate in randomized controlled clinical trials. A recent study suggests that even in patients with a substantial genetic susceptibility for developing nephrolithiasis coffee, milk, and perhaps tea might also be protective against stone formation.

    This approach, directed at both specific and nonspecific risk factor reduction, was shown to decrease frequency of recurrent stone formation and reduce the number of cystoscopies, surgeries, and hospitalizations.

B. Uric acid stones. Therapy for uric acid stones is directed at the three major risk factors for uric acid lithiasis (decreased urine pH, decreased urine volume, and hyperuricosuria). First, urine volume should be increased to 2 to 3 L per day. Second, urine should be alkalinized to a pH of 6.5 using potassium citrate. The starting dose is 30 mEq twice daily to be titrated upward according to urinary pH. More than 80 to 100 mEq is rarely required. Sodium alkali therapy should be avoided, because it may result in hypercalciuria. In one study of 12 patients, alkali therapy resulted in a dissolution of stones within a period of 3 weeks to 5 months. Increases in urinary pH above 6.5 should be avoided because of the increased risk of calcium phosphate stone formation at high urinary pH. If first morning void urine remains acidic, acetazolamide (250 mg) can be added at bedtime.

    If hyperuricosuria is present, dietary purine consumption should be reduced. Allopurinol should only be used when stones recur despite fluid and alkali administration, or if uric acid excretion is above 1,000 mg per day. When allopurinol is administered for massive uric acid overproduction, adequate hydration must be maintained to avoid the precipitation of xanthine crystals.

C. Struvite-carbonate stones. Open surgical removal was formerly the treatment of choice for staghorn struvite-carbonate calculi. The recurrence rate, however, 6 years after surgery is 27%, and UTI persists in 41%. A second pyelolithotomy carries substantial morbidity. More recently, the combination of percutaneous nephrolithotomy and extracorporeal shock wave lithotripsy has decreased morbidity substantially and is now the treatment modality of choice. Total stone elimination remains a challenge, because of the inability to remove small, bacteria-containing particles that act as nidi for further crystal growth. After complete removal, chronic culture-specific antimicrobial agents are indicated as prophylaxis against recurrent infection. If a struvite-carbonate stone is not removed in its entirety, the patient will continue to have recurrent UTI, and the stone will regrow. Stone growth in most patients with residual fragments progresses despite antibiotic treatment. It can be slowed by reducing the bacterial population, but cure with antibiotics alone is remote. Urease inhibitors, such as acetohydroxamic acid, reduce urinary saturation of struvite-carbonate and prevent stone growth and may, on occasion, cause dissolution of existing stones. These agents, however, are associated with a variety of severe complications including hemolytic anemia, thrombophlebitis, and nonspecific neurologic symptoms (e.g., disorientation, tremor, and headache) and best avoided if possible.

D. Cystine stones. Water is the hallmark of cystinuria treatment. The required dose is based on the patient's urinary cystine excretion. A urine output of at least 4 L per day is often required to reduce recurrent stone formation in patients with severe cystinuria. Two 8-oz glasses of water should be ingested every 4 hours. When patients void during the night, they should drink two glasses of water. Urine can be periodically examined for cystine crystals to assess adequacy of fluid intake. Caution should be exercised in interpreting urinary cystine concentrations in treated patients. Cystine excretion may be underestimated due to precipitation in the sample. In addition, many cystine assays employ steps that disrupt cysteine-thiol bonds releasing cysteine bound to therapeutic agents, discussed further in the following text, such as D-penicillamine, α-mercaptopropionylglycine or captopril. The released cysteine can dimerize and form cystine overestimating the amount of free cystine in the urine. These therapeutic agents can also interfere with cystine assays because they contain an active thiol group. Cystine excretion is related to sodium intake and some advocate salt restriction to reduce urinary cystine excretion. In addition, methionine is a substrate for cystine production and fish, red meat, poultry, and dairy products are rich sources of methionine.

Urinary alkalinization may be of some benefit. The dissociation constant of cystine is 6.5. As a result, a pH of 7.5 is required for 90% of cystine to exist in the ionized form. At this pH, calcium phosphate stone formation risk is increased. As a result, alkalinization should be viewed as an ancillary measure. The goal should be to keep monitored urinary pH in the 6.5 to 7.0 range. Potassium citrate is the agent of choice and is preferable to sodium-containing alkali because ECF volume expansion increases cystine excretion.

If these measures are ineffective, then either D-penicillamine, α-mercaptopropionylglycine, or captopril can be tried. These compounds are thiols that bind preferentially to cysteine, forming compounds that are more soluble than cysteine-cysteine dimers (cystine). α-Mercaptopropionylglycine causes fewer complications than D-penicillamine. D-Penicillamine also binds pyridoxine, and therefore pyridoxine (50 mg per day) should be administered to prevent deficiency. Zinc supplements can usually prevent the anosmia and loss of taste that often occurs with D-penicillamine. Captopril has fewer side effects than D-penicillamine or α-mercaptopropionylglycine, but may be less effective in reducing urinary cystine.

Suggested Readings

Bichler KH, Eipper E, Naber K, et al. Urinary infection stones. *Int J Antimicrob Agents* 2002;19:488–498.

Borghi L, Schianchi T, Meschi T, et al. Comparison of two diets for the prevention of recurrent stones in idiopathic hypercalciuria. *N Engl J Med* 2002;346:77–84.

Coe FL, Evan A, Worcester E. Kidney stone disease. *J Clin Invest* 2005;115:2598–2608.

Delvecchio FC, Preminger GM. Medical management of stone disease. *Curr Opin Urol* 2003;13:229–233.

Evan A, Lingeman J, Coe FL, et al. Randall's plaque: pathogenesis and role in calcium oxalate nephrolithiasis. *Kidney Int* 2006;69:1313–1318.

Frick KK, Bushinsky DA. Molecular mechanisms of primary hypercalciuria. *J Am Soc Nephrol* 2003;14:1082–1095.

Gettman MT, Segura JW. Struvite stones: diagnosis and current treatment concepts. *J Endourol* 1999;13:653–658.

Maalouf NM, Cameron MA, Moe OW, et al. Novel insights into the pathogenesis of uric acid nephrolithiasis. *Curr Opin Nephrol Hypertens* 2004;13:181–189.

Moe OW. Kidney stones: pathophysiology and medical management. *Lancet* 2006;367: 333–344.

Moe OW, Bonny O. Genetic hypercalciuria. *J Am Soc Nephrol* 2005;16:729–745.

Pak CYC, Odvina CV, Pearle MS, et al. Effect of dietary modification on urinary stone risk factors. *Kidney Int* 2005;68:2264–2273.

Reynolds TM. ACP best practice no 181: chemical pathology clinical investigation and management of nephrolithiasis. *J Clin Pathol* 2005;58:134–140.

Shekarriz B, Stoller ML. Cystinuria and other noncalcareous calculi. *Endocrinol Metab Clin North Am* 2002;31:951–977.

Taylor EN, Curhan GC. Diet and fluid prescription in stone disease. *Kidney Int* 2006; 70:835–839.

7

THE PATIENT WITH URINARY TRACT INFECTION

Marilyn E. Levi and L. Barth Reller

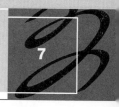

$\mathcal{U}$rinary tract infections (UTIs) are some of the most common infections experienced by humans, exceeded in frequency among ambulatory patients only by respiratory and gastrointestinal infections. Bacterial infections of the urinary tract are the most common cause of both community-acquired and nosocomial infections for patients admitted to hospitals in the United States.

The prognosis and management of UTIs depend on the site of infection and any predisposing factors.

I. **DEFINITIONS.** Some definitions are necessary because infection of the urinary tract may result from microbial invasion of any of the tissues extending from the urethral orifice to the renal cortex. Although the infection and resultant symptoms may be localized at one site, the presence of bacteria in the urine (bacteriuria) places the entire urinary system at risk of invasion by bacteria.

A. **Significant bacteriuria** is defined as the presence of 100,000 or more colony-forming units (CFU) of bacteria per milliliter of urine, although smaller colony counts can be of diagnostic importance, particularly in young women, where 1,000 bacteria per CFU may be associated with cystitis or acute urethral syndrome.

B. **Anatomic location.** The first useful distinction is between upper (kidney) and lower (bladder, prostate, and urethra) UTIs. Infections confined to the bladder (cystitis), the urethra (urethritis), and the prostate (prostatitis) commonly cause dysuria, frequency, and urgency. Pyelonephritis is the nonspecific inflammation of the renal parenchyma; acute bacterial pyelonephritis is a clinical syndrome characterized by chills and fever, flank pain, and constitutional symptoms caused by the bacterial invasion of the kidney. Chronic pyelonephritis has a histopathology that is similar to tubulointerstitial nephritis, a renal disease caused by a variety of disorders such as chronic obstructive uropathy, vesical ureteral reflux (reflux nephropathy), renal medullary disease, drugs and toxins, and possibly chronic or recurring renal bacteriuria.

C. **Recurrence of UTI** is the result of either relapse or reinfection; making this distinction is clinically important. Reinfection is a recurring infection due to a different microorganism, which is usually drug susceptible. Most recurring episodes of cystourethritis are due to reinfection. Relapse is a return of infection due to the same microorganism, which often is drug resistant. Most relapses occur after treatment of acute pyelonephritis or prostatitis. Finally, asymptomatic bacteriuria is an important clue to the presence of parenchymal infection somewhere in the urinary tract; however, the importance of the infection and the need for treatment depend on the age, sex, and underlying condition of the patient.

D. **Complicated and uncomplicated UTIs.** For the clinician, another important distinction is made between uncomplicated and complicated infections. An uncomplicated infection is an episode of cystourethritis following bacterial colonization of the urethral and bladder mucosae in the absence of upper tract disease. This type of infection is considered *uncomplicated* because sequelae are rare and exclusively due to the morbidity associated with reinfections in a subset of women. Complicated UTIs may occur with pregnancy, diabetes, immunosuppression, structural abnormalities of the urinary tract, symptoms lasting for more than 2 weeks, and previous pyelonephritis. Young women constitute a subset of patients with pyelonephritis (acute uncomplicated pyelonephritis) who often respond well to therapy and may also have a low incidence of sequelae. In contrast, complicated infections include those involving parenchyma (pyelonephritis or prostatitis) and frequently occur in the setting of obstructive uropathy or after instrumentation. Episodes may be refractory to therapy, often resulting in relapses, and occasionally leading to significant sequelae such as sepsis, metastatic abscesses, and, rarely, acute renal failure.

   E. Several authors have proposed a **clinical classification** for the practicing clinician.

      1. Asymptomatic bacteriuria
      2. Acute uncomplicated cystitis in women
      3. Recurrent infections in women
      4. Acute uncomplicated pyelonephritis in women
      5. Complicated UTIs in both sexes
      6. Catheter-associated UTIs

II. RISK FACTORS AND PATHOGENESIS. Early recognition and possible prevention depend on an understanding of the pathogenesis and epidemiology of UTIs. In Figure 7-1 the major risk periods of life for symptomatic UTIs are shown; the increasing prevalence of asymptomatic bacteriuria that accompanies aging is apparent. Much has been learned about the risk factors for UTIs. Associations have been established between UTI and age; pregnancy; sexual intercourse; use of diaphragms, condoms, and spermicides, particularly Nonoxynol-9; delayed postcoital micturition; menopause; and a history of recent UTI. Factors that do not seem to increase the risk include diet, use of tampons, clothing, and personal hygiene, including directions of cleansing after defecation and bathing practices. Studies on pathogenesis have elucidated specific interactions between the host and microbes that are causally related to bacteriuria. Bacteria in the enteric flora periodically gain access to the genitourinary tract. How such bacteria actually migrate from the gastrointestinal tract to the periurethra is not known; close proximity of the anus in women is a likely factor. The subsequent bacterial colonization of uroepithelial cells is the biological phenomenon that sets the stage for persistent

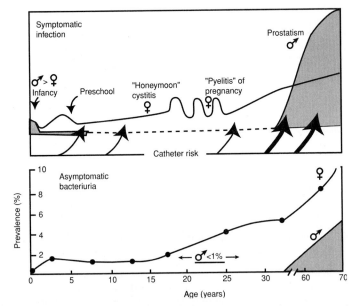

Figure 7-1. Frequency distribution of symptomatic urinary tract infections and prevalence of asymptomatic bacteriuria by age and sex (male, *shaded area;* female, *line*). (Modified from Jawetz's original concept. From Kunin CM. *Detection, prevention and management of urinary tract infections,* 4th ed. Philadelphia: Lea & Febiger, 1987. Reprinted with permission.)

bacteriuria. The colonization of the periurethra often precedes the onset of bladder bacteriuria. P-fimbriated strains of *Escherichia coli* adhere to uroepithelial cells, in which glycolipids function as receptors in women who secrete blood group antigens. *E. coli* that encode for the type 1 pilus, which contains the adhesin FimH, recognizes multiple cell types associated with cystitis, sepsis, and meningitis. Immunocompromised patients may become infected with less virulent *E. coli* strains. Opposing colonization are several host factors, most notably acid pH, normal vaginal flora, and type-specific cervicovaginal antibodies.

After periurethral colonization, uropathogens gain access to the bladder through the urethra, to the kidneys through the ureters, and to the prostate through the ejaculatory ducts. The urethra and ureterovesical junction are mechanical barriers that prevent ascension. Besides instrumentation and mechanical obstruction, however, factors promoting ascent of bacteria are not as well understood. In the bladder, organisms multiply, colonize the bladder mucosa, and invade the mucosal surface. Although urine adequately supports the growth of most uropathogens, the bladder has several mechanisms that prevent bacteriuria: (a) a mucopolysaccharide (urine slime) layer covers the bladder epithelium and prevents colonization; (b) Tamm-Horsfall protein, which is a component of uromucoid, adheres to P fimbriae and prevents colonization; and (c) urine flow and bladder contraction serve to prevent stasis and colonization. Bladder bacteriuria sets the stage for subsequent migration to the kidneys, where organisms such as P-fimbriated *E. coli* adhere to renal tubular cells. In fact, outside the setting of obstructive nephropathy, this strain of *E. coli* is the most common cause of pyelonephritis. With obstruction, however, bacterial adherence is ostensibly unimportant. Other host factors that prevent a renal infection are a high urine osmolality, high ammonium concentration, phagocytes, and increased urine flow rate.

In the presence of a urethral catheter, defense mechanisms against bacterial–epithelial cell interactions are impaired both by disruption of the protective glycosaminoglycan layer of the bladder as well as by the formation of biofilm on the catheter. Microorganisms in the biofilm are protected from antibiotics, host defenses, and mechanical flushing. Effective therapy ultimately requires removal of the catheter.

Pathogens colonizing indwelling urinary catheters often have reduced virulence, for example, *E. coli* strains lacking P fimbriation, which accounts for the low incidence of febrile UTIs and bacteremia.

Chronic urinary catheters are associated with lower tract obstruction due to catheter blockage with encrustation and urinary tract stones and may be complicated by scrotal abscesses, epididymitis, and prostatitis. The incidence of bladder cancer may be increased with prolonged catheter use that exceeds 10 years as in patients with spinal cord injuries.

III. CLINICAL SETTING

A. **Asymptomatic bacteriuria** is especially common in women, as evidenced by a minimum prevalence of 2% to 4% in young and 10% in elderly women and a 3 to 4 times higher prevalence of asymptomatic bacteriuria in diabetic women compared to their nondiabetic counterparts. The higher incidence of asymptomatic bacteriuria in diabetic women is attributed to lower urinary cytokine and leukocyte concentrations and enhanced adherence to uroepithelial cells of *E. coli* that express type 1 fimbriae.

The cumulative prevalence of asymptomatic bacteriuria in women increases approximately 1% per decade throughout life. Of note, this phenomenon has been observed in different ethnic groups and geographic locations. In contrast to women, the occurrence of asymptomatic bacteriuria in men is rare until after the age of 60 years, at which time the prevalence increases per decade and often approaches the rate in elderly women. For example, in noncatheterized, institutionalized elderly men, the prevalence of bacteriuria exceeds 20%. Prostatic hypertrophy and increased likelihood of instrumentation are thought to account for the bacteriuria of older men. Moreover, differences between men and women in the rates of bacteriuria have been attributed to the shorter female urethra and its proximity to the vaginal and rectal mucosae and the abundant microbial flora of these areas. Patients in long-term care facilities have an increased risk of asymptomatic bacteriuria as do patients with spinal cord injuries owing to intermittent catheters, sphincterotomies, or condom catheters.

Bacteriuria related to indwelling catheters increases at a rate of 3% to 10% per day and is predominantly asymptomatic. In the absence of UTI symptoms, a positive urine culture for 10^5 CFU per mL of bacteria is consistent with asymptomatic catheter-associated bacteriuria. Asymptomatic catheter-associated candiduria is defined as 10^3 per mL of yeast. The incidence of significant morbidity with asymptomatic bacteriuria and candiduria is low, and antimicrobial therapy is not recommended while the catheter is present.

B. Symptomatic UTIs occur in all age-groups. Among newborns and infants, boys are affected more often than girls. When the urinary tract is the source of neonatal sepsis, serious underlying congenital anomalies are frequently present. During childhood, persistent bacteriuria, with or without repeated symptomatic episodes, occurs in a small group (less than 2%) of school-aged girls. Such girls, and also school-aged boys with bacteriuria, should have a urologic evaluation to detect correctable structural abnormalities when UTIs are documented. Sexually active women have a markedly increased risk of episodes of cystitis. *E. coli* is the predominant organism in 75% to 90% of cases, whereas *Staphylococcus saprophyticus* is found in 5% to 15%, primarily in young women. The remainder of cases are due to *enterococci* and aerobic gram-negative rods, such as *Klebsiella* species and *Proteus mirabilis*.

In the absence of prostatitis, bacteriuria and symptomatic UTIs are unusual in men. In fact, asymptomatic prostatitis is very common in men presenting with febrile UTIs. More recently, uropathogenic strains of *E. coli* have been recognized as causes of cystitis in young men at risk because of homosexuality and anal intercourse, lack of circumcision, or having a partner with vaginal colonization with such P-fimbriated *E. coli*. At any age, both sexes may develop symptomatic infections in the presence of risk factors that alter urinary flow.

1. **Obstruction to urine flow**
   a. **Congenital anomalies**
   b. **Renal calculi**
   c. **Ureteral occlusion (partial or total)**
2. **Vesicoureteral reflux**
3. **Residual urine in bladder**
   a. **Neurogenic bladder**
   b. **Urethral stricture**
   c. **Prostatic hypertrophy**
4. **Instrumentation of urinary tract**
   a. **Indwelling urinary catheter**
   b. **Catheterization**
   c. **Urethral dilation**
   d. **Cystoscopy**

IV. CLINICAL FEATURES

A. Acute urethral syndrome. The cardinal symptoms of frequency and dysuria occur in more than 90% of ambulatory patients with acute genitourinary tract infections. One-third to one-half of all patients with frequency and dysuria, however, do not have significant bacteriuria, although most have pyuria. These patients have acute urethral syndrome, which can mimic both bladder and renal infections. Vaginitis, urethritis, and prostatitis are common causes of the acute urethral syndrome. Although certain signs and symptoms help to differentiate these clinical entities, a classic UTI can be definitively diagnosed only by quantitative cultures of urine.

1. **Vaginitis.** Approximately 20% of women in the United States have an episode of dysuria each year, and one-half of these seek medical care. The presence of an abnormal vaginal discharge (leukorrhea) and irritation make vaginitis the likely cause of dysuria, unless a concomitant UTI can be confirmed by culture. *Candida albicans*, the most common specific cause of vaginitis, can be demonstrated readily by culture or by finding yeast cells in a Gram-stained smear of vaginal secretions or in a saline preparation with potassium hydroxide

added. Trichomoniasis can be documented with a saline preparation that shows the motile protozoa of *Trichomonas vaginalis*. Nonspecific vaginitis most often is associated with *Gardnerella vaginalis*. A clue to this diagnosis is the presence of many small gram-negative bacilli that adhere to vaginal epithelial cells.

2. **Urethritis.** Acute urinary frequency, dysuria, and pyuria in the absence of vaginal symptoms favor a diagnosis of urethritis or UTI rather than vaginitis. *Chlamydia trachomatis* is a common cause of the acute urethral syndrome in women, as well as nonspecific urethritis in men. *Neisseria gonorrhoeae* is also a widespread cause of urethritis and dysuria. The diagnosis and treatment of gonorrhea are now well standardized. Low colony count (100 to 1,000 CFU) infections with coliforms are now a recognized cause of urethritis in symptomatic young women with pyuria. Herpes simplex virus, usually type 2, is another sexually transmitted agent that can cause severe dysuria through ulcerations in close proximity to the urethral orifice. The diagnosis of herpes progenitalis can be confirmed by finding giant multinucleated transformed cells in epidermal scrapings stained with Wright's stain (Tzanck smear), by isolating the virus in tissue culture, or by direct fluorescent antibody test.

3. **Prostatitis.** Prostatitis is a common affliction in men that causes dysuria and urinary frequency in middle-aged and younger men more frequently than UTIs do. In addition, more than 90% of men with febrile UTIs have asymptomatic prostatitis manifested by elevated prostate-specific antigens (PSAs) and prostate volume. The PSA may remain elevated for up to 12 months. Prostate syndromes have classically been divided into four clinical entities: (a) acute bacterial prostatitis, (b) chronic bacterial prostatitis, (c) nonbacterial prostatitis, and (d) prostatodynia.

   a. **Acute bacterial prostatitis** is easily distinguished from the other prostatitis syndromes by its acute characteristics. The patient often appears acutely ill, with the sudden onset of chills and fever, urinary frequency and urgency, dysuria, perineal and low back pain, and constitutional symptoms. Rectal examination should not be performed because of the risk of precipitating sepsis, but it may disclose an exquisitely tender, hot, and swollen prostate gland. Microscopical examination of the urine usually displays numerous white blood cells. Urine culture is usually positive for enteric gram-negative bacteria (especially *E. coli*); gram-positive bacteria (*staphylococci* and *enterococci*) are less frequently isolated.

   b. **Chronic bacterial prostatitis.** A hallmark of chronic prostatitis is relapsing UTIs. Urinary frequency, dysuria, nocturia, and low back and perineal pain are the usual symptoms, although patients may have a minimum of symptoms between UTIs. The patient is often afebrile, does not appear acutely ill, and may have an unremarkable prostate examination. A proposed mechanism to explain the migration of bacteria into the prostate is by reflux of urine and bacteria into the prostatic ducts from the urethra. This syndrome is distinguished from other forms of chronic prostatitis by displaying an initial negative midstream urine examination and culture; after prostate massage, however, the urine displays a positive microscopical examination for white blood cells, and a uropathogen can be cultured (see section V). Nonbacterial prostatitis is the most common form of chronic prostatitis. It mimics chronic bacterial prostatitis clinically and displays inflammatory cells on post–prostate massage specimens. However, bacteriologic cultures of urine and prostatic secretions are sterile. The etiology is unknown, but some evidence exists for an infectious etiology involving organisms that are difficult to culture.

   c. **Prostatodynia** has also been referred to as *chronic noninflammatory prostatitis*. Clinically, it presents with symptoms similar to other forms of chronic prostatitis. It is distinguished by the absence of inflammatory cells or uropathogens from all specimens.

B. **UTIs.** Despite the mimicking syndromes, a presumptive diagnosis of infections of the urinary tract can be established economically by analyzing urine in patients with characteristic, albeit nonspecific, signs and symptoms. Acute uncomplicated UTIs occur mainly in women of childbearing age. The presenting features are only suggestive of the site of infection. Patients with bacterial cystourethritis, as distinct from urethritis caused by a sexually transmitted disease (STD) pathogen, will have had prior episodes, experienced symptoms for less than 1 week, and will experience suprapubic pain.

V. LABORATORY DIAGNOSIS
A. Urine specimens for culture
1. **Indications.** The diagnosis of UTI, from simple cystitis to complicated pyelonephritis with sepsis, can be established with absolute certainty only by quantitative cultures of urine. The major indications for urine cultures are:
   a. **Patients with symptoms or signs of UTIs**
   b. **Follow-up of recently treated UTI**
   c. **Removal of indwelling urinary catheter**
   d. **Screening for asymptomatic bacteriuria during pregnancy**
   e. **Patients with obstructive uropathy and stasis before instrumentation**
2. When universally applied, the first two indications may not be the most cost-effective approach to diagnosing UTIs in nonpregnant, young-adult women. These individuals present with dysuria, urgency, and pyuria due to an uncomplicated episode of cystourethritis, with organisms usually susceptible to a variety of antimicrobial agents, or due to an STD pathogen such as *gonococcus* or *chlamydia*. Moreover, because the beneficial outcome of therapy is to minimize morbidity rather than prevent life-threatening complications, laboratory costs and use of resources can be minimized if pretreatment cultures are not ordered in this clinical setting. Therefore, women with symptoms consistent with simple uncomplicated lower tract disease and a positive urine dipstick can be treated without obtaining a urine culture. Additionally, if symptoms completely resolve, posttreatment cultures also are unnecessary for patients with uncomplicated infections.
3. **Methods.** Urine specimens must be cultured promptly within 2 hours or be preserved by refrigeration or a suitable chemical additive (e.g., boric acid sodium formate preservative). Acceptable methods of collection are:
   a. **Midstream urine voided into a sterile container after careful washing (water or saline) of external genitalia (any soap must be rinsed away)**
   b. **Urine obtained by single catheterization or suprapubic needle aspiration of the bladder**
   c. **Sterile needle aspiration of urine from the tube of a closed catheter drainage system (do not disconnect tubing to get specimen)**
4. Not acceptable, because of constant contamination and the impossibility of quantitative counts, are tips from indwelling urinary catheters and urine obtained randomly, without adequate patient preparation. The clean-voided, midstream technique of collection is preferred whenever possible to avoid the risk of introducing infection at the time of catheterization, a hazard in elderly patients confined to bed, in men with condom catheters, and in diabetic patients with dysfunctional bladders. Because contamination is exceedingly rare in circumcised men, a clean-catch, midstream specimen is unnecessary in such patients. Occasionally, suprapubic aspiration of the bladder is necessary to verify infection. This technique has been most helpful in obtaining specimens from possibly septic infants and from adults in whom repeated clean-voided specimens have yielded equivocal colony counts on culture.
5. **The usual microbial pathogens** isolated from patients with UTIs are listed in Table 7-1. Results of cultures highly depend, however, on the clinical setting in which bacteriuria occurs. For example, *E. coli* is found in the urine of 80% to 90% of patients with acute uncomplicated cystitis and acute uncomplicated pyelonephritis. Many patients with staghorn calculi of the kidneys harbor urea-splitting *Proteus* organisms in their urine. *Klebsiella*, *Pseudomonas aeruginosa*, and *Enterobacter* infections are commonly acquired in the hospital. The presence of *Staphylococcus aureus* in the urine most often

TABLE 7-1 Microbial Pathogens of Kidney and Bladder

Organism	Uncomplicated cystitis: young women[a] (%)	Pyelonephritis: outpatient, women[b] (%)	UTI: men[c] (%)	Bacteremic UTIs[d] (%)	Nosocomial UTIs[e] (%)
Gram-negative bacteria					
Escherichia coli	79	86	41	54	29
Klebsiella pneumoniae	3	4	3	9	8
Proteus	2	3	6	8	4
Enterobacter	0	0	1	2	4
Pseudomonas aeruginosa	0	0	NS	3	9
Gram-positive bacteria					
Staphylococcus saprophyticus	11	3	NS	0	0
Staphylococcus aureus	0	1	1	13	
Staphylococcus not aureus	0	0	5	1	5
Enterococci	2	0	5	6	13
Other bacteria	0	4	19	4	15
Mixed infections	3	3	18	2	NS
Yeast	0	0	0	3	13

NS, not stated; UTIs, urinary tract infections.
[a]Data from 607 episodes of cystitis; from Stamm WE. Urinary tract infections. In: Root RK, ed. *Clinical infectious diseases: a practical approach*, 1st ed. New York: Oxford University Press, 1999.
[b]Eighty-four episodes from Stamm 1992 and 54 nonhospitalized women; from Pinson AG, Philbrock JT, Lindbeck GH, Schorling JB, eds. Management of acute pyelonephritis in women: a cohort study. *Am J Emerg Med* 1994;12:271–278.
[c]Data from 223 outpatient males with symptoms; from Pead L, Maskell R. Urinary tract infections in adult men. *J Infect* 1981;3:71–78.
[d]185 Cases (excluding five cases of *Candida albicans*); from Ackermann RJ, Monroe PW. Bacteremic urinary tract infections in older people. *J Am Geriat Soc* 1996;44:927–933.
[e]90% Catheter-associated infections, 1991 experience at the University of Iowa (900-bed hospital); from Bronsema DA, Adams JR, Pallares R, Wenzel RP. Secular trends in rates and etiology of nosocomial urinary tract infections at a university hospital. *J Urol* 1993;150:414–416.

103

is a clue to concomitant staphylococcal bacteremia, unless an underlying risk factor exists. Microorganisms in young men are similar to the organisms that cause uncomplicated infections in women. *Enterococci* and coagulase-negative *staphylococci* are more common in elderly men, most likely representing recent instrumentation or catheterization. *C. albicans* is rarely encountered, except in patients with indwelling catheters, nosocomial UTIs, or relapsing infections after multiple courses of antibiotic therapy. Most urinary catheter-related infections originate from the patient's colonic flora with long-term catheterization exceeding 28 days. Multidrug-resistant organisms such as *Providencia stuartii*, *Pseudomonas* spp., *Proteus* spp., *Morganella* spp., and *Acinetobacter* spp. are found more frequently owing to antibiotic exposure. In addition, polymicrobial bacteriuria is found in up to 95% of urine cultures from patients with long-term catheter use. Although the likely microorganism and usual susceptibility patterns are sufficient to guide the initial empiric therapy of uncomplicated cystitis, adequate treatment of acute bacterial pyelonephritis and complicated UTIs necessitates precise therapy based on isolation of the causative bacterium and standardized antimicrobial susceptibility testing using the disk-diffusion or the broth-dilution or agar-dilution methods.

B. Interpretation of urine cultures. Organisms residing in the distal urethra and on pubic hairs contaminate voided, clean-catch specimens. This bacterial contamination must be distinguished from "true infection" or "significant bacteriuria" in urine cultures. Quantitative bacteriology makes this distinction. Because quantitation of bacteriuria is so important clinically, methods for culture of urine must enable the CFU number of a potential pathogen per milliliter of urine to be assessed. The standard procedure involves the use of calibrated bacteriologic loops that deliver a known volume of urine to the surface of agar plates. Proper plating techniques achieve isolated colonies that can be enumerated accurately. A satisfactory alternative for the diagnosis of uncomplicated UTIs is the dip slide method, which is particularly well suited to quantitative urine cultures in smaller clinics. Rapid methods based on filtration and colorimetry, bioluminescence, growth kinetics, and biochemical reactions are used increasingly to screen urine specimens for the presence of bacteria. The sensitivities of these rapid assays are in the range of 10^4 to 10^5 CFU per mL. The simplest screen is the paper-strip test for detection of leukocyte esterase and nitrite in first morning urine specimens. However, these methods are not a substitute for standard cultures in symptomatic patients with complicated UTIs.

    1. Colony counts. In Figure 7-2, a basic guide to the interpretation of quantitative cultures of urine is shown. Colony counts greater than 10^5 CFU per mL in properly collected and transported specimens usually indicate infection. Colony counts of 10^3 or fewer CFU per mL from untreated patients are uncommon with true UTIs, except in symptomatic young women with pyuria and urethritis, in whom colony counts of *E. coli* as low as 10^3 may be interpretable if the urine was obtained by single catheterization. Intermediate counts, especially with mixed flora, usually imply poor collection or delayed transport and culture. Brisk diuresis may transiently reduce an otherwise high colony count.

    2. Suprapubic needle aspiration. Any growth from urine obtained by suprapubic needle aspiration may be important. Use of a 0.01-mL quantitative loop for culturing aspirated urine permits the detection of as few as 100 CFU per mL. Two or more colonies (less than or equal to 200 CFU per mL) of the same microorganism ensure the purity of growth from such specimens and permit standardized antimicrobial susceptibility testing. Similar criteria should be used for patients who are receiving antimicrobials at the time of culture. Except in unusual circumstances, the isolation of diphtheroids, α-hemolytic *streptococci*, and *lactobacilli* indicates contamination of the urine specimen with vaginal or periurethral flora.

    3. Prostatic secretions. In men, the distinction between a urinary source and a prostatic focus of infection must be made. The procedure for obtaining voided urine and expressed prostatic secretions in partitioned segments that enable

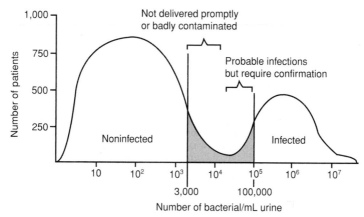

Figure 7-2. Results of quantitative bacterial counts from cultures of urine specimens. (From Brumfitt W, Percival A. Pathogenesis and laboratory diagnosis of nontuberculous urinary tract infection: a review. *J Clin Pathol* 1964;17:482. Reprinted with permission.)

proper interpretation is diagrammed in Figure 7-3. Leukocytes (greater than 10 to 15 white blood cells per high-power field) and lipid-laden macrophages are seldom observed in the expressed prostatic secretion of healthy men. These agents signify prostatic inflammation. Therefore, a prostatic focus of infection should be considered when a significant step-up of pyuria or colony counts occurs in the prostate specimens. A UTI of prostatic origin is indicated by colony counts of 10^5 or more CFU per mL of the same microorganism in all four specimens. Both urologists and primary care physicians underuse this procedure. In one study, a two-step procedure involving microscopical examination and culture of pre– and post–prostate massage urine specimens compared favorably to this four-step procedure. This simplified approach was able to arrive at a similar diagnosis in 91% of patients. Further trials are needed to evaluate this approach, which may improve physician use.

C. **Microscopic examination of urine.** Procedures for the microscopical examination of urine are poorly standardized; nonetheless, visualization of bacteria, leukocytes, and epithelial cells in urine can provide some useful information and enable the clinician to make a presumptive diagnosis of UTI. The advantages of microscopical analysis are immediate availability and low cost. The disadvantages, depending on the method, are lack of sensitivity, specificity, or both. Only properly collected and processed specimens for quantitative urine cultures can provide definitive diagnosis. The microscopical examination can be done on either unspun urine or the centrifuged sediment. A critical comparison of these two techniques is not available. The presence of squamous epithelial cells and mixed bacterial flora indicates contamination and the need for a repeat specimen.

   1. **Unspun urine.** When fresh, unspun urine from patients with significant bacteriuria (greater than 10^5 CFU per mL) is examined microscopically ($\times 1,000$), 90% of specimens show one or more bacteria, and 75% of specimens show one or more white blood cells per oil-immersion field. The best assessment of pyuria is the finding of approximately 10 white blood cells per mm^3 of unspun urine examined in a counting chamber.

   2. **Centrifuged sediment.** After 10 mL of urine is centrifuged in a standard 15-mL conical tube for 5 minutes at 2,500 revolutions per minute in a clinical centrifuge, three or four drops of the sediment are examined under a coverslip at high power ($\times 400$) in diminished light. Patients with significant bacteriuria usually show bacilli in the urinary sediment whereas only approximately 10% of patients with fewer than 10^5 CFU per mL show bacteria. Approximately

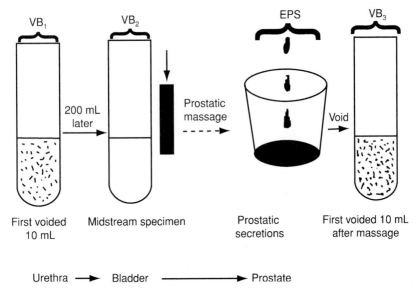

Figure 7-3. Localization of infection with segmented cultures of the lower urinary tract in men. VB_1 is the first 10 mL of voided urine, and VB_2 is the midstream specimen of urine obtained before prostatic massage. Subsequently, the expressed prostatic secretions (EPS) are collected before the final voided urine specimen (VB_3). When the bacterial colony counts in the urethral culture exceed by 10-fold or more those of the midstream and prostatic cultures, the urethra is the source of the infection. The diagnosis is bacterial prostatitis if the quantitative counts of the prostatic specimens exceed those of the urethral and midstream samples. (From Meares EM, Stamey TA. Bacteriologic localization patterns in bacterial prostatitis and urethritis. *Invest Urol* 1968;5:492. Reprinted with permission.)

60% to 85% of patients with significant bacteriuria have 10 or more white blood cells per high-power field in the sediment of midstream voided urine; however, approximately 25% of patients with negative urine cultures also have pyuria (10 or more white blood cells per high-power field), and only approximately 40% of patients with pyuria have 10^5 or more bacteria per mL of urine by quantitative culture. The principal pitfall is false-positive pyuria owing to leukocytes from a contaminating vaginal discharge.

3. **Gram's stain.** A simple Gram-stained smear of unspun urine or spun sediment can enhance the specificity of the test, because morphology and stain characteristics aid in identifying the likely pathogen and in targeting empiric therapy.

4. **Pyuria.** Although the presence of pyuria in a midstream specimen has low predictive value for significant bacteriuria, pyuria is a sensitive indicator of inflammation. Therefore, pyuria may be more accurate than bacteriuria in distinguishing a "true infection" from contamination: 95% of patients with pyuria have a genitourinary tract infection; however, pyuria cannot distinguish a bacterial UTI from acute urethral syndrome. In addition to a UTI, any of the causes of acute urethral syndrome (see section IV.A) can result in pyuria. For example, tuberculosis is a cause of pyuria with negative routine urine cultures, although mycobacterial cultures are positive in 90% of instances. Analgesic nephropathy, interstitial nephritis, perinephric abscess, renal cortical abscess, disseminated fungal infection, and appendicitis may also result in pyuria.

D. **Biochemical tests for bacteriuria.** Two metabolic capabilities shared by most bacterial pathogens of the urinary tract are use of glucose and reduction of nitrate to nitrite; these are properties of all *enterobacteriaceae*. Because small amounts of glucose and nitrate are normally present in urine, the presence of significant numbers of bacteria in urine results in the absence of glucose and presence of nitrite. Dipstick devices are commercially available for both types of testing. Studies with nitrite-indicator strips show that 85% of women and children with culture-confirmed significant bacteriuria show positive results if three consecutive morning urine specimens are tested. A morning urine specimen is preferred for the nitrite test because most bacteria take 4 to 6 hours to convert nitrate to nitrite. A negative nitrite test may be observed in patients taking diuretics or with organisms that do not produce nitrate reductase (*Staphylococcus* species, *Enterococcus* species, and *P. aeruginosa*). The sensitivity of the glucose-use test is approximately 90% to 95% in patients without diabetes mellitus. Both biochemical tests have fewer than 5% false-positive results. Therefore, these biochemical tests can be used by patients or parents, after proper instruction, to determine when quantitative cultures are needed in the management of recurrent episodes of UTI. Spectrum bias in the use of dipsticks must be avoided. Dipsticks should only be used for patients with symptoms suggestive of UTI (i.e., high pretest probability of UTI), and not for asymptomatic screening, as in pregnancy.

E. **Localization of the site of infection.** The site of infection within the urinary tract has great therapeutic and prognostic importance. Upper UTI (pyelonephritis) indicates a much greater likelihood of underlying uropathy (e.g., congenital anomalies, renal stones, ureteral occlusion, vesicoureteral reflux, neurogenic bladder, or prostatic hypertrophy) or previous instrumentation (see section III.B). Relapses with the same, often multiple–antibiotic-resistant bacteria are common with pyelonephritis or chronic bacterial prostatitis. Treatment is long (minimum 10 to 14 days) and may be arduous. On the other hand, cystitis rarely is complicated, and treatment can be short (single dose or 3-day) and usually is easy. No ready way exists to distinguish between upper and lower UTIs by simple laboratory tests. The difficulty in making this distinction reliably on clinical grounds alone has been discussed (see section IV.B). Older, indirect methods (e.g., serum antibodies, urine concentration test, and urinary β-glucuronidase activity) are neither sensitive nor specific. Direct methods for localization (e.g., ureteral catheterization, renal biopsy, and the bladder washout technique) are hazardous, expensive, or both. Eradication of bacteriuria with single-dose or short-course (3-day) antibiotic therapy in symptomatic patients with uncomplicated disease is a practical method for presumptive localization of infection to the bladder or urethra.

F. **Radiography and other diagnostic procedures: indications.** The principal role of radiographic and urologic studies for patients with UTIs is to detect vesicoureteral reflux, renal calculi, and potentially correctable lesions that obstruct urine flow and cause stasis. Uncomplicated reinfections (cystitis and urethritis) in women who respond to short-course antimicrobial therapy are not an indication for radiographic and cystoscopic investigation of the urinary tract. Radiologic and urologic evaluation should be considered in all children with a first episode of UTIs (except for school-aged girls). Special emphasis should be on the early detection of urologic abnormalities in all young children and boys with a first infection, as well as any child with pyelonephritis or a complicated course. A review of studies evaluating diagnostic imaging in children with UTIs expressed the need for better outcome-based research in this area. Radiologic and urologic evaluation should be considered in adults with UTIs. In the past, all UTIs in males were considered complicated. The conventional recommendation that all males presenting with initial UTIs undergo urologic evaluation to identify predisposing anatomic or functional abnormalities is still followed. However, several studies have indicated that only approximately 20% of men have previously unidentified abnormalities. Some sexually active males are at a higher risk for cystitis (homosexual males, males with a partner who harbors a uropathogen, uncircumcised males). The value of urologic evaluation in this high-risk group, with a single episode of cystitis and an uncomplicated course, is not known. In general, urologic evaluations are recommended in the following situations: (a) males with first episode, (b) all patients with a complicated infection or bacteremia, (c) suspected obstruction or renal stones, (d) hematuria following infection, (e) failure to respond to appropriate antibiotic therapy, and (f) patients with recurrent infections.

Some experts recommend the evaluation of all patients with pyelonephritis. The radiologic evaluation of a subgroup of patients with pyelonephritis (young and otherwise healthy women who respond well to therapy) may have a low diagnostic yield. In one study, only 1 of 25 young women with uncomplicated pyelonephritis had a surgically correctable etiology, and 2 of 25 had focal abnormalities that resolved on a follow-up ultrasonography. This has led others to recommend a diagnostic evaluation in young women with uncomplicated pyelonephritis after the second recurrence, or at any time, if a complicating course is present. The ease in obtaining a noninvasive test (ultrasonography) has increased radiologic evaluations for most patients admitted with pyelonephritis.

Ultrasonography with a plain film of the abdomen has replaced the intravenous pyelogram (IVP) as the initial radiologic studies for most adults. For a detailed evaluation of the ureterovesical junction, bladder, and urethra, a voiding cystourethrogram and measurement of the residual urine after voiding may be necessary. If vesicoureteral reflux is present after acute infection has been treated, a urologist should be consulted. Cystoscopy may be warranted. Renal calculi can usually be detected on a plain radiograph of the abdomen. An IVP confirms the presence and the location of calculi, detects radiolucent stones (fewer than 10% of renal calculi), and discloses the degree of obstruction and dilation. Ordinarily, radiographic studies should not be performed within 6 weeks of acute infections.

Gram-negative bacilli have the ability to impede ureteral peristalsis, and transient abnormalities of the IVP are common with acute pyelonephritis. These include hydroureter, vesicoureteral reflux, diminished pyelogram, loss of renal outline, and renal enlargement. Acute pyelonephritis with an obstructed ureter is a surgical emergency, and a perinephric abscess also requires surgical drainage. These complications, however, are best detected initially by ultrasonography and by computed tomography (CT), respectively. To avoid radiocontrast-induced acute renal failure, excretory urography and other radiocontrast studies should be avoided whenever possible in patients with a serum creatinine above 1.5 mg per dL, diabetes mellitus, dehydration, or advanced age.

VI. TREATMENT OF UTI

A. Principles of underlying therapy and follow-up. To successfully treat a UTI, the clinician must have knowledge of microbial susceptibility and mechanisms of resistance, pharmacokinetics and pharmacodynamics, and status of host defenses. First, most uropathogens are susceptible to a wide range of antibiotics; however, resistant gram-negative bacteria frequently are seen with indwelling catheters, in immunocompromised patients, and in patients with relapsing bacteriuria. Second, most antibiotics are filtered by the kidney and therefore achieve a urinary concentration that is many times higher than the minimum inhibitory concentration. Third, although most antibiotics achieve adequate concentration in renal tissue, only tetracyclines, trimethoprim-sulfamethoxazole, and fluoroquinolones achieve any reasonable concentration in the prostate. Finally, patients with systemic or local abnormalities in host defenses usually develop a renal infection that is refractory to therapy. In this case, antibiotics that achieve adequate serum concentrations and are bactericidal are preferable to bacterial static agents. The basic caveats for the effective management of UTIs are outlined here.

1. **Asymptomatic patients** should have colony counts greater than or equal to 100,000 per mL on at least two occasions before treatment is considered.
2. Unless symptoms are present, **no attempt should be made to eradicate bacteriuria** until catheters, stones, or obstructions are removed.
3. Selected patients with chronic bacteriuria may benefit from suppressive therapy.
4. A patient who develops **bacteriuria as a result of catheterization** should have treatment to reestablish a sterile urine after the removal of catheter.
5. **Antimicrobial agents used for treatment** should be the safest and least expensive agents to which the causative microorganisms are susceptible.

6. **Efficacy of treatment** should be evaluated by urine culture 1 week after completion of therapy, except in nonpregnant adult women who respond to therapy for uncomplicated cystitis and uncomplicated pyelonephritis.

B. **Antimicrobial agents**

1. **β-Lactams.** The increasing antimicrobial resistance observed in *E. coli* makes amoxicillin and ampicillin less attractive choices for empiric therapy in the patient with a complicated UTI, unless *enterococcus* is strongly considered to be the etiologic agent. Amoxicillin has replaced oral ampicillin due to improved bioavailability and less frequent dosing. Amoxicillin is effective for uncomplicated cystitis, but short-course therapy (single-dose and 3-day regimens) has generally been less effective than trimethoprim-sulfamethoxazole or fluoroquinolones given for a similar duration. Cefixime and cefpodoxime are oral third-generation cephalosporins with enhanced activity against enteric gram-negative bacteria, longer serum half-life, and less frequent dosing than first-generation cephalosporins. Parenteral β-lactams are generally reserved for more complicated infections. Ceftriaxone is a third-generation cephalosporin with good activity against most community-acquired gram-negative enteric bacteria (except *P. aeruginosa*). Ceftazidime and cefepime are examples of cephalosporins with good activity against many gram-negative bacteria, including *P. aeruginosa*.

2. **Nitrofurantoin** is active against many uropathogens, including *E. coli, S. saprophyticus,* and *Enterococcus faecalis.* Some gram-negative bacteria are resistant to nitrofurantoin (*Klebsiella, Enterobacter,* and *Pseudomonas* species), making it a less than ideal agent for the empiric therapy of complicated UTIs. No clinically significant increase in resistance has been observed. However, this drug is significantly less active than fluoroquinolones and trimethoprim-sulfamethoxazole against non–*E. coli* aerobic gram-negative rods and is inactive against *Proteus* and *Pseudomonas* species. The major role of nitrofurantoin in therapy includes the treatment of uncomplicated cystitis and as an alternative agent for cystitis caused by *E. faecalis.* The oral adult dose for both crystalline and macrocrystalline preparations is 50 to 100 mg every 6 hours for 7 days. Although a 3-day regimen is successful in many patients with uncomplicated cystitis, one clinical trial found nitrofurantoin to be less effective than a 3-day regimen of trimethoprim-sulfamethoxazole. Patients with renal insufficiency (creatinine clearance less than 60 mL per minute) should not receive this agent. Nitrofurantoin has been used in pregnancy [U.S. Food and Drug Administration (FDA) category B], although it is contraindicated in nursing mothers, pregnant women near term, and newborns (in whom it is associated with hemolytic anemia). Suppressive therapy has been successful in some patients, although concern for less common reactions (e.g., peripheral neuropathy, pneumonitis, and hepatitis) may limit long-term use.

3. **Trimethoprim-sulfamethoxazole and trimethoprim.** Trimethoprim-sulfamethoxazole has a wide spectrum of activity against many uropathogens. However, lack of clinical activity against *enterococci* and *P. aeruginosa,* as well as increased resistance by some enteric gram-negative bacteria (*Klebsiella* species, *Enterobacter* species), makes trimethoprim-sulfamethoxazole a less than ideal agent for the treatment of complicated UTIs. In addition, resistance patterns tabulated by microbiology laboratories show trimethoprim-sulfamethoxazole resistance variability depending on locale; an 18% incidence of resistance is present in the southeastern and western United States for women with acute cystitis who have had a UTI in the last 6 months. Therefore, some authorities recommend the use of trimethoprim-sulfamethoxazole only if (a) the local resistance pattern is less than 20%, (b) no sulfa allergy exists, and (c) no recent antibiotic use is present. Of interest, despite a 30% resistance prevalence in some locales, at least half of the women treated with trimethoprim-sulfamethoxazole have 80% to 85% clinical and microbiologic cures.

    Trimethoprim-sulfamethoxazole is well tolerated in most patients. Adverse effects due to sulfonamides are well described and include gastrointestinal symptoms, transient elevation in the serum creatinine, and hematologic and dermatologic reactions. Sulfonamides displace warfarin and hypoglycemic agents from albumin thereby potentiating these drug effects. Trimethoprim-sulfamethoxazole is highly effective for the prophylaxis and therapy for uncomplicated cystitis and for therapy of uncomplicated pyelonephritis. A randomized trial with four different 3-day drug regimens in women with uncomplicated acute cystitis found a 3-day regimen of trimethoprim-sulfamethoxazole was the most cost effective. Complicated UTIs, especially catheter-associated infections and nosocomial UTIs, should have *in vitro* susceptibility testing performed. Trimethoprim-sulfamethoxazole has been used in pregnancy, but it is not FDA-approved for pregnant women. Other agents such as amoxicillin, nitrofurantoin, and cephalosporins are preferred.

Trimethoprim alone is preferred over trimethoprim-sulfamethoxazole by some experts for the prophylaxis and treatment of uncomplicated cystitis because its efficacy is similar and the side effects fewer (because of the absence of sulfamethoxazole). This agent should not be used alone for the therapy of complicated UTIs.

Trimethoprim monotherapy also achieves good prostate concentrations and is an alternative to fluoroquinolones depending on the susceptibility pattern of the bacteria.

4. Multiple **fluoroquinolones** are now available for clinical use (Tables 7-2 and 7-3). These agents achieve very high concentrations in the urine and renal tissue, easily exceeding the minimal inhibitory concentration of most uropathogens. Fluoroquinolones should not be used as first-line agents for the therapy of uncomplicated cystitis because of concern for the development of resistance and because of the cost. However, their antimicrobial spectrum and generally low side effect profile make them excellent choices for empiric therapy of complicated UTIs. Among current agents within this antimicrobial class, no particular drug has demonstrated superior clinical efficacy for the therapy of patients with UTIs. An exception is moxifloxacin, which does not achieve adequate urinary concentrations and should be avoided in the treatment of UTIs. Fluoroquinolones should not be used for enterococcal UTIs (only 60% to 70% susceptible), during pregnancy or in children (until further information is available). Aluminum- and magnesium-containing antacids and iron-, calcium-, and zinc-containing preparations should not be administered with oral fluoroquinolones due to a significant decrease in absorption. In general, these agents are well tolerated by most patients. The most common adverse effects are gastrointestinal and on the central nervous system, but these infrequently lead to drug discontinuation. Photosensitivity may limit the use of some of these agents (e.g., lomefloxacin, sparfloxacin). Many of these agents are available for both parenteral and oral administration. Conversion from parenteral to oral therapy (step-down therapy) should be considered for patients who are clinically stable and tolerating oral medications. The excellent bioavailability of these drugs, good clinical success with oral therapy, and the high cost of parenteral therapy due to intravenous catheter–related complications and cost of intravenous preparations are all good reasons for considering oral therapy.

C. Treatment of asymptomatic bacteriuria

1. **Pregnancy** increases the risk of UTI complications. The rate of prematurity in children born to women who have bacteriuria during pregnancy is increased, and 20% to 40% of these patients develop pyelonephritis. Successful therapy in these patients with bacteriuria decreases the risk of symptomatic infection by 80% to 90%. Therefore, all women should be screened twice during gestation for asymptomatic bacteriuria. All patients with bacteriuria should be treated for 7 days, with follow-up cultures to identify relapses. Long-term prophylaxis offers no advantage over close surveillance. In selecting therapy, the risk to the fetus should be considered. Short-acting sulfonamides or amoxicillin for 7 days usually suffices, because almost all these infections are caused by susceptible

TABLE 7-2 Oral Antimicrobial Agents Commonly Used for Treatment of Urinary Tract Infections

	Adult dose	Comment
Miscellaneous agents		
Trimethoprim	100 mg every 12 hr	Prophylaxis, uncomplicated cystitis
Trimethoprim-sulfamethoxazole	160 mg/800 mg every 12 hr	Uncomplicated cystitis; cost-effective
Nitrofurantoin	50–100 mg every 6 hr	Prophylaxis, uncomplicated cystitis
Tetracycline	250–500 mg every 6 hr	Prophylaxis
β-lactams[a]		
Amoxicillin	250–500 mg every 8 hr	During pregnancy, enterococcal infections
Cephalexin or cephradine	250 mg every 6 hr	During pregnancy, uncomplicated cystitis
Cefixime	200 mg every 12 h/400 mg every 24 hr	Step-down therapy[a]
Cefpodoxime	100–200 mg every 12 hr	Step-down therapy[a]
Fluoroquinolones		
Norfloxacin	400 mg every 12 hr	Low-serum drug levels
Ciprofloxacin	250–500 mg every 12 hr	First "systemic" fluoroquinolone
Lomefloxacin	400 mg every 24 hr	Skin photosensitivity reactions
Enoxacin	400 mg every 12 hr	P-450 drug interactions[b]
Ofloxacin	200–400 mg every 12 hr	Generally replaced by levofloxacin
Levofloxacin	250–500 mg every 24 hr	L-isomer of ofloxacin

Comments for miscellaneous agents and β-lactams relate to role in therapy. The role of fluoroquinolones has been for treatment of complicated UTIs and as an alternative agent for uncomplicated cystitis. Because these agents have not been rigorously compared, comments are related to general spectrum of activity, side effect profile, and drug interactions.
[a]Short-course therapy for uncomplicated cystitis has generally been less effective than the use of trimethoprim-sulfamethoxazole or fluoroquinolones for a similar duration. The general role of extended-spectrum oral cephalosporins (cefixime, cefpodoxime) has been for the treatment of complicated UTIs (alternative agent) and for intravenous to oral step-down therapy.
[b]Enoxacin is a potent inhibitor of P-450 hepatic isoenzymes. (Inhibition of hepatic isoenzymes causes an elevation of serum levels of theophylline and caffeine.)

E. coli. Tetracyclines (FDA category D), trimethoprim (FDA category C), and fluoroquinolones (FDA category C) should be avoided.

2. **Children.** Asymptomatic bacteriuria in preschool- and school-aged girls may signify underlying vesicoureteral reflux. Moreover, vesicoureteral reflux, when combined with recurring bacteriuria, can result in progressive renal scarring. Therefore, in this at-risk population, asymptomatic bacteriuria should routinely be detected and treated, with follow-up urologic evaluations after 6 weeks.

3. **General population.** Asymptomatic bacteriuria in men and nonpregnant women, a common condition in the elderly, does not appear to cause renal damage in the absence of obstructive uropathy or vesical ureteral reflux. Prospective randomized studies of therapy for asymptomatic bacteriuria in the elderly have been recently reviewed. Of five clinical trials reviewed, three studies had very small sample sizes, and one nonblinded study displayed a nonstatistical significant decrease in symptomatic infections. The largest randomized trial failed to demonstrate any significant difference in mortality between treated and untreated patients. Therefore, repeated attempts to clear

	TABLE 7-3	**Intravenous Antimicrobial Agents Commonly Used for Treatment of Urinary Tract Infections (Utis)**

	Adult dose	Comment
β-lactams		
Ampicillin	1–2 g every 4 hr	*Enterococcus faecalis;* usually combined with gentamicin
Ceftriaxone	1 g every 12–24 hr	Pyelonephritis
Ceftazidime	1–2 g every 8–12 hr	Complicated UTI, including *Pseudomonas aeruginosa*
Cefepime	1–2 g every 12 hr	Complicated UTI, including *Pseudomonas aeruginosa*
Aztreonam	1 g every 8–12 hr	Penicillin-allergic patient
Fluoroquinolones[a]		
Ciprofloxacin	200–400 mg every 12 hr	—
Ofloxacin	200–400 mg every 12 hr	Generally changed to levofloxacin
Levofloxacin	500 mg every 24 hr	—
Miscellaneous agents		
Trimethoprim-sulfamethoxazole	160 mg/800 mg every 12 hr	Prophylaxis, uncomplicated cystitis
Vancomycin	1 g every 12 hr	Methicillin-resistant *Staphylococcus aureus;* serious enterococcal infection in the penicillin-allergic patient
Gentamicin	4–7 mg/kg every 24 hr	Serious gram-negative infection
	1.5–2.0 mg/kg every 8 hr	Older dosing schedule; for enterococcus combined with ampicillin

[a]Because oral fluoroquinolones have excellent bioavailability and cost approximately 20% as much as parenteral fluoroquinolones, conversion from intravenous to oral therapy should be done when the patient is clinically stable.

the bacteriuria with antimicrobial agents seem unwarranted; they may only select for more resistant microorganisms and create a need for more toxic and costly antibiotics should the patient subsequently develop symptoms. Treatment of asymptomatic catheter-associated UTIs should be avoided due to the risk of developing a reservoir of resistant organisms.

4. **Miscellaneous.** Instrumentation of the genitourinary tract should be avoided in patients with asymptomatic bacteriuria or, if necessary, done under the cover of prophylactic antimicrobial therapy. Treatment of asymptomatic catheter-associated bacteriuria is recommended only for (a) patients undergoing urologic surgery or implantation of a prosthesis, (b) part of a treatment plan to control a virulent organism predominant in a treatment unit, (c) patients at risk for serious infectious complications, such as immunosuppressed individuals, and (d) treatment of pathogens associated with a high risk for bacteremia, such as *Serratia marcescens.*

D. **Treatment of uncomplicated cystitis.** Acute cystitis and low colony-count coliform urethritis are almost exclusively diseases of women, mostly sexually active women between the ages of 15 and 45 years. Although reinfection is common, complications are rare.

1. **Short-course therapy.** Appreciable evidence exists that infections truly confined to the bladder or urethra respond as well to single-dose or short-course (3-day) therapy as to conventional therapy for 10 to 14 days. Indeed, response to single-dose or short-course therapy implies a lower UTI. Reviews of short-course

therapy have concluded that 3-day regimens are more effective than single-dose therapy. One randomized trial evaluated four different 3-day drug regimens in women with uncomplicated acute cystitis. A 3-day regimen of trimethoprim-sulfamethoxazole was more effective than a 3-day regimen of nitrofurantoin. Cure rates for cefadroxil (66%) and amoxicillin (67%) were not statistically different from the cure rate for trimethoprim-sulfamethoxazole (82%). The 3-day regimen of trimethoprim-sulfamethoxazole was the most cost-effective regimen. IDSA guidelines recommend the use of oral 3-day regimens including trimethoprim-sulfamethoxazole or a fluoroquinolone. This variety of treatments is an important breakthrough in the management of uncomplicated cystitis and coliform urethritis, because all patients were treated formerly with the standard 10 to 14 days of therapy. Diabetic women with uncomplicated infections (i.e., with normal urinary tracts) may also be treated with a 3-day course of antibiotic therapy. Posttreatment urine cultures are not required unless symptoms persist. Formal urologic imagings, such as ultrasonography, IVP, and CT, are not needed in most cases because correctable abnormalities are rarely found.

2. **Seven-day regimen.** A longer course of therapy for cystitis should be considered in patients with complicating factors that lead to a lower success rate and a higher risk of relapse. These complicating factors include a history of prolonged symptoms (more than 7 days), recent UTI, diabetic patients with abnormal urinary tracts, age older than 65 years, and use of a diaphragm. Importantly, the elderly frequently have concurrent renal bacteriuria; therefore, short-course therapy should not be used.

3. **Symptomatic pyuria without bacteriuria** in an otherwise healthy young person suggests chlamydial or gonococcal urethritis. The importance of documenting these infections as well as screening for other STDs (e.g., human immunodeficiency virus infection, syphilis), and the necessity of counseling about STD risk reduction cannot be understated. Recent guidelines suggest that either a single dose of azithromycin or a 7-day course of doxycycline is effective for chlamydial urethritis. Therapy for gonococcal urethritis includes a single dose of ceftriaxone or cefixime, or a fluoroquinolone combined with therapy for chlamydial infection.

E. **Management of recurrent cystitis (reinfections).** Ten percent to 20% of women develop recurrent UTIs within several months. Some infections are related to inadequate antimicrobial therapy. It is common, however, for women whose periurethral and vaginal epithelial cells avidly support attachment of coliform bacteria to have recurrent episodes of cystitis in the absence of recognized structural abnormalities of the urinary tract. A recent prospective study of UTIs in young women identified recent use of a diaphragm and spermicide such as Nonoxynol-9, recent sexual intercourse, and a history of recurrent infection as risk factors for infection.

1. **Antimicrobial strategies.** Strategies for managing the disease of women with frequent episodes of cystitis include (a) postcoital prophylaxis, (b) continuous low-dose prophylaxis, (c) patient self-administered therapy, and (d) consideration of contraception or barrier methods against STDs without the use of vaginal spermicides. Postcoital prophylaxis is most helpful for patients who associate recurrent UTIs with sexual intercourse. In these women, a single dose of an antimicrobial after sexual intercourse or thrice weekly at bedtime has been shown to significantly reduce the frequency of episodes of cystitis from an average of 3 per patient-year to 0.1 per patient-year. Women with frequent recurrent infections (more than three UTIs per year) are offered these prophylactic regimens. Women with fewer than three UTIs per year can be offered self-administered treatment. Multiple antimicrobial agents have demonstrated efficacy in prophylaxis and self-administered therapy. Some of these regimens include nitrofurantoin, 50 or 100 mg; trimethoprim, 100 mg; trimethoprim-sulfamethoxazole, 40 mg per 200 mg; and cephalexin, 250 mg. Fluoroquinolones and cephalosporins are also effective but are more expensive. Although antimicrobial prophylaxis is effective and usually safely tolerated

for months to years, single-dose therapy for acute cystitis makes prophylaxis more expensive and possibly more hazardous for most patients because of alterations in fecal and vaginal bacterial flora. Indeed, self-administration of a single-dose regimen at the onset of symptoms has proved to be as cost effective as prophylaxis.

2. **Nonantimicrobial prophylaxis issues.** Encouraging women to practice regular and complete emptying of the bladder may help prevent recurrent cystitis. Postcoital emptying of the bladder has also been widely recommended, although one prospective study failed to demonstrate any relationship with recurrent infections. Moreover, several theoretic preventive measures relate to the use of an alternative contraceptive method: to use a properly fitted diaphragm, to void frequently when wearing a diaphragm, and to limit diaphragm use to the recommended 6 to 8 hours after intercourse. In postmenopausal women, intravaginal administration of estriol can reduce recurrent UTIs by modifying the milieu for vaginal flora. Cranberry juice (300 mL per day) was effective in decreasing asymptomatic bacteriuria with pyuria in postmenopausal women. The small difference in symptomatic UTIs was not statistically significant.

F. **Treatment of acute bacterial pyelonephritis.** The occurrence of flank pain, chills and fever, and nausea and vomiting with or without dysuria suggests acute bacterial pyelonephritis. In this clinical setting, blood cultures and quantitative cultures of urine should be obtained. Whether ambulatory patients should be admitted to the hospital for treatment depends in part on a subjective assessment of toxicity, likely compliance with therapy, and the home situation. When the assessment is doubtful, the patient should be treated in the hospital, at least until a clear response to therapy has occurred. This policy also applies to patients with known underlying uropathies because complications are more common in these patients.

1. **Outpatient therapy.** Recommendations for therapy of uncomplicated pyelonephritis are outlined in Table 7-4. Fluoroquinolone or trimethoprim-sulfamethoxazole is the drug of choice for initial therapy of pyelonephritis in outpatients. Local susceptibility patterns will influence the choice for initial therapy. After culture results and susceptibility tests are available, a full 10- to 14-day course of antimicrobial therapy may be completed with the least expensive drug to which the patient's microorganism is susceptible.

2. **Inpatient therapy.** Patients who require admission to the hospital should be treated initially with a third-generation cephalosporin or a fluoroquinolone (intramuscular or intravenous), or gentamicin or tobramycin (1.5 to 2.0 mg per kg every 8 hours or 4.0 to 7.0 mg per kg every 24 hours, with appropriate alteration of the dose interval if the serum creatinine exceeds 1 mg per dL) if the urine shows gram-negative bacilli on microscopical examination. If gram-positive cocci are seen in the urine, intravenous ampicillin (l g every 4 hours) should be given in addition to the aminoglycoside, to cover the possibility of enterococcal infection while the results of urine and blood cultures and antimicrobial susceptibility tests are pending. If no complications ensue and the patient becomes afebrile, the remaining days of a 10- to 14-day course can be completed with oral therapy. However, persistent fever, persistent bacteriuria in 48 to 72 hours, or continual signs of toxicity beyond 3 days of therapy suggest the need for an evaluation to exclude obstruction, metastatic focus, or the formation of a perinephric abscess. The urinary tract is a common source of sepsis and bacteremic shock in patients with underlying uropathies. As with other patients in septic shock, intravenous fluids must be given to maintain adequate arterial perfusion, which usually results in a urinary output in excess of 50 mL per hour. Failure to respond to seemingly appropriate therapy suggests the possibility of undrained pus. Examination by ultrasonography or CT may disclose an obstructed ureter or perinephric abscess, both of which require surgical drainage.

G. **Management of recurrent renal infections (relapses).** Chronic bacterial pyelonephritis is one of the most refractory problems in clinical medicine; relapse rates are as high as 90%. The entity is a heterogeneous one with multiple underlying factors.

TABLE 7-4   Recommendations for Therapy for Urinary Tract Infections

Infection	Group	Medication	Duration
Uncomplicated cystitis	Young women	Trimethoprim-sulfamethoxazole, trimethoprim, fluoroquinolone[a]	3 d
Cystitis	Women with risk factors including recent UTI, symptoms >7 d, diaphragm use, age older than 65 yr, diabetic patients with abnormal GU structures	Trimethoprim-sulfamethoxazole, trimethoprim, fluoroquinolone, nitrofurantoin, cephalosporins	7 d
	Pregnant women	Amoxicillin, cephalosporins[b], nitrofurantoin, sulfonamides, trimethoprim-sulfamethoxazole[c]	7 d
Acute uncomplicated pyelonephritis	Women (outpatient)	Fluoroquinolone, trimethoprim-sulfamethoxazole, oral cephalosporin[d]	10–14 d
	Women (inpatient)	Fluoroquinolone[e], ceftriaxone, ampicillin plus gentamicin[f], trimethoprim-sulfamethoxazole	14 d
Complicated infection	Outpatient	Fluoroquinolone	10–14 d
	Inpatient	Fluoroquinolone[e], cephalosporins[g], ampicillin plus gentamicin[f]	14 d

GU, genitourinary; UTI, urinary tract infection.
[a] Oral fluoroquinolones are listed in Table 7-2; they offer no significant advantage over trimethoprim-sulfamethoxazole in women with uncomplicated cystitis.
[b] Oral cephalosporins: cephradine, cephalexin.
[c] Trimethoprim-sulfamethoxazole has been used in pregnancy, but it has not been approved by the U.S. Food and Drug Administration for pregnant patients.
[d] Oral cephalosporins with an extended spectrum: cefpodoxime, loracarbef.
[e] Fluoroquinolones available for intravenous administration are listed in Table 7-3.
[f] Increasing ampicillin resistance among many enteric bacteria, including *Escherichia coli*, limits ampicillin as a single agent for complicated UTIs. If enterococcus is not likely, then a fluoroquinolone or a parenteral third- or fourth-generation cephalosporin is recommended.
[g] Some examples of parenteral cephalosporins are listed in Table 7-3.
(Adapted from Falagas ME. Practice guidelines: urinary tract infections. *Infect Dis Clin Pract* 1995;4:241–257; Kunin CM. *Detection, prevention, and management of urinary tract infections*, 5th ed. Philadelphia: Lea & Febiger, 1997; Stamm WE. Urinary tract infections. In: Root RK, ed. *Clinical infectious diseases: a practical approach*, 1st ed. New York: Oxford University Press, 1999.)

1. **Risk factors.** To improve the success rate, it is of utmost importance that any correctable lesion be repaired, that obstructions to urine flow be relieved, and that foreign bodies (e.g., indwelling urinary catheters or renal staghorn calculi) be removed if possible. If the risk factors cannot be corrected, long-term eradication of bacteriuria is almost impossible. To attempt eradication in such instances leads only to the emergence of more resistant strains of bacteria or fungi; consequently, the physician must be resigned to treating symptomatic episodes of infection and suppressing bacteriuria in selected patients.

2. **Acute symptomatic infection.** The treatment of the acute symptoms and signs of UTI in a patient with chronic renal bacteriuria is the same as for patients with acute bacterial pyelonephritis. Urine cultures to detect a possible change in antimicrobial susceptibility of the infecting microorganism are important. Toxic patients also should have blood cultures.

3. **Prolonged treatment.** Some patients with relapsing bacteriuria after 2 weeks of therapy respond to 6 weeks of antimicrobial therapy. This is especially true of patients with no underlying structural abnormalities. Men may require 6 to 12 weeks of antibiotic therapy for febrile UTIs because more than 90% have associated asymptomatic prostatitis. Patients who fail the longer therapy, who have repeated episodes of symptomatic infection, or who have progressive renal disease despite corrective measures are candidates for suppressive chemotherapy.

4. **Suppressive therapy.** To reduce the colony counts in their urine, patients selected for suppressive therapy should have 2 to 3 days of specific high-dose antimicrobial therapy, to which their infecting bacteria are susceptible. The preferred agent for long-term suppression is methenamine mandelate, 1 g four times daily in adults. To be most effective, the pH of the urine should be maintained below 5.5; this can be accomplished with ascorbic acid, 500 mg two to four times daily. Alternatively, the dosage of methenamine mandelate alone can be increased to 8 g or even 12 g per day. The dosage should be adjusted to the minimum amount required to keep the urine free of bacteria. To avoid metabolic acidosis, the dosage of methenamine mandelate must be reduced in patients with renal insufficiency, in whom 2 g per day may suffice. In these patients, methenamine mandelate should not be used at all unless the creatinine clearance exceeds 10 mL per minute. Alternative therapy is trimethoprim-sulfamethoxazole (160 mg/800 mg tablets twice daily) or nitrofurantoin (50 to 100 mg once or twice daily).

5. **Prognosis.** Although a common cause of appreciable morbidity, UTIs do not play a major role in the pathogenesis of end-stage renal disease. Patients who come to renal dialysis or transplantation because of chronic bacterial pyelonephritis almost always have an underlying structural defect. Most often, the lesion is chronic atrophic pyelonephritis associated with vesicoureteral reflux that started in infancy. The role of surgical correction of vesicoureteral reflux is not clear despite years of debate; what is certain, however, is the importance of meticulous control of infection in children to prevent progressive renal scarring and renal failure by early adulthood.

H. **Treatment of prostatitis**

1. **Acute bacterial prostatitis** is commonly accompanied by acute cystitis, which enables the recovery of its causative pathogen by culture of voided urine. Massage of an acutely inflamed prostate gland often results in bacteremia; therefore, this procedure should be avoided unless the patient is already receiving effective antibiotic therapy. Antimicrobial selection depends on the susceptibility pattern of the causative bacteria and the ability of the drug to achieve concentrations in the prostate that exceed the minimum inhibitory concentrations of the bacteria. The drug of choice most commonly is either the combination of trimethoprim-sulfamethoxazole (cotrimoxazole) or a fluoroquinolone; treatment, however, must be based ultimately on an accurate microbiological diagnosis. β-Lactam antibiotics should be avoided because of the low concentrations achieved in prostatic tissue and lower cure rates. Treatment should be given for 30 days to prevent chronic bacterial prostatitis. After acute symptoms

subside, a suitable oral antibiotic can be given in full dose for at least 30 days. Urethral catheterization should be avoided. If acute urinary retention develops, drainage should be by suprapubic needle aspiration or, if prolonged bladder drainage is required, by a suprapubic cystostomy tube, placed while the patient is under local anesthesia.

2. **Chronic bacterial prostatitis.** The hallmark of chronic bacterial prostatitis is relapsing UTI. It is most refractory to treatment. Although erythromycin with alkalinization of the urine has been effective against susceptible gram-positive pathogens, most instances of chronic bacterial prostatitis are caused by gram-negative enteric bacilli. Cotrimoxazole or a fluoroquinolone is the drug of choice. Approximately 75% of patients improve, and 33% are cured with 12 weeks of cotrimoxazole therapy (160 mg/800 mg twice daily). For patients who cannot tolerate cotrimoxazole or a fluoroquinolone, nitrofurantoin, 50 or 100 mg once or twice daily, can be used for long-term (6 to 12 months) suppressive therapy.

3. The therapy for **nonbacterial chronic prostatitis** is difficult because an exact etiology has not been identified. Owing to a concern for *C. trachomatis, Ureaplasma urealyticum,* and other fastidious and difficult to culture organisms, many experts recommend a 6-week trial of a tetracycline or erythromycin. Symptomatic therapy with nonsteroidal anti-inflammatory drugs (NSAIDs) and α-receptor blockers has also been used.

I. **Recommendations for the care of urinary catheters.** Urinary catheters are valuable devices for enabling drainage of the bladder and while they may be associated with asymptomatic bacteruria, their use is also associated with an appreciable risk, associated with an appreciable risk of infection in the urinary tract, specifically pyelonephritis. In addition, bacteremia and sepsis are recognized complications.

On August 1, 2007, the Centers for Medicare and Medicaid Services issued a decision to implement a modification to the Inpatient Prospective Payment System whereby additional payment for the complication or comorbidity of a catheter-related UTI will not be reimbursed. Therefore, it is imperative that guidelines for the prevention and expeditious treatment of catheter-related UTIs be enforced. In addition, documentation of an existing UTI at the time of admission is recommended.

For a single (in-and-out) catheterization, the risk is small (12%), though this prevalence is much higher in diabetic and elderly women. Intermittent catheterization is a safe alternative for patients in four situations: (a) children with neurogenic bladders (such as spina bifida), (b) uncontrolled reflex detrusor contraction resulting in incontinence in women, (c) chronic urinary retention due to ineffective or absent detrusor contraction, and (d) bladder outlet obstruction in men who are not surgical candidates.

In the absence of outlet obstruction, condom catheters are an alternative method of urinary drainage that has a lower incidence of bacteriuria.

Bacteriuria occurs in virtually all patients with indwelling urinary catheters within 3 to 4 days unless placement is done under sterile conditions and a sterile, closed drainage system is maintained (Fig. 7-4). The use of a neomycin-polymyxin irrigant does not prevent catheter-associated infections. To decrease the incidence of catheter-associated UTIs, use of suprapubic catheters, condom drainage systems, or intermittent catheters may be preferable in appropriate patients. Explicit recommendations for the prevention of catheter-associated UTIs, formulated by the Centers for Disease Control and Prevention, are as follows:

1. **Indwelling urinary catheters should be used only when absolutely necessary.** They should never be used solely for nurse or physician convenience and be removed as soon as possible. Duration of catheter use is the most important risk factor for the development of bacteriuria.

2. **Catheters should be inserted only by adequately trained personnel.** If practical, a team of individuals should be given responsibility for catheter insertion and maintenance.

3. **Urinary catheters should be aseptically inserted using proper sterile technique and the following sterile equipment:** gloves, a fenestrated drape,

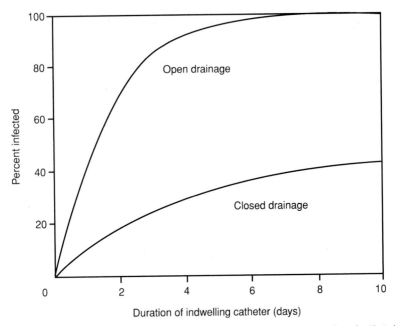

Figure 7-4. Prevalence of bacteriuria in catheterized patients according to duration of catheterization and type of drainage system. (From Fass RJ, Klainer AS, Perkins RL. Urinary tract infection: practical aspects of diagnosis and treatment. *JAMA* 1973;225:1509. Reprinted with permission.)

sterile sponges and an iodophor solution for periurethral cleansing, a lubricant jelly, and an appropriately sized urinary catheter. After insertion, catheters should be properly secured to prevent movement and urethral traction.

4. **Once- or twice-daily perineal care for catheterized patients** should include cleansing of the meatal-catheter junction with an antiseptic soap; subsequently, an antimicrobial ointment may be applied.

5. **A sterile closed drainage system should always be used.** The urinary catheter and the proximal portion of the drainage tube should not be disconnected (thereby opening the closed system) unless it is required for irrigation of an obstructed catheter. Sterile technique must be observed whenever the collecting system is opened and catheter irrigation is done. A large-volume sterile syringe and sterile irrigant fluid should be used and then discarded. If frequent irrigations are necessary to ensure catheter patency, a triple-lumen catheter that permits continuous irrigation within a closed system is preferable.

6. **Small volumes of urine for culture can** be aspirated from the distal end of the catheter with a sterile syringe and 21-gauge needle. The catheter must first be prepared with tincture of iodine or alcohol. Urine for chemical analyses can be obtained from the drainage bag in a sterile manner.

7. **Nonobstructed gravity flow must be maintained at all times.** This requires emptying the collecting bag regularly, replacing poorly functioning or obstructed catheters, and ensuring that collection bags always remain below the level of the bladder.

8. **All closed collecting systems contaminated by inappropriate technique, accidental disconnection, leaks, or other means should be immediately replaced.**

9. **Routine catheter change is not necessary** in patients with urinary catheterization of less than 2 weeks' duration, except when obstruction, contamination,

or other malfunction occurs. In patients with chronic indwelling catheters, replacement is necessary when concretions can be palpated in the catheter or when malfunction or obstruction occurs.

   10. Catheterized patients should be separated from each other whenever possible and should not share the same room or adjacent beds if other arrangements are available. Separation of patients with bacteriuria and those without it is particularly important.

   These guidelines should be adhered to meticulously, and the use of indwelling urinary catheters should be kept to a responsible minimum.

J. Catheter-associated infections. Catheter-associated bacteriuria should only be treated in the symptomatic patient. When the decision to treat a patient with a catheter-associated infection is made, removal of the catheter is an important aspect of therapy. If an infected catheter remains in place, relapsing infection is very common. The interaction between the organisms and catheter (foreign body) cause the organism to form a biofilm or area in which antibiotics are unable to completely eradicate these organisms. Recommendations for empiric therapy are similar to recommendations for complicated UTIs (Table 7-4). The choice of empiric therapy is based on an initial Gram's stain of the urine, local susceptibility patterns, host factors, and the patient's recent antibiotic use. The final choice of an antibiotic and duration of therapy should be based on the identification and susceptibility of the etiologic agent and the host's response to therapy. Patients who respond rapidly to therapy may be treated for 7 days although making firm conclusions about duration of therapy is very difficult.

   Patients with candiduria may fall into several different clinical categories. Otherwise healthy patients with asymptomatic candiduria often require only a urinary catheter change and may not require antifungal therapy. On the other end of the spectrum is the immunocompromised host, in whom candiduria may represent disseminated infection. The patient with disseminated candidiasis requires systemic therapy with either fluconazole or amphotericin B or a liposomal preparation of amphotericin. General recommendations for treating patients with candiduria and without evidence of disseminated infection include the removal of the urinary catheter and discontinuation of antibiotics. Antifungal options include either fluconazole (200 mg the first day, then 100 mg for 4 days), continuous bladder irrigation with amphotericin B (50 mg per 1,000 mL of sterile water through a three-way catheter for 5 days), or low-dose intravenous therapy with amphotericin (0.3 mg per kg in a single dose). Occasionally, longer systemic therapy with oral 5-fluorocytosine, intravenous amphotericin B, or both is required.

Suggested Readings

Ang BSP, Telenti A, King B, et al. Candidemia from a urinary source: microbiological aspects and clinical significance. *Clin Infect Dis* 1993;17:662–666.

Domingue GJ, Hellstrom WJG. Prostatitis. *Clin Microbiol Rev* 1998;11:604–613.

Edelstein H, McCabe RE. Perinephric abscess: modern diagnosis and treatment in 47 cases. *Medicine (Baltimore)* 1988;67:118–131.

Fihn SD. Acute uncomplicated urinary tract infection in women. *N Engl J Med* 2003; 349:259–266.

Fisher JF, Newman CL, Sobel JD. Yeast in the urine: solutions for a budding problem. *Clin Infect Dis* 1995;20:183–189.

Fowler JE Jr, Pulaski ET. Excretory urography, cystography, and cystoscopy in the evaluation of women with urinary-tract infection. *N Engl J Med* 1981;304:462–465.

Godfrey KM, Harding MD, Zhanel GG, et al. Antimicrobial treatment in diabetic women with asymptomatic bacteriuria. *N Engl J Med* 2002;347:1576–1583.

Gupta K, Hooton TM, Roberts PL, et al. Patient-initiated treatment of uncomplicated recurrent urinary tract infections in young women. *Ann Intern Med* 2001;135: 9–16.

Hooton TM, Fihn SD, Johnson C, et al. Association between bacterial vaginosis and acute cystitis in women using diaphragms. *Arch Intern Med* 1989;149:1932–1936.

Hooton TM, Scholes D, Hughes JP, et al. A prospective study of risk factors for symptomatic urinary tract infection in young women. *N Engl J Med* 1996;335:468–474.

Hooton TM, Winter C, Tiu F, et al. Randomized comparative trial and cost analysis of 3-day antimicrobial regimens for treatment of acute cystitis in women. *JAMA* 1995; 273:41–45.

Kincaid-Smith P, Becker G. Reflux nephropathy and chronic atrophic pyelonephritis: a review. *J Infect Dis* 1978;138:774–780.

Krieger JN. Complications and treatment of urinary tract infections during pregnancy. *Urol Clin North Am* 1986;13:685–693.

Kunin CM. *Detection, prevention, and management of urinary tract infections,* 5th ed. Philadelphia: Lea & Febiger, 1997.

Kunin CM, Chin QF, Chambers S. Indwelling urinary catheters in the elderly: relation of "catheter life" to formation of encrustations in patients with and without blocked catheters. *Am J Med* 1987;82:405–411.

Lachs MS, Nachamkin I, Edelstein PH, et al. Spectrum bias in the evaluation of diagnostic tests: lessons from the rapid dipstick test for urinary tract infection. *Ann Intern Med* 1992;117:135–140.

Lipsky BA, Baker CA. Fluoroquinolone toxicity profiles: a review focusing on new agents. *Clin Infect Dis* 1999;28:352–364.

Neuhauser MM, Weinstein RA, Rydman R, et al. Antibiotic resistance among gram-negative bacilli in US intensive care units: implications for fluoroquinolone use. *JAMA* 2003;289:885–888.

Nickel JC. The Pre and Post Massage Test (PPMT): a simple screen for prostatitis. *Tech Urol* 1997;3:38–43.

Nicolle LE. Asymptomatic bacteriuria in the elderly. *Infect Dis Clin North Am* 1997; 11:647–662.

Nicolle LE, Bradley S, Colgan R, et al. Infectious diseases society of american guidelines for the diagnosis and treatment of asymptomatic bacteriuria in adults. *Clin Infect Dis* 2005;40:643–654.

Nicolle LE, Bjornson J, Harding GK, et al. Bacteriuria in elderly institutionalized men. *N Engl J Med* 1983;309:1420–1425.

Nicolle LE, Harding GK, Preiksaitis J, et al. The association of urinary tract infection with sexual intercourse. *J Infect Dis* 1982;146:579–583.

Silverman DE, Stamey TA. Management of infection stones: the Stanford experience. *Medicine (Baltimore)* 1983;62:44–51.

Stamm WE. Guidelines for prevention of catheter-associated urinary tract infections. *Ann Intern Med* 1975;82:386–390.

Stamm WE, Counts GW, Wagner KF, et al. Antimicrobial prophylaxis of recurrent urinary tract infections: a double-blind, placebo-controlled trial. *Ann Intern Med* 1980;92:770–775.

Stapleton A, Latham R, Johnson C, et al. Postcoital antimicrobial prophylaxis for recurrent urinary tract infection: a randomized, double-blind, placebo-controlled trial. *JAMA* 1990;264:703–706.

Stapleton A, Stamm WE. Prevention of urinary tract infection. *Infect Dis Clin North Am* 1997;11:719–733.

Strom BL, Collins M, West SL, et al. Sexual activity, contraceptive use and other risk factors for symptomatic and asymptomatic bacteriuria: a case-control study. *Ann Intern Med* 1987;107:816–823.

Talan DA, Klimberg IW, Nicolle LE, et al. Once daily, extended release ciprofloxacin for complicated urinary tract infections and acute uncomplicated pyelonephritis. *J Urol* 2004;171(2):734–739.

Tenke P, Kovacs B, Bjerklund Johansen TE, et al. European and Asian guidelines on management and prevention of catheter-associated urinary tract infections. *Int J Antimicrob Agents* 2008;31 (Suppl 1):68–78.

Ulleryd P. Febrile urinary tract infection in men. *Int J Antimicrob Agents* 2003; 22:S89–S93.

Velasco M, Horcajada JP, Mensa J, et al. Decreased invasive capacity of quinolone-resistant Escherichia coli in patients with urinary tract infections. *Clin Infect Dis* 2001; 33:1682–1686.

Velasco M, Martinez JA, Moreno-Martinez A, et al. Blood cultures for women with uncomplicated acute pyelonephritis: are they necessary? *Clin Infect Dis* 2003;37: 1127–1130.

Wald HL, Kramer AM. Nonpayment for harms resulting from medical care: catheter-associated urinary tract infections. *J Am Med Assoc* 2007;298(23):2782–2784.

Warren JW. Catheter-associated urinary tract infections. *Infect Dis Clin North Am* 1997; 11(3):609–622.

Warren JW, Abrutyn E, Hebel JR, et al. Infectious Diseases Society of America (IDSA). Guidelines for antimicrobial treatment of uncomplicated acute bacterial cystitis and acute pyelonephritis in women. *Clin Infect Dis* 1999;29:745–758.

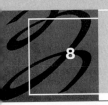

THE PATIENT WITH HEMATURIA, PROTEINURIA, OR BOTH, AND ABNORMAL FINDINGS ON URINARY MICROSCOPY

8

Sharon G. Adler and Kenneth Fairley

I. **URINE ANALYSIS.** A urine sample is usually easy to obtain, and it can be studied by very simple techniques on the ward or in the physician's office. Examination of the urine is one of the most rewarding steps in clinical medicine. Not only does it uncover renal parenchymal and urinary tract disease that eludes detection by other methods of investigation but it also frequently points to a specific diagnosis. Almost every patient with parenchymal renal disease shows abnormal findings on urine microscopy, an increase in urine protein, or both. Urine microscopy reveals abnormalities in many patients with renal disease who have no significant proteinuria. Many renal diseases that require treatment are first suspected on the basis of urinary findings—in particular, infections, glomerulonephritis, and interstitial nephritis.

A. **Method of collection of urine specimens.** The method of collecting a urine sample is of critical importance when the specimen is to be examined microscopically. For dipstick testing, the sample should be examined promptly for accurate results. Urine pH may change with time after collection, and contaminating bacteria multiply and convert nitrate to nitrite, causing a false-positive test result for bacteriuria. At low specific gravity (less than 1.010), cells lyse and casts form less readily. Casts also dissolve in alkaline urine.

   1. **Midstream urine collection.** In collecting urine for microscopical examination, avoiding contamination with bacteria, squamous cells, and leukocytes is important. Contamination is very common in women, in whom contaminating cells and bacteria arise in the vagina and vulval area. The important points in collecting a good midstream urine sample are shown in Table 8-1. Although bacteria are often detected on microscopy, infection is best proved by culture, which also allows the antibiotic sensitivity of infecting organisms to be determined. Special media are required for the culture of some organisms, such as the tubercle bacillus, *Mycoplasmas*, anaerobic organisms, and yeasts. Culture results are reported as colony-forming units (CFUs) per mL of urine; the significance of a count depends on the method of collection (Table 8-2).

   2. A catheter specimen in women is best collected as a **midcatheter specimen** using a short open-ended catheter. At least 200 mL must pass through the catheter to flush out contaminating urethral contents before the specimen is collected. Conventional "side hole" catheters push urethral contents into the bladder before urine can run out, and critical bacterial counts are 30-fold higher using a conventional catheter than those obtained on urine collected with an open-ended catheter.

   3. **Suprapubic aspiration.** A fine lumbar puncture needle with stylet in place is passed through sterilized suprapubic skin directly into a full bladder. Uncontaminated urine can then be aspirated.

B. **Dipstick testing.** Dipstick testing of urine provides a rapid determination of urine pH, specific gravity, and the presence of protein, blood (hemoglobin), leukocytes, nitrites, glucose, and bile. Dipsticks are less sensitive in detecting pyuria and bacteriuria.

   The method of screening for proteinuria is the examination of a randomly excreted urine sample by dipstick. Tetrabromophenol is buffered to a pH of 3, and this results in a yellow-to-green color that changes with increasing protein concentration. False-positive dipstick results for proteinuria are seen when urine pH is greater than or equal to 8 and when the patient is excreting metabolites of penicillins, aspirin, or oral hypoglycemic agents in the urine. Standard dipsticks for

TABLE 8-1	Guidelines for Collecting Midstream Urine Sample

Women
   When possible use a vaginal tampon
   Hold labia well separated during collection of the specimen
   Gently cleanse the periurethral area from anterior to posterior with several moistened gauze
      squares
Men
   Hold the retracted foreskin back throughout the collection
   Clean the urethral meatus with moist gauze
   If urethral or prostatic infection is suspected:
      The first 10 mL of voided urine reflects urethral infection (it also includes bladder contents)
      The midstream urine collected, as mentioned earlier, reflects the bladder contents
      Prostatic fluid, if available, reflects prostatic infection most accurately
      The first 10 mL of urine voided after prostatic massage provides information on infection
         in prostatic secretions (it also includes bladder contents)

In both sexes, at least 200 mL should be passed before a midstream urine specimen is collected without interruption of the flow of urine.

protein fail to detect very small quantities of abnormal albuminuria (e.g., microalbuminuria) and are relatively insensitive to even large amounts of nonalbumin protein. To alleviate the first of these shortcomings, dipsticks capable of detecting microalbuminuria are currently available and may be useful, when used properly, as a screening test to identify patients with diabetes mellitus and incipient nephropathy or to detect patients with a high risk of coronary artery and/or cerebrovascular disease. However, positive results from these dipsticks require confirmation by an enzyme-linked immunosorbent assay (ELISA) test. Dipsticks that are more sensitive to nonalbumin proteins are under development. Currently, a 24-hour urine collection is required to detect such proteins.

    Urine color varies with its concentration and with the presence of drugs such as phenazopyridine (Pyridium), phenindione, and multivitamin tablets, and of blood, bile, porphyrin, melanin, and homogentisic acid. Some of these color changes may be mistaken for hematuria. Dipstick examination of the urine accurately determines the presence of hemoglobin, which depends on the oxidation of orthotolidine by cumene hydroperoxide, although cross-reactivity with myoglobin does occur. Although the microscopic examination of urine for erythrocytes provides far more information about the underlying renal lesion, a dipstick is quick, simple, and provides quantitative information. The Ames N Multistix and Boehringer nephron

TABLE 8-2	Influence of Collection Technique on Accuracy of Detection of Urine Abnormalities

Collection technique	Hematuria	Pyuria	Significant bacteriuria (CFU/mL)	Fastidious microorganisms
Midstream urine	Excellent	Fair[a]	>100,000	Poor
Open-ended catheter	Good	Very good	>1,000	Good
Suprapubic aspiration	Poor	Excellent	>1	Excellent

CFU, colony-forming unit.
[a]Depends on collection technique.

tests provide sensitive and specific methods of detecting microscopical hematuria. Ascorbic acid, a strong reducing agent, prevents the chemical reaction in dipsticks that detects hemoglobin and is the cause of many false-negative test results. In the case of a low–specific-gravity urine (below 1.010), lysis of erythrocytes leads to false-negative microscopy, but the dipsticks provide a positive test result.

C. **Microscopic analysis.** In the United States, urine is characteristically examined using a standard light microscope to make a semiquantitative estimate of the frequency of the formed elements in the urine by counting their number per high-power field. More quantitative measures can be obtained by examining the urine on a coverslipped counting chamber rather than on a plain glass slide. The counting-chamber method is more accurate, largely because it eliminates the error introduced by the variability of the depth of the layer of urine on the slide, which occurs as a function of viscosity. The accuracy of the microscopic examination can also be enhanced by using phase-contrast microscopy, which allows for more sensitivity in the observation of morphologic detail. If a phase-contrast microscope is unavailable, staining the urine sediment with Sternheimer-Malbin stain may also enhance visualization of cellular elements using a standard light microscope.

Most large clinical laboratories now perform the microscopic examination of the urine with automated analyzers utilizing flow cytometry. These accurately quantify urine elements such as epithelial, red and white blood cells, but a qualitative morphologic assessment is not performed. Therefore, a distinction between dysmorphic glomerular hematuria and eumorphic hematuria of lower tract origin still requires manual examination. In addition, the assessments of bacteriuria, crystalluria, budding yeast, and cellular as well as noncellular casts are still better evaluated manually than by automated analyzers.

1. **Hematuria.** A large amount of blood present in the urine is obvious to the naked eye. The red blood cell count in such cases is always well above 10^6 cells per mL. The morphology and quantitation of the urinary erythrocytes are two of the most important investigations in clinical nephrology. They not only provide information about the underlying cause but also assist in determining the nature of investigations required. Because the recognition that glomerular bleeding can be determined by the appearance of erythrocytes on phase-contrast microscopy, prompt assessment of the number and morphology of urinary erythrocytes has assumed new significance. In the case of crescentic glomerulonephritis, which can be suspected when red blood cell casts and large numbers of dysmorphic erythrocytes are seen on urine microscopy, the physician is alerted to the urgent need for biopsy confirmation and appropriate treatment.

   A high count of glomerular erythrocytes (more than 10^6 red blood cells per mL) has both prognostic and therapeutic implications, because it suggests the presence of crescents on renal biopsy. If 4+ dipstick testing for heme is present, immediate urine microscopy is indicated to determine the nature and hence the source of erythrocytes, and, if possible, the count per milliliter. The source of erythrocytes can be determined by measuring their size and by examining their morphology. After centrifuging the urine specimen, if a red pellet results, adequate numbers of erythrocytes are present to measure their volume in an automated counter of the type customarily used for complete blood counts (CBCs). If the urinary erythrocyte mean corpuscular volume is less than 72 fL, a glomerular bleeding source is likely.

   The best method for assessing erythrocyte morphology is phase-contrast microscopy. If bright-field illumination is used, many erythrocytes will not be correctly identified. In particular, those that have lost their hemoglobin staining are not seen, a common occurrence in an acid urine. The small and distorted erythrocytes characteristic of glomerular bleeding may also be missed. Characteristic dysmorphic erythrocytes, which indicate that hematuria is arising in glomeruli, are illustrated in Figure 8-1. These vary considerably in size, shape, and hemoglobin content, and many bizarre forms are present. Normal urine contains up to 8,000 glomerular erythrocytes per mL in a centrifuged specimen and 13,000 per mL in uncentrifuged urine. Erythrocytes arising from a

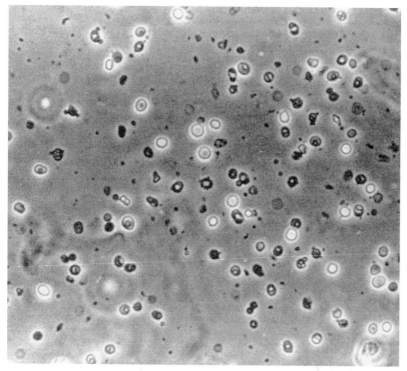

Figure 8-1. Erythrocytes, showing the wide variation in size, shape, and hemoglobin content, in the urine of a patient with glomerulonephritis (phase-contrast microscopy). (From Fairley KF. Urinalysis. In: Schrier RW, Gottschalk CW, eds. *Diseases of the kidney*, 4th ed. Boston: Little, Brown and Company, 1988. Reprinted with permission.)

nonglomerular source are uniform in size and shape but may show some "ghost cells," cells that are losing their hemoglobin (Fig. 8-2). The latter change occurs particularly in an acid urine.

2. **Urinary casts.** Casts are formed from Tamm-Horsfall glycoprotein, which is synthesized and secreted in the ascending limb of the loop of Henle and distal convoluted tubules.

   a. Physiologic casts. Hyaline casts are transparent and cylindrical and are seen in the urine of healthy subjects. Their presence does not indicate renal disease. Granular casts are semitransparent cylinders with refractile granules of uncertain origin. These, too, are present in individuals without renal disease. The number of hyaline and granular casts in urine may be increased by fever, exercise, and volume depletion.

   b. Pathologic casts. Casts may contain cellular material (erythrocytes, leukocytes, tubular cells, bacteria, or fungi), fibrin, lipids, bile, and crystals.

   The most important cellular cast is that composed of erythrocytes (Fig. 8-3). This indicates glomerular bleeding, as do erythrophagocytic cells. Large numbers of erythrocyte casts also increase the likelihood of crescents in glomeruli. Casts composed of polymorphonuclear leukocytes usually indicate renal parenchymal infection. These may also be seen in acute interstitial nephritis and occasionally in glomerular lesions, where numerous polymorphonuclear leukocytes are in glomeruli. Casts may also contain all varieties of mononuclear leukocytes and may include tubular epithelial cells from all segments of the nephron. In nephrotic

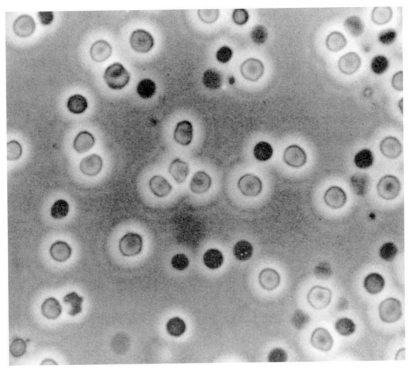

Figure 8-2. Nonglomerular bleeding, showing two populations of cells (phase-contrast microscopy). (From Fairley KF. Urinalysis. In: Schrier RW, Gottschalk CW, eds. *Diseases of the kidney*, 4th ed. Boston: Little, Brown and Company, 1988. Reprinted with permission.)

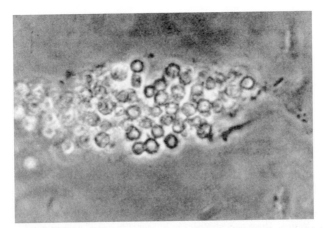

Figure 8-3. An erythrocyte cast in an acid urine, composed of red cells from which much of the hemoglobin has disappeared. (From Fairley KF. Urinalysis. In: Schrier RW, Gottschalk CW, eds. *Diseases of the kidney*, 4th ed. Boston: Little, Brown and Company, 1988. Reprinted with permission.)

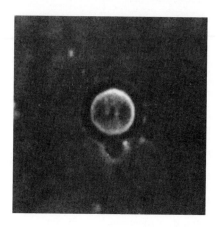

Figure 8-4. A cholesterol ester spherulite approximately the same size as an erythrocyte. (From Fairley KF. Urinalysis. In: Schrier RW, Gottschalk CW, eds. *Diseases of the kidney*, 4th ed. Boston: Little, Brown and Company, 1988. Reprinted with permission.)

syndrome, all casts usually contain fat particles and some contain oval fat bodies. Because the fat bodies consist of cholesterol esters, they can be easily identified by their "Maltese cross" birefringence (Figs. 8-4 and 8-5). Many fat bodies, however, are composed of fat particles too small to show crosses, and these appear as a faint glow in polarized light.

Crystals in casts are commonly present in patients who are taking triamterene. The crystals disappear when the urine is alkalinized or the drug is discontinued. Crystals may also occasionally be present in casts in patients with hypercalcemia or hyperuricosuria, or as an isolated finding.

Broad waxy casts signify chronic renal disease. These typically have a very sharp border and are easily seen with bright-field illumination. They do not dissolve in alkaline urine.

3. **Leukocytes and nucleated cells in the urine.**   Normal midstream urine contains up to 2,000 nucleated cells per mL, and most of these are leukocytes. Normal bladder urine obtained by needle aspiration contains very low counts of leukocytes (mean, 283 per mL, with only 2 of 25 urine samples containing more than 1,000 per mL). In one author's (Kenneth Fairley) laboratory, the mean count in a midstream specimen in the same subjects performed at the same time was 2,018 leukocytes per mL, even when meticulous care was taken to avoid contamination. The additional cells in the midstream sample presumably arise in the urethra.

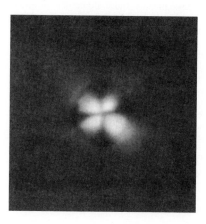

Figure 8-5. The particle in Figure 8-4, when viewed with polarized light, shows the classic "Maltese cross." (From Fairley KF. Urinalysis. In: Schrier RW, Gottschalk CW, eds. *Diseases of the kidney*, 4th ed. Boston: Little, Brown and Company, 1988. Reprinted with permission.)

An increase in the leukocyte count in the urine most commonly implies infection. Infected urines show an increase in leukocytes in more than 90% of cases. When pyuria is present without bacteriuria, three-fourths of patients show an underlying urinary tract abnormality.

Sterile pyuria may be seen in tuberculosis, renal papillary necrosis, acute interstitial nephritis, urate nephropathy, glomerulonephritis, and polycystic disease of the kidney. It may also be present in patients with calculi and in a variety of other urinary tract abnormalities. Before a diagnosis of sterile pyuria is made, fastidious organisms such as ureaplasmas, anaerobic bacteria such as *Gardnerella vaginalis*, and chlamydia should be sought in an appropriate specimen using special culture techniques.

When it is difficult to distinguish leukocytes from renal tubular epithelial cells, a drop of acetic acid makes it easier to recognize the lobed nuclei of polymorphonuclear leukocytes. Staining the cells also distinguishes them.

4. **Renal tubular cells.** Large numbers of renal tubular cells are found in the urine in acute tubular necrosis and acute interstitial nephritis. Acute interstitial nephritis can be distinguished by a much higher count of leukocytes (more than 15,000 per mL) and a higher total nucleated cell count (more than 75,000 per mL) than are seen in acute tubular necrosis. Eosinophils are present in the urine in most cases of interstitial nephritis, in counts above 5,000 per mL; these are rare in acute tubular necrosis. Eosinophils in the urine are best seen with Hansel's stain, which, unlike Wright's stain, is not pH dependent.

Nucleated cells are also present in the urine in glomerulonephritis, particularly crescentic glomerulonephritis, in which total cell counts, leukocytes, and renal tubular cells are present in higher numbers than in noncrescentic glomerulonephritis. Glomerular epithelial cells identified by monoclonal antibody staining for podocyte-specific proteins such as nephrin are also present in a much higher percentage of urines from patients with crescentic glomerulonephritis than from those with noncrescentic glomerulonephritis.

5. **Crystals.** Although crystals of calcium oxalate and uric acid may be seen in normal urine samples, large, bizarre crystals of any type, including calcium oxalate and uric acid, usually indicate increased urinary excretion and may indicate calculous disease. Cystine crystals are always abnormal and indicate cystinuria.

II. HEMATURIA

A. **Localization and differential diagnosis.** An abnormal quantity of erythrocytes in the urine can either be due to a glomerular disorder or to nonglomerular bleeding. Glomerular bleeding should be suspected if any of the following are present: dysmorphic urinary erythrocytes, erythrocytes with mean corpuscular volume less than 72 fL, red blood cell casts, and concomitant proteinuria, especially higher than 1 g per day. In Table 8-3, an asterisk denotes those glomerular disorders that frequently manifest hematuria. Nonglomerular hematuria is characterized by the presence of isomorphic urinary erythrocytes with a mean corpuscular volume of more than 72 fL in the absence of red blood cell casts or significant proteinuria. The further localization of nonglomerular bleeding can be suggested by the three-glass test. In this procedure, patients with macroscopic hematuria urinate 10- to 15-mL aliquots of urine each into three containers. A urethral site of bleeding is suggested if the hematuria predominates in the first 10 mL, whereas a bladder origin is implied if most of the blood is in the final aliquot. Upper tract bleeding is characterized by hematuria in all three collection vessels. The differential diagnosis of nonglomerular proteinuria is outlined in Table 8-4. Many of these disorders are either characterized by or occasionally present with hematuria.

B. **Clinical evaluation and treatment.** Patients with hematuria may present with quantities of blood visible to the naked eye (macroscopic or gross hematuria) or visible only by microscopic examination (microscopic hematuria). The initial evaluation of the patient with gross or microscopic hematuria should include those steps outlined earlier to distinguish glomerular from nonglomerular causes. If a

TABLE 8-3   Causes of Glomerular Proteinuria

"Primary" glomerular disorders
  Minimal change, mesangial proliferative (IgA, IgM[a]), focal and segmental
  glomerulosclerosis,[a] membranous, membranoproliferative,[a] crescentic[a]
Hereditary
  Alport's syndrome,[a] Fabry's disease,[a] nail-patella syndrome[a]
Infectious
  Bacterial,[a] viral,[a] fungal,[a] protozoal,[a] and helminthic[a] causes, including bacterial
  endocarditis,[a] poststreptococcal glomerulonephritis,[a] visceral abscesses,[a] secondary
  syphilis,[a] hepatitis B and C,[a] human immunodeficiency virus,[a] malaria[a]
Metabolic
  Diabetes mellitus
Immunologic
  Systemic lupus erythematosus,[a] mixed connective tissue disease, Sjögren's syndrome,
  Henoch-Schönlein purpura,[a] Wegener granulomatosis,[a] microscopic polyarteritis
  nodosa,[a] Goodpasture's syndrome,[a] cryoglobulinemia[a]
Medications
  Penicillamine, gold- or mercury-containing compounds, lithium, nonsteroidal
  anti-inflammatory drugs, angiotensin-converting enzyme inhibitors, heroin[a]
Neoplasms
  Multiple myeloma[a]; colon, lung, or breast carcinoma; lymphoma; leukemia
Miscellaneous
  Sickle cell disease,[a] allergies,[a] immunizations,[a] cirrhosis,[a] immunotactoid
  glomerulopathy,[a] amyloidosis,[a] reflux nephropathy,[a] congenital nephrotic syndrome

IgA, immunoglobulin A; IgM, immunoglobulin M.
[a]Denotes glomerular disorders that frequently present with hematuria.

TABLE 8-4   Causes of Tubular Proteinuria

Hereditary
  Polycystic kidney disease, medullary cystic disease
Infectious
  Pyelonephritis, tuberculosis
Metabolic
  Diabetes mellitus, hyperuricemia, uricosuria, hypercalcemia, hypercalciuria, hypokalemia,
  oxalosis, cystinosis
Immunologic
  Sjögren's syndrome, renal transplant rejection, drug hypersensitivity, sarcoidosis
Toxic
  Analgesic abuse, radiation nephritis, lithium, heavy metals (lead, cadmium, mercury),
  Balkan nephritis, cyclosporine, cisplatinum, aminoglycosides
Anatomic
  Obstruction, ureterovesical reflux, medullary sponge kidney
Miscellaneous
  Multiple myeloma, amyloidosis, sickle cell disease, medullary sponge kidney

glomerular cause is suspected, patients should be further evaluated as described in section III.C.

For patients who have been determined to have nonglomerular hematuria, the differential diagnosis outlined in Table 8-4 may be narrowed by obtaining a relevant history and physical examination. The history and review of systems should include questions regarding passage in the urine of stones, tissue, or blood clots; frequent urinary tract infections (UTIs); episodic gross hematuria; fever; weight loss; medication or drug use, particularly oral contraceptives or analgesics; dysuria; tuberculosis; diabetes mellitus; trauma; coagulation disorders; and family history of renal disease. Pertinent aspects of the physical examination should include auscultation for renal bruits, palpation of the prostate for nodules or prostatitis, and palpation of the abdomen for enlarged kidneys indicative of polycystic kidney disease.

Table 8-5 outlines a suggested diagnostic approach to the patient with nonglomerular hematuria. Initial laboratory studies should include a CBC, international normalized ratio (INR), prothrombin time, and partial thromboplastin time to rule out coagulopathy and hemoglobinopathy. A serum chemistry panel is useful to determine the level of renal function and to rule out the presence of hypercalcemia,

TABLE 8-5   **A Diagnostic Approach in the Patient with Nonglomerular Hematuria**

Urinary findings
No erythrocyte casts
Urinary RBC of normal morphology
Proteinuria <1 g/d/1.73 m^2
Urinary RBC >72 fL
↓

Urine culture and sensitivity, acid-fast bacteria × 3	Diagnostic → → →	Urinary tract infection
Prostate examination		Tuberculosis
Cytology		Tumors
↓		
Nondiagnostic		
↓		
Intravenous urography (or ultrasonography)	Diagnostic → → →	Cystic disorders
		Intrarenal tumors
		Calculi
↓		Papillary necrosis
Nondiagnostic		Trauma/fracture
		Medullary sponge kidney
↓		Horseshoe kidney
Cystoscopy/retrogrades	Diagnostic → → →	Urethral lesions
		Cystitis
↓		Collecting system/bladder tumors
Nondiagnostic		
↓		
Angiography	Diagnostic → → →	Ureteral varices
		Aneurysm
		Arteriovenous malformation

RBC, red blood cells.

hyperuricemia, and hyperglycemia. Urine should be cultured for bacterial and mycobacterial infection and, if clinically suspected, mycoplasma or other more fastidious organisms. Once a UTI has been excluded, an examination of the urinary tract anatomy should be undertaken to define the bleeding site. In the presence of normal or near-normal glomerular filtration rate (GFR), intravenous urography remains the most useful diagnostic radiologic procedure available for defining renal anatomy. It should disclose the presence of renal cysts (hereditary and acquired); calculi; papillary necrosis; medullary sponge kidney; renal, pelvic, and ureteral tumors; and ureteral strictures. In the event of a nondiagnostic intravenous urographic study, cystoscopy can be performed to more definitively examine the bladder for the presence of tumors or infectious (inflammatory/interstitial) cystitis and the urethra for the presence of urethritis, strictures, or both. A nondiagnostic cystoscopic examination can be followed, if clinically indicated, by arteriography to pursue the possibility that hematuria is secondary to ureteral varices or aneurysms, arteriovenous malformations, or the loin pain hematuria syndrome.

The treatment of hematuric states is entirely dependent on the underlying cause of erythrocyturia. The reader is therefore referred to textbooks of internal medicine, nephrology, and urology for detailed coverage of these topics. In this section, however, UTIs are discussed briefly, because they are commonly encountered by the general practitioner as well as by the specialist.

The most common presentation with UTI is dysuria and frequency in a woman of childbearing years. The urine may show macroscopic or heavy nonglomerular microscopic hematuria, as well as pyuria and bacteriuria. Some have recently advocated that even in patients with diabetes, pyuria without clinical signs or symptoms of infection should not be treated with antibiotics. In those in whom treatment is indicated, a single dose of an appropriate antibiotic (e.g., 2 g of amoxicillin or ampicillin) cures the infection in 80% of cases. Antibiotic resistance may be responsible for some treatment failure (e.g., ampicillin-resistant *Escherichia coli*). However, unresponsiveness to treatment may be an indication for further investigation, because a high percentage of those who do not respond to a single dose show abnormalities on further investigation by imaging techniques, such as intravenous urography. Failure to respond to treatment may also suggest an upper rather than lower UTI.

UTI in a child or a man should always be investigated, because of the high incidence of underlying abnormalities. Infection in the presence of an underlying urinary tract abnormality usually requires longer courses of treatment. Eradicating the infection without removing the abnormality may be impossible in some cases, notably with infected stones or staghorn calculi.

III. PROTEINURIA

A. Biochemical evaluation. Although not specific for glomerular disease, an abnormal amount of protein excreted in the urine is a cardinal manifestation of disease in virtually all patients with glomerulonephritis. Fever, exercise, hyperglycemia, and severe hypertension can transiently increase proteinuria.

To precisely quantitate and qualitatively analyze the amount and composition of urinary proteins, an examination of a 24-hour collection of urine is usually required. The collection method involves emptying the bladder and discarding the first urine on the morning of collection, and scrupulously collecting all subsequent urine for the next 24 hours. The final urine at the end of the 24-hour period is also kept as part of the collection. If the urine is refrigerated during the 24-hour period, no preservative is required. If refrigeration is unavailable, a preservative such as acetic acid (or a cup of vinegar) can be added to the collection vessel.

Quantification of the 24-hour urine creatinine should be performed to ensure that a complete collection was submitted. The normal 24-hour urine protein excretion in the adult ranges from 30 to 130 mg. Children and adolescents may excrete as much as twice this amount. In female patients under steady-state conditions of renal function, the 24-hour urinary excretion of creatinine should equal approximately 15 to 20 mg per kg of ideal body weight; in male patients, the excretion should be approximately 18 to 25 mg per kg. Accurate quantitative methods of protein excretion by precipitation include the sulfosalicylic acid precipitation test, the micro-Kjeldahl method, Esbach's picric acid–citric acid reagent, and the biuret method. Results are expressed either as grams excreted in 24 hours or as a ratio of protein to creatinine excretion.

In the initial evaluation and/or the follow-up of patients with heavy proteinuria (e.g., when assessing responsiveness to therapy), the urinary protein–creatinine concentration ratio or urinary albumin–creatinine concentration ratio are useful substitutes for repeated full 24-hour urine collections. Normal spot urinary protein–creatinine ratios on random samples generally fall below 0.2 (assuming that both the protein and the creatinine concentrations are expressed in mg per dL units). Values higher than 3 suggest the presence of nephrotic-range proteinuria. Normal spot urinary albumin–creatinine ratios on random samples generally fall below 0.03 (assuming that both the albumin and the creatinine concentrations are expressed in mg per dL units).

Qualitative assessments of urinary protein composition are often a valuable addition to the quantitative examination. Urine protein electrophoresis (UPEP) separates urinary proteins on the basis of molecular weights into five peaks: albumin and α_1, α_2, β, and γ globulins. Normally, urinary proteins are composed of filtered proteins from plasma (50%) and proteins that are secreted into the urine from urinary tract cells (50%). Of the filtered proteins, albumin is the most abundant, representing approximately 15% of the total urinary protein. This is followed by immunoglobulins (Igs) (5%), light chains (5%), β_2 microglobulin (less than 0.2%), and other plasma proteins (25%). Of the secreted proteins, Tamm-Horsfall protein enters the urine after synthesis in the tubular cells of the ascending limb of the loop of Henle. It is the single most abundant protein in normal urine, accounting for 50% of the total urinary protein.

UPEP and immunoelectrophoresis (IEP) can be helpful in identifying the nature of proteins present in the urine. Immunofixation may be more sensitive than either of the two latter methods. Examining the urine for Bence-Jones proteinuria by seeking urinary precipitates at $45°$C to $55°$C that redissolve at a higher temperature is a less sensitive method than are UPEP, IEP, and immunofixation for identifying overflow proteinuria. It is essentially only of historical interest.

B. Pathophysiologic classification of proteinuria. Given the diverse sources of urinary proteins and the implication of source for the site of pathology, proteinuria is classified into three major categories reflecting pathogenesis.

1. **Overflow proteinuria** is due to the filtration by the normal glomerulus of an abnormally large amount of small molecular weight protein present in serum whose filtration exceeds the capacity of normal tubules for reabsorption. This occurs in monoclonal gammopathies (such as multiple myeloma), in intravascular hemolysis (hemoglobinuria), and in rhabdomyolysis (myoglobinuria). Overflow proteinuria can be identified by an abnormal peak or "spike" on the UPEP. For example, a "spike" occurring in the γ region (or, less commonly, in the α_2 or β region) suggests the presence of a monoclonal gammopathy. Further identification of the protein can be accomplished by performing IEP or immunofixation.

2. **Tubular proteinuria** is found in both acute and chronic injuries involving the renal tubulointerstitial region. Usually quantitatively less than 2 g per day, tubular proteinuria is derived from three sources. First, injured tubules fail to completely reabsorb small molecular weight proteins filtered by the glomerulus, such as β_2 microglobulin and amylase. Second, injured tubules secrete brush border components and cellular enzymes, such as N-acetylglucosamine and lysozyme, into the urine. Finally, with tubulointerstitial injury, Tamm-Horsfall protein may be secreted into the urine in greater amounts by the tubular cells of the ascending limb of the loop of Henle and the distal nephron. UPEP, IEP, and immunofixation may also aid in distinguishing glomerular from tubular proteinuria. The overwhelming predominance of albumin rather than globulins on a UPEP suggests the presence of glomerular proteinuria. A quantitative comparison of the urinary albumin and β_2 microglobulin levels performed by IEP or other

immunologic techniques (including immunoprecipitation, immunodiffusion, or radioimmunoassay) may also be helpful in this regard. A urinary albumin to β_2 microglobulin ratio of 10:1 suggests the presence of tubular proteinuria, whereas in glomerular proteinuria, this ratio usually exceeds 1,000:1. In normal urine, the albumin to β_2 microglobulin ratio ranges from 50:1 to 200:1.

3. **Glomerular proteinuria** occurs when injury to the glomerulus results in an ultra-filtrate characterized by a fractional increase in the clearance of serum proteins. In some forms of glomerulonephritis, this is due to changes in the size-selective properties of the glomerular capillary wall that allow the passage of larger molecular weight proteins or even of cells (e.g., in crescentic glomerulonephritis). In other forms, this has been ascribed to changes in the charge-selective properties of the glomerular capillary wall that enhance the ultrafiltration of negatively charged albumin (e.g., minimal change nephropathy), although the existence of the charge-selective barrier at the level of the glomerular capillary wall has recently come into question. Some glomerular disorders are characterized by changes in both size and charge selectivity (e.g., diabetic nephropathy). Mesangial injury may also induce proteinuria, perhaps by interfering with normal mesangial clearance functions.

Glomerular proteinuria is composed predominantly of albumin and, when quantitatively large (i.e., more than 3.0 to 3.5 g per day, or more than 2 g per day per m^2), it is said to be in the nephrotic range. The nephrotic syndrome consists of a pentad of nephrotic-range proteinuria, hypoalbuminemia, hyperlipidemia, lipiduria, and edema. With the exception of minimal change glomerulopathy, the occurrence of heavy proteinuria in glomerular disorders is associated with a higher risk for progressive renal insufficiency.

4. **Other types of proteinuria.** Two forms of proteinuria do not fit easily into the classification described earlier. Benign orthostatic proteinuria is typically found in tall adolescents and occurs when the patient is in the lordotic position. Protein is found in the urine collected on retiring and in the morning after the patient has been ambulant, but not in the overnight specimen collected immediately on rising. No abnormality should be present in the urine sediment, and proteinuria should not exceed 1 g per day. In one-half of these patients, proteinuria disappears within 10 years; however, in a small proportion, overt renal disease develops in later life. Finally, functional, transient proteinuria may be associated with such diverse causes as cardiac failure, fever, or heavy exercise. It disappears within hours of cessation of exercise and with resolution of the disease process. Proteinuria after marathon running may be as heavy as 5 g per L of urine.

C. **Clinical evaluation and treatment.** The most important first step in the development of an appropriate differential diagnosis and subsequent treatment plan for patients with proteinuria is classification of the urinary protein.

1. **Classification of proteinuria**

   a. **Overflow proteinuria.** The presence of overflow is suggested by a disparity characterized by a small amount of proteinuria demonstrated by dipstick and a disproportionately larger amount measured on a 24-hour collected specimen. This is most often due to excretion of monoclonal light chains, which can be confirmed by IEP or immunofixation. Identification of a monoclonal Ig in the urine should stimulate diagnostic testing for multiple myeloma, amyloidosis, or a lymphoproliferative disorder. Hemoglobinuria and myoglobinuria can also cause overflow proteinuria. However, these are readily identifiable, because in these conditions the dipstick for blood is strongly positive, whereas the microscopical examination of urine demonstrates few or no red blood cells. This finding should stimulate an evaluation for hemolysis and for rhabdomyolysis.

   b. **Tubular proteinuria.** A wide range of conditions can cause tubulointerstitial injury (Table 8-4). An investigation of tubular proteinuria should begin with a detailed history regarding other affected family members (to rule out polycystic kidney disease); prescribed or over-the-counter medication use (analgesic nephropathy); frequent UTIs (reflux); flank pain; passage of renal stones; skin rash, arthralgias, arthritis (drug hypersensitivity, rheumatological immune diseases); dry mouth or eyes (Sjögren's syndrome); occupational or recreational exposure to potential toxins; and manifestations of systemic disease. Physical findings confirmatory of disorders in the differential diagnosis listed in Table 8-4 should be sought. These might include palpably enlarged kidneys (polycystic kidney disease), band keratopathy (hypercalcemia, hyperparathyroidism), skin rash (systemic lupus, drug hypersensitivity), arthritis (gout, lupus, rheumatoid arthritis), or oral mucosal lead line (lead toxicity). Laboratory tests including CBC with examination of the peripheral smear; measurements of serum creatinine, urea nitrogen, glucose, calcium, phosphorus, uric acid, and potassium; and urine culture are adjunctive information to the history, physical examination, urinalysis, and quantitative urine studies in focusing the differential diagnosis. Positive or negative results in these areas may suggest the need for further tests, which may include renal ultrasonography (polycystic kidney disease, renal stones, obstruction); urine, serum, or hemoglobin electrophoresis (monoclonal gammopathy, sickle cell disease, or trait); urine culture and sensitivity (pyelonephritis, renal tuberculosis); serum angiotensin-converting enzyme level (sarcoidosis); intravenous urography (medullary sponge kidney); or serum lead levels (lead toxicity). Although some tubulointerstitial disorders have characteristic histomorphologic features (medullary cystic disease, amyloidosis, myeloma kidney, hypokalemia), the microscopic appearance of most tubulointerstitial disorders lacks uniquely distinguishing characteristics. Renal biopsy is therefore used infrequently in the diagnosis of patients with tubulointerstitial disease. Therapy for the tubulointerstitial disorders is dependent on the underlying cause.

c. **Glomerular proteinuria.** When proteinuria is characterized by a disproportionate amount of albumin, a glomerular origin is implied. Mild transient proteinuria, especially associated with acute and reversible disease, is usually of little long-term significance. However, heavy and sustained proteinuria suggests a more serious disorder. Because the differential diagnosis is large, and many of the implicated disorders are uncommon, consultation with a nephrologist is recommended during the initial evaluation and treatment.

Patients with constant heavy proteinuria require close diagnostic scrutiny. Glomerular proteinuria in this group is often categorized either as nonnephrotic (less than 3.5 g per day per 1.73 m^2 body surface area) or nephrotic (more than 3.5 g per day per 1.73 m^2 body surface area). This somewhat arbitrary division of patients into those with lesser and greater amounts of urinary protein is justified by two major observations. First, patients with nonnephrotic proteinuria tend to have a better prognosis with regard to renal function than do patients with heavier proteinuria. As a result, an aggressive diagnostic or therapeutic approach may not be immediately indicated. Therefore, after a search for underlying causes discernible by history, physical examination, and serologic assessment (see section III.D.), therapy including the use of antiproteinuric agents such as angiotensin-converting enzyme inhibitors (ACEis) with or without angiotensin receptor blockers (ARBs), and follow-up to observe the course of the renal function and degree of proteinuria may be indicated in individual patients before consideration of renal biopsy and the use of potentially risky immunosuppressive therapeutic regimens. Second, the morbidity and prognosis of patients with heavier proteinuria is conferred not only by the patient's renal functional outcome but also by the pathophysiologic consequences of heavy proteinuria (e.g., the nephrotic syndrome).

The nephrotic syndrome is defined by the presence of more than 3.5 g of proteinuria per 1.73 m^2 of body surface area per day, hypoalbuminemia, hyperlipidemia, lipiduria, and edema. Heavy proteinuria induces enhanced tubular reabsorption and catabolism of proteins leaked into the glomerular ultrafiltrate, thereby contributing to hypoproteinemia. Sodium and water retention, with resultant edema, occurs secondary to hypoproteinemia in some patients and as a direct result of glomerular injury in others. Hypoproteinemia and an associated decrement in plasma oncotic pressure may stimulate apolipoprotein synthesis in the liver, causing hyperlipidemia and lipiduria. It is postulated that in nephrotic disorders that are resistant to therapy and persist for many years, hyperlipidemia may contribute to accelerated atherosclerosis. Heavy proteinuria also predisposes to hypercoagulability. Variable losses of antithrombin III, protein S, and protein C have been described in some but not all nephrotic patients. Other urinary losses may variably induce subtle abnormalities of function in some patients with nephrotic syndrome, including losses of Ig and complement (predisposition to infection), thyroid-binding globulin (low total thyroxine, normal thyroid-stimulating hormone), and vitamin D (hypovitaminosis, hypocalcemia, and secondary hyperparathyroidism). Individuals with heavy proteinuria express the complications of nephrotic syndrome variably, further reflecting differences in urinary protein losses, dietary intake, and genetic predisposition.

D. **The differential diagnosis of heavy proteinuria.** Once proteinuria is determined to result from glomerular injury, an underlying disorder should be sought. The very large number of differential diagnoses outlined in Table 8-3 can be narrowed substantially by obtaining a detailed history, physical examination, and appropriate serologic testing. The history should cover the following important details: the presence of diabetes; deafness; similarly affected family members (suggestive of Alport's nephropathy or other familial nephritis); ethnicity (IgA nephropathy is frequent in Asians and infrequent in African-Americans); presence of fever; travel; medication use; transfusions, drug abuse, sexual orientation and partners [human immunodeficiency virus (HIV), hepatitis, syphilis]; arthritis, arthralgias, malar or skin rash, oral ulcers, alopecia [systemic lupus erythematosus (SLE) and other immune or hypersensitivity disorders]; hemoptysis (Goodpasture's disease, Wegener's granulomatosis); sinusitis, sterile otitis (Wegener's granulomatosis); paresthesias, angiokeratomas, dyshidrosis, focal neurologic deficits (Fabry's disease); weight loss, cough, breast mass (malignancy and secondary membranous nephropathy); allergies; childhood or adolescent UTIs (focal sclerosis secondary to reflux nephropathy); and episodes of gross or persistent microhematuria (IgA nephropathy, thin basement membrane nephropathy). The physical examination should be directed at establishing whether systemic disease is present and whether the nephrotic syndrome or its complications are present. All adult patients with abnormal proteinuria should also have, at a minimum, a chest x-ray; CBC; serum and UPEP or immunofixation; serum chemistry panel, including tests of renal and hepatic function; and a measurement of serum albumin, total protein, total and low- and high-density lipoprotein cholesterol, triglycerides, glucose, and calcium levels. For patients older than 40 years, age and gender-appropriate cancer screening should also be performed. Additional serologic testing may be warranted, depending on the presence or absence of hematuria and the results of the aforementioned studies. Such additional tests include, but are not limited to, antinuclear and antidouble stranded DNA antibodies (lupus); antineutrophil cytoplasmic antibody (ANCA), antiproteinase 3 and anti-myeloperoxidase (anti-MPO) antibodies (Wegener's granulomatosis and other vasculitic syndromes); C3 and C4 (may be low in endocarditis, poststreptococcal glomerulonephritis, lupus, membranoproliferative glomerulonephritis (MPGN), cryoglobulinemia); antihyaluronidase, anti-DNase B, antistreptolysin O (poststreptococcal glomerulonephritis); antiglomerular basement membrane antibody (Goodpasture's disease); rheumatoid factor (endocarditis, cryoglobulinemia, rheumatoid arthritis; hepatitis C); serum cryoglobulins; angiotensin-converting enzyme (sarcoidosis); glycosylated hemoglobin; serologic testing for syphilis; hepatitis B antigens and antibody; recombinant immunoblot testing and viral load for hepatitis C; and ELISA/Western blot for human immunodeficiency virus. In the spirit of cost-consciousness, these tests should not be routinely ordered in all patients with glomerular proteinuria. Rather, a thoughtful synthesis of the history and physical examination should guide the selection of appropriate tests among those listed (and potentially others not mentioned).

A renal biopsy should be considered if no underlying disorder emerges as a cause for glomerular proteinuria after a thorough evaluation. In addition, renal biopsy is indicated when a secondary cause has been identified and a histologic examination of the renal tissue would help guide therapy, as is often the case for SLE.

IV. **THERAPY.** The treatment of glomerular disorders falls into three categories: treatment of the underlying systemic disease, general management of the nephrotic syndrome, and therapies for specific glomerular diseases.

A. **Treatment of underlying systemic disease.** Owing to the large number of entities that potentially cause glomerulonephritis, the reader is referred to a textbook of internal medicine or nephrology for their treatment. However, special mention should be made of diabetes mellitus. Data suggest that glycemic control, tight blood pressure control (less than 130/80 mmHg), and ACEi and/or ARBs are useful in preventing or forestalling the development of overt diabetic nephropathy in patients with diabetes mellitus. These also have been shown to have a favorable impact on serum creatinine levels, progression to end-stage renal disease, and overall mortality in patients with diabetic nephropathy.

1. **General management of the nephrotic syndrome.** The treatment of edema due to the nephrotic syndrome begins with sodium restriction and diuretics. Care should be taken to avoid inducing a state of marked prerenal azotemia.

Many strategies have been advocated to decrease heavy proteinuria. Nonsteroidal anti-inflammatory drugs (NSAIDs) reportedly produce a decrease in proteinuria in some patients, along with a smaller decrement in GFR. Despite their utility in a few patients, however, the overall impact of NSAIDs in substantially diminishing proteinuria for most patients with nephrosis is disappointingly small. ACEi and ARBs are also useful to decrease proteinuria, and their efficacy has been tested both in patients with diabetic nephropathy and in patients with the idiopathic nephrotic syndrome. Combinations of these agents may be additive in limiting proteinuria. Many months may elapse between ACEi and/or ARB initiation and the achievement of the maximal decrement in proteinuria from that dose, a phenomenon that suggests more than hemodynamic change as its mechanism of action. Proteinuria may also be reduced by lowering patients' mean arterial pressure to levels below 92 mm Hg, independent of the class of antihypertensive agents used to achieve this target. Finally, dietary protein restriction in the range of 0.6 to 0.8 g per kg per day has been suggested, both to slow the rate of loss of renal function and as a further means of diminishing proteinuria. The efficacy of angiotensin blockade, the conflicting supporting data for the efficacy of low-protein diets, and concerns regarding nutritional safety in patients with heavy proteinuria (i.e., more than 10 g per day) have made stringent dietary protein restriction less frequently prescribed in recent years. Nevertheless, patients with heavy proteinuria should probably be advised to eat a diet close to the recommended daily allowance of protein, which is 0.8 g protein per kg body weight, and at least to avoid high-protein diets.

The hyperlipidemia of the nephrotic syndrome may contribute to accelerated atherosclerosis. Use of the 3-hydroxy-3-methylglutaryl–coenzyme A (HMG-CoA) reductase inhibitors (statins) or agents such as gemfibrozil often lower serum low-density lipoprotein cholesterol and triglyceride levels substantially in patients with nephrotic syndrome. However, they should not be used together because of the increased risk of rhabdomyolysis. Statins may also induce modest decrements in proteinuria. For the patient with venous or, less commonly, arterial thrombosis or pulmonary emboli, long-term anticoagulation for the duration of the nephrotic syndrome is recommended.

2. **Therapies for specific glomerular diseases.** The so-called primary glomerular disorders fall into essentially seven histologic categories: minimal change glomerulopathy, IgM mesangial proliferative glomerulonephritis, focal and segmental glomerulosclerosis (FSGS), IgA nephropathy, membranous nephropathy, MPGN, and crescentic glomerulonephritis. From a therapeutic standpoint, the first three are often considered as a group, and the latter four are considered separately. Because these latter four disorders are relatively uncommon and

therapies often involve the use of potentially toxic drugs, referral to a nephrologist is advised.

a. **Minimal change glomerulopathy — IgM mesangial proliferation glomerulonephritis — focal and segmental glomerulosclerosis.** If the nephrotic syndrome is present, conservative general care as described in section IV.A.1 may be appropriate as an adjunct to specific therapy. These glomerular disorders are variably responsive to high-dose prednisone (1 mg per kg, maximum, 80 mg). More than 90% of children with minimal change glomerulopathy have a complete remission of proteinuria within 2 months of starting steroid therapy. In adults, this figure is approximately 80% to 90%. Patients with FSGS who have underlying genetic mutations are unlikely to be responsive to prednisone, and some have suggested that genetic testing should precede a therapeutic trial. However, genetic testing is not generally available to most clinicians at this time. This may explain why response rates for the latter two disorders are not high (approximately 40% to 50% and 20% to 30%, respectively). Extending the duration of high-dose prednisone to 4 to 6 months may accrue as many as 10% to 15% additional complete remissions. Prednisone should then be slowly tapered over approximately 4 months. Relapse, steroid dependence, or both can be treated with the addition of cytotoxic agents (e.g., cyclophosphamide or chlorambucil), cyclosporine A, or possibly mycophenolate mofetil, depending on the severity of the nephrotic syndrome and the level of renal function. Treatment of prednisone-resistant patients is controversial.

b. **IgA nephropathy (Berger's disease).** This is the most common form of primary glomerular disease in the world. It is particularly prevalent in Asia, Australia, and Mediterranean Europe and rare in African-Americans. Originally thought to be benign, it is now apparent that the condition progresses to end-stage renal disease in 20% to 40% of patients affected. Occasionally, reversible acute renal failure has been noted, particularly in association with gross hematuria. It may, rarely, be complicated by the presence of crescents; some of these patients have myeloperoxidase-antineutrophil cytoplasmic antibodies (MPO-ANCA) antibodies and respond poorly to immunosuppressive medications. Clinically, IgA nephropathy may be confused with a benign familial disorder, thin basement membrane nephropathy, because the presenting manifestation of each is predominantly glomerular hematuria. These two entities may be distinguished by a family history of hematuria (occasional in IgA nephropathy, frequent in thin basement membrane nephropathy), the presence of abnormal proteinuria (frequent in IgA nephropathy, uncommon in thin basement membrane nephropathy), and renal biopsy (no glomerular Ig present in thin basement membrane nephropathy, but mesangial IgA in Berger's disease). No therapeutic regimen is agreed upon to clearly affect outcome in IgA nephropathy, although there is support in different geographic locations for warfarin and dipyridamole with or without cyclophosphamide, omega-3 fatty acids, ACEi with or without ARBs, long-term steroids, and steroids with cytotoxic agents, the latter particularly for those with progressive renal insufficiency. Rituximab therapy for IgA nephropathy is under investigation.

c. **Membranous nephropathy.** Two-thirds of patients with this disorder either have a spontaneous remission or have stable or very slowly progressive renal insufficiency. Therefore, the majority do well with conservative therapy (including ACEi and ARBs) directed at minimizing progression associated with proteinuira. For patients at high risk for progression (e.g., those with heavy proteinuria hypertension, diminished GFR, male gender, or tubulointerstitial fibrosis on renal biopsy), specific therapy may be indicated. In this setting, steroids with a cytotoxic agent (either chlorambucil or cyclophosphamide) appear to be preferable to steroids alone in inducing a timely complete or partial remission. Cyclosporine A has been shown to be of benefit in a randomized trial; the benefit of mycophenolate mofetil remains anec-dotal. In patients with minimal mesangial proliferation and small amounts of mesangial IgA deposition, steroids may induce rapid remissions similar to those observed in minimal change disease.

d. **MPGN.** Hepatitis C is the most common cause of MPGN type I. Definitive therapy is uncertain, but a combination of interferon-α and ribavirin (or pegylated interferon-α with ribavirin) may be indicated. Side effects due to ribavirin increase when the GFR falls below 50 mL per minute. Steroids and cytotoxics may increase viral load, and should be used only for the cryoglobulinemic vasculitis complications of hepatitis C. Some investigators controversially suggest that children with MPGN type I (mesangial and subendothelial deposits) benefit from steroid therapy. Initial enthusiasm for the use of aspirin and dipyridamole has waned. No therapy is effective for MPGN type II (dense-deposit disease).

e. **Crescentic glomerulonephritis.** When glomerulonephritis is accompanied by crescents, a nephrologic emergency is present, due to the propensity for rapid progression to end-stage renal disease. Early diagnosis and implemen-tation of therapy are essential to preserve renal function. After excluding poststreptococcal glomerulonephritis, three classes of crescentic glomeru-lonephritis are recognized. The reader is referred to a textbook of nephrology for the treatment of type I (antiglomerular basement membrane nephritis or Goodpasture's syndrome) and type III (pauci-immune glomerulonephritis, such as Wegener's granulomatosis or microscopic polyangiitis). Type II (immune complex–mediated glomerulonephritis) is treated initially with intravenous methylprednisolone sodium succinate (Solu-Medrol), followed by high-dose oral prednisone usually with a cytotoxic agent such as cyclophos-phamide. Because of the relative rarity of the syndrome, no randomized controlled trials have proved that additional benefits accrue from the use of cytotoxic agents. However, largely due to the clear-cut benefits of cyclophos-phamide in types I and III and plasmapheresis in type I, some investigators have recommended their use in type II.

Suggested Readings

Addis T. The number of formed elements in the urinary sediment of normal individuals. *J Clin Invest* 1926;2:409.

Birch DF, Fairley KF, Whitworth JA, et al. Urinary erythrocyte morphology in the diagnosis of glomerular hematuria. *Clin Nephrol* 1983;20:78.

Fairley KF, Birch DF. Haematuria: a simple method for identifying glomerular bleeding. *Kidney Int* 1982;21:105.

Gadehold H. Quantitative estimation of cells in the urine. *Acta Med Scand* 1968;183:309.

Godfrey K, Harding M, Zhanel GG, et al. Manitoba Diabetes Urinary Tract Infection Study Group. Antimicrobial treatment in diabetic women with asymptomatic bacteriuria. *N Engl J Med* 2002;347:1576–1583.

Haver MH. *Urinary sediment: a textbook atlas.* Chicago: American Society of Pathologists, 1983.

Kim M, Corwin H. Urinalysis. In: Schrier RW, ed. *Diseases of the kidney and urinary tract,* 8th ed. Philadelphia: Lippincott Williams & Wilkins, 286–297.

Kincaid-Smith P, Whitworth JA, eds. *The kidney,* 2nd ed. Oxford, UK: Blackwell Science, 1987.

Murphy BM, Fairley KF, Birch DF, et al. Culture of mid catheter urine collected via an open-ended catheter: a reliable guide to bladder bacteriuria. *J Urol* 1984;131:19.

Nakao N, Yoshimura A, Morita H, et al. Combination of treatment of angiotensin II receptor blocker and angiotensin-converting enzyme inhibitor in nondiabetic renal disease (COOPERATE): a randomised controlled trial. *Lancet* 2003;361:117–124.

Ottiger C, Huber AR. Quantitative urine particle analysis: integrative approach for the optimal combination of automation with UF-100 and microscopic review with KOVA cell chamber. *Clinical Chemistry* 2003;49:617–623.

Ruggenenti P, Gaspari F, Perna A, et al. Cross-sectional longitudinal study of spot morning urine protein: creatinine ratio, 24-hour urine protein excretion rate, glomerular filtration rate, and end-stage renal failure in chronic renal disease in patients without diabetes. *BMJ (Clinical Research Edition)* 1998;316(7130):504.

Scherberich JE. Urinary proteins of tubular origin: basic immunochemical and clinical aspects. *Am J Nephrol* 1990;10(Suppl 1):43.

Waller KV, Ward KM, Mahan JD, et al. Current concepts in proteinuria. *Clin Chem* 1989;35:755.

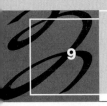

THE PATIENT WITH GLOMERULONEPHRITIS OR VASCULITIS

Joshua M. Thurman and Alexander Wiseman

I. **OVERVIEW.** The glomerular diseases are defined by their clinical presentations and the histologic findings on renal biopsy. Glomerular diseases can also be categorized as primary processes in which the disease process is confined to the kidney, or as secondary processes in which a systemic disease impacts the kidney. Most of these diseases are autoimmune in nature. Injury to the kidney may be caused by the deposition of immune complexes within the glomeruli or by autoantibodies directed against antigens present within the kidney. The small vessels of the kidney and the glomerular capillaries are also frequently the target of small vessel vasculitides.

Clinically, the presence of a glomerular disease should be considered when proteinuria is present; glomerulonephritis and vasculitis should be considered when hematuria and/or proteinuria are present. Therefore, the approach to the patient with possible glomerular disease should begin with an assessment of the protein excretion in the urine and a microscopic analysis of the urine for dysmorphic red blood cells and/or red blood cell casts.

II. **PROTEINURIA.** Although a number of conditions, such as interstitial nephritis, can cause proteinuria, the quantity of nonglomerular proteinuria is typically less than 1 g on a 24-hour urine collection. Clinically and therapeutically relevant glomerular diseases are associated with proteinuria of greater than 1.5 to 3 g per day, and the absence of proteinuria essentially excludes clinically significant glomerular disease.

   A. **Evaluation of proteinuria.** A number of methods are utilized to assess the presence and degree of proteinuria.

   1. **The 24-hour urine collection.** When done properly, the 24-hour urine collection provides the most accurate measure of urinary protein excretion. This method involves emptying the bladder and discarding the first morning urine, then collecting all urine for the subsequent 24 hours, including the first morning void the following day. The urine should be refrigerated during the collection period. If this is not possible, one cup of vinegar can be added to the collection container to act as a preservative. To ensure adequate collection, a 24-hour total creatinine excretion should be obtained on the same sample. In females under steady-state conditions of renal function, the 24-hour urinary excretion of creatinine should equal approximately 15 to 20 mg per kg of ideal body weight; in males, the excretion should be 18 to 25 mg per kg of ideal body weight.

   2. **Urine dipstick test.** As a rapid screen for the presence of albuminuria, commercially available dipsticks can provide the clinician a gross estimate of the presence and degree of proteinuria. Quantification of proteinuria, however, must be performed using a 24-hour urine collection or alternatively, multiple early morning spot urine collections for the calculation of the protein to creatinine ratio.

   3. **Urine sulfosalicylic acid (SSA) test.** The urine dipstick detects albuminuria, but not smaller molecular weight proteins such as immunoglobulin light chains. The urine SSA test detects the presence of all proteins in the urine, including light chains. A positive SSA test result with a normal dipstick indicates the presence of nonalbumin proteins in the urine as might occur with multiple myeloma.

   4. **Urine protein–creatinine ratio.** A urinary protein–creatinine concentration ratio on the first voided morning urine sample can be used as a quick assessment of proteinuria, and it can be useful as a substitute for repeated full 24-hour urine collections to assess responsiveness to therapy. The normal 24-hour urine

protein excretion in the adult can range from 30 to 130 mg, whereas children and adolescents may excrete as much as twice this amount. Assuming that the average individual excretes approximately 1 g of creatinine per day, normal spot urinary protein–creatinine ratios on random samples generally fall below 0.2 (mg protein per mg creatinine), whereas values greater than 3 suggest the presence of nephrotic-range proteinuria. This ratio should not be used as a substitute for an initial 24-hour collection in cases in which glomerulonephritis is considered or in cases in which the creatinine generation is likely greater than 1 g per day (e.g., in individuals with large muscle mass).

B. Classification of proteinuria. As mentioned earlier, a number of nonglomerular diseases can lead to proteinuria. When proteinuria is identified, it is important to identify whether it is glomerular or nonglomerular in origin, because the treatments for these conditions are dramatically different. In general, proteinuria can be classified into three major categories.

1. Overflow proteinuria. Overflow proteinuria is caused by the filtration of an abnormally large amount of small molecular weight proteins from the serum that exceeds the capacity of the tubules for reabsorption. Diseases associated with overflow proteinuria include rhabdomyolysis (myoglobinuria), intravascular hemolysis (hemoglobinuria), and multiple myeloma (light chains). Evaluation of overflow proteinuria may be aided by urine protein electrophoresis (UPEP), which separates urinary proteins into five peaks based on the molecular weights of the proteins. The peaks include albumin and α_1, α_2, β, and γ globulins. For example, an abnormal peak or "spike" occurring in the γ region (or, less commonly, in the α_2 or β region) suggests the presence of a monoclonal gammopathy.

2. Tubular proteinuria. In contrast to overflow proteinuria, in which normal tubular reabsorption is overwhelmed by an abnormally large amount of filtered proteins, tubular proteinuria is caused by damage to the renal tubulointerstitial region, which leads to a failure to reabsorb small molecular weight proteins. Under normal conditions, the small amount of urinary protein is composed of filtered proteins from plasma (50%) and proteins that are secreted into the urine from urinary tract cells (50%). Filtered proteins include small amounts of albumin (approximately 15% of the total urinary protein), immunoglobulins (5%), light chains (5%), β_2 microglobulin (less than 0.2%), and other plasma proteins (25%). The most prevalent tubular protein (and the most abundant protein in normal urine) is Tamm-Horsfall protein, which enters the urine after synthesis in the tubular cells of the ascending limb of the loop of Henle and is secreted into the urine. Under conditions of tubulointerstitial injury, up to 1 to 2 g per day of filtered and secreted proteins may be found in the urine. Increases in tubular proteinuria may occur by three mechanisms. First, injured tubules are unable to reabsorb the small molecular weight proteins normally filtered by the glomerulus, such as β_2 microglobulin. Second, brush border components and cellular enzymes such as N-acetylglucosamine and lysozyme are secreted into the urine under conditions of tubular injury. Lastly, increased amounts of Tamm-Horsfall protein may be secreted into the urine by injured tubular cells of the ascending limb of the loop of Henle and the distal nephron. When the source of proteinuria is unclear, UPEP and immunoelectrophoresis (IEP) can be utilized to aid in diagnosis. In glomerular proteinuria, a UPEP demonstrates primarily albumin rather than globulins, whereas tubular proteinuria demonstrates a predominance of small molecular weight proteins. IEP can quantify the relative amounts of protein in the urine if a definitive spike is not present on UPEP. A urinary albumin to β_2 microglobulin ratio of 10:1 is indicative of tubular proteinuria, in contrast to glomerular proteinuria, in which this ratio usually exceeds 1,000:1. In comparison, in normal urine, the albumin to β_2 microglobulin ratio ranges from 50:1 to 200:1.

3. Glomerular proteinuria. Glomerular proteinuria results from injury to the glomerulus, leading to an increase in filtered proteins. This injury may result in changes in the *size*-selective properties of the GBM, allowing the passage of larger molecular weight proteins or even of cells (as in crescentic glomerulonephritis), or may result in changes in the *charge*-selective properties of the glomerular basement membrane (GBM), permitting the ultrafiltration of negatively charged albumin (as in minimal change nephropathy). Glomerular injury may lead to a combination of defects in both size and charge selectivity (as in diabetic nephropathy). Finally, mesangial injury may also induce proteinuria through mechanisms that are not clear, perhaps by interfering with normal mesangial clearance functions.

As described earlier, glomerular proteinuria is characterized by the preponderance of albumin compared to smaller molecular weight proteins. Generally, the greater the degree of proteinuria the worse the renal prognosis. In this regard, nephrotic-range proteinuria, defined by significant proteinuria greater than 3.0 to 3.5 g per day, often requires specific therapeutic intervention based on the underlying disease.

4. **Other proteinuria.** Although most forms of proteinuria may be classified into overflow, tubular, or glomerular sources, two additional causes of proteinuria exist that do not fall into these categories. Benign orthostatic proteinuria is proteinuria of less than 1 g per day without other urinary abnormalities; this is typically found in tall adolescents. When split urine collections are performed (a 12-hour overnight collection and 12-hour daytime collection), protein is found only in the daytime collection. The condition is considered to be benign and often disappears in adulthood; however, in a very small proportion, overt renal disease develops in adulthood. Proteinuria can occur with cardiac failure, fever, or heavy exercise. It is transient and disappears within hours of cessation of exercise or with recovery from the disease process. Table 9-1 lists the most common causes of nonglomerular proteinuria.

C. **Clinical assessment of proteinuria.** The clinical approach to a patient with proteinuria identified on a screening test (such as a urine dipstick or spot urine protein measurement) should be tailored to assess the presence of concurrent renal injury and the potential for future renal damage. A 24-hour urine protein measurement and a serum creatinine measurement should be obtained, and the urine should be evaluated for the presence of red blood cells and casts (described in section III.A). If renal function is normal, no red cells are present, and proteinuria is less than 200 mg per day, the renal injury sustained from a potential low-grade glomerular disease is minimal, and the risk of future renal injury is low if diabetes and/or hypertension are not present. Proteinuria in the range of 200 mg per day to 2 g per day with no hematuria and normal renal function may be caused by

TABLE 9-1	Common Causes of Nonglomerular Proteinuria

Overflow	Tubular	Other
Rhabdomyolysis	Polycystic kidney disease	Benign orthostatic
Hemoglobinuria	Pyelonephritis	proteinuria
Monoclonal gammopathy	Obstruction	Transient proteinuria
(light chain deposition	Vesicoureteral reflux	(cardiac failure, fever,
disease)	Medications (chronic lithium	heavy exercise)
	exposure, analgesic nephropathy,	
	aminoglycosides)	
	Metabolic defects (oxalosis,	
	cystinosis, hypercalcemia,	
	hypercalciuria, hyperuricemia)	
	Trace metals (lead, mercury,	
	cadmium)	

glomerular lesions but also may be related to tubular abnormalities; investigation should be directed accordingly, because a glomerular disease in this clinical scenario carries a good prognosis if blood pressure is adequately controlled. Proteinuria greater than 2 to 3 g per day needs further evaluation for the presence of glomerular injury regardless of renal function. This evaluation is outlined in section IV. Any presentation in which red blood cell casts or dysmorphic red blood cells are present, regardless of the degree of renal function or proteinuria, must be further evaluated for the presence of a glomerulonephritis or vasculitis.

III. **HEMATURIA.** The pathognomonic finding of glomerular injury is the presence of dysmorphic red blood cells or red blood cell casts in the urine. This finding is a hallmark of glomerular capillary injury and limits the differential diagnosis significantly. However, care must be taken to rule out other causes of hematuria, which produce red blood cells in the urine that are of normal morphology and do not form casts (typical of lower urinary tract abnormalities, e.g., bladder cancer) and positive dipstick hematuria in the absence of red blood cells due to myoglobinuria or hemoglobinuria.

   A. **Evaluation and classification of hematuria.** The initial evaluation is typically provoked either by macroscopic hematuria (visible discoloration of the urine) or by incidental findings on a dipstick. Similar to the evaluation of proteinuria, hematuria can either be due to a glomerular disorder or to a nonglomerular source. Glomerular bleeding should be suspected if dysmorphic urinary red blood cells, red blood cell casts, and proteinuria are present. Nonglomerular hematuria is characterized by the presence of isomorphic urinary erythrocytes without red blood cell casts or significant proteinuria. Hematuria secondary to nonglomerular causes can be differentiated by the three-glass test. In this procedure, an initial stream, midstream, and endstream sample of urine (10 to 15 mL each) is collected in three separate containers. A urethral site of bleeding is likely if the hematuria predominates in the initial sample, whereas a bladder origin is suggested if hematuria is predominately identified in the final sample. Ureteral and renal sources are suspected if hematuria is present in all three-collection samples.

   B. **Clinical assessment of hematuria.** The initial evaluation of the patient with gross or microscopic hematuria should be focused on differentiating glomerular from nonglomerular causes. If microscopy suggests a glomerular cause, with dysmorphic red blood cells and red blood cell casts, patients should be further evaluated for renal dysfunction and glomerulonephritis as described in section IV. Nonglomerular hematuria typically entails an evaluation for the possibility of a urogenital malignancy, infection, stone, or cystic disease. In this regard, the history and review of systems should focus on the frequency and nature of hematuria (gross or microscopic), pain, burning with urination, increased frequency of urination, fever, weight loss, and passage of stones. Medications that may lead to hematuria should be reviewed, including oral contraceptives and analgesics, particularly in patients with diabetes. Other causes of hematuria, including trauma, coagulation disorders, and family history of renal disease should be considered. The physical examination can identify certain causes of hematuria, such as renal bruits suggestive of arteriovenous fistulae; an enlarged prostate or nodules suggestive of hypertrophy, prostatitis, or malignancy; or enlarged kidneys on abdominal palpation, suggestive of polycystic kidney disease.

   The diagnostic evaluation of nonglomerular hematuria should include urine culture for bacterial infection, and if suspected, mycobacterial and mycoplasma infection. Once a urinary tract infection (UTI) has been excluded, the urinary tract anatomy should be evaluated through radiologic imaging or direct visualization to rule out malignancy, stone disease, and hereditary renal disease. The upper tract (the kidneys and ureters) can be evaluated by either a renal ultrasonography, computed tomography (CT), or intravenous pyelography (IVP), whereas the lower tract (bladder and urethra) is best evaluated by cystoscopy. Urine cytology can serve as an additional test to screen for the abnormal cellularity suggestive of urogenital malignancy. At the discretion of a urologist, a combination of the above-mentioned tests should be performed in the patient with unexplained hematuria.

In the presence of a normal or near-normal glomerular filtration rate (GFR), intravenous urography is the most useful diagnostic radiologic procedure available for defining renal anatomy. It should disclose the presence of renal cysts (hereditary and acquired); calculi; papillary necrosis; medullary sponge kidney; renal, pelvic, and ureteral tumors; and ureteral strictures. In the event of a nondiagnostic intravenous urographic study, cystoscopy can be performed to more definitively examine the bladder for the presence of tumors or infectious (inflammatory/interstitial) cystitis and the urethra for the presence of urethritis, strictures, or both. A nondiagnostic cystoscopic examination can be followed, if clinically indicated, by arteriography to pursue the possibility that hematuria is secondary to ureteral varices or aneurysms, arteriovenous malformations, or the loin pain hematuria syndrome.

IV. **GLOMERULAR HEMATURIA AND/OR PROTEINURIA.** Once the evaluation of hematuria and/or proteinuria lead the clinician to consider a glomerular disease as the most likely etiology, further clinical information can assist in the classification of the renal disorder before invasive testing. Although it is often difficult to predict the histologic pattern of injury in a patient with glomerular disease, one can first consider if a pattern of injury exists that may be segregated based on two general clinical presentations—the nephritic syndrome and the nephrotic syndrome—to assist in serologic testing.

A. **The nephritic syndrome.** This clinical syndrome typically presents with clinical findings of hematuria, proteinuria, and dysmorphic red blood cells and/or red blood cell casts. The proteinuria can range from 200 mg per day to heavy proteinuria (greater than 10 g per day). Clinically, it is accompanied by hypertension and edema. Renal insufficiency is common and typically progressive. The term *rapidly progressive glomerulonephritis (RPGN)* refers to diseases with a nephritic syndrome that lead to a rapid deterioration in renal function, defined as a doubling of serum creatinine or a 50% decrease in GFR over 3 months or less.

B. **The nephrotic syndrome.** This clinical syndrome also presents with proteinuria and edema, but unlike the nephritic syndrome, proteinuria is the most prominent feature (greater than 3.5 g per 1.73 m^2 per day). Dysmorphic red blood cells and casts are typically absent [exceptions do exist: focal segmental glomerulosclerosis (FSGS) usually presents with nephrotic-range proteinuria but can also present with hematuria]. Additional features of the nephrotic syndrome include hypercholesterolemia and hypoalbuminemia (serum albumin less than 3.0 mg per dL). The diseases that cause the nephrotic syndrome can lead to chronic, progressive renal injury, but typically are more indolent than diseases that present as a nephritic syndrome.

Once the clinical pattern has been identified, the clinician must consider if there is a systemic process that may be causing the proteinuria. Tables 9-2 and 9-3 list systemic diseases that present with a nephritic or nephrotic syndrome, respectively, and also highlight key laboratory findings that may aid in an initial diagnosis. In the absence of evidence of systemic disease, the clinician must consider primary (or isolated) glomerular diseases in the differential diagnosis. Histologically, the primary diseases can often not be distinguished from the injury pattern seen in systemic diseases.

C. **Clinicopathologic correlation**

The pathologic diagnosis of glomerular diseases incorporates the histologic pattern defined by light microscopy, immunofluorescent staining for immunoglobulins and complement proteins, and examination of the glomerular ultrastructure by electron microscopy. The primary glomerular diseases are listed in Table 9-4, with the prominent histologic findings on biopsy that define the disorder. There is a general correlation between the pattern of histologic injury and the clinical presentation. Conversely, the clinical findings can suggest the underlying pathologic process, although definitive diagnosis requires a biopsy.

The nephritic syndrome is usually caused by glomerular inflammation and manifests with an "active" urine sediment. Immune complexes which deposit in the mesangium or in the subendothelial space [membranoproliferative

TABLE 9-2	Systemic Diseases that Cause Glomerular Injury and a Nephritic Clinical Presentation	

Disease	Specific examples	Laboratory findings
Infections	Hepatitis C (B less commonly)	Low C3, hepatitis C Ab, hepatitis C viral PCR, cryoglobulins
	Poststreptococcal GN	Low C3, anti-streptolysin Ab
	Bacterial endocarditis	Low C3, positive blood cultures
	Methicillin resistant *staphylococcal aureus* (MRSA) infection	Low C3, positive blood cultures
Autoimmune diseases	SLE	Low C3, ANA, anti-dsDNA Ab
	Goodpasture's syndrome	Anti-GBM Ab
Vasculidities	Wegener's granulomatosis	c-ANCA
	Churg-Strauss syndrome	p-ANCA
	Henoch-Shönlein purpura	IgA in skin biopsy
	Polyarteritis nodosa	ANCA in 20% (c- or p-ANCA)
	Mixed cryoglobulinemia	Rheumatoid factor, low C4
Thrombotic microangiopathy	Scleroderma renal crisis	Anti-Scl-70
	Thrombotic thrombocytopenic purpura	Low platelets, hemolysis
	Hemolytic uremic syndrome	Low platelets, hemolysis, *Escherichia coli* enteritis
	Malignant hypertension	

ANA, antinuclear antibody; anti-dsDNA Ab, anti double-stranded DNA antibody; ANCA, antineutrophil cytoplasmic antibody; GN, glomerulonephritis; Ig, immunoglobulin; SLE, systemic lupus erythematosus.

glomerulonephritis (MPGN), immunoglobulin (Ig) A nephropathy, and many forms of lupus nephritis] generate inflammatory mediators that have access to the circulation and can cause an influx of inflammatory cells. Glomerular endothelial injury is also caused by autoantibodies to the glomerular basement membrane (anti-GBM), and with necrotizing injury of the glomerular capillaries as occurs in the antineutrophil cytoplasmic antibody (ANCA)-mediated vasculidites. These processes also cause a nephritic pattern of disease and frequently present with glomerular crescents and an RPGN. In patients with anti-GBM disease, immunofluorescence microscopy reveals a linear pattern of IgG (and occasionally IgA or IgM) along the glomerular capillaries. In contrast, immunoglobulin is not seen in renal vasculitis, a pattern referred to as *pauci-immune*.

Diseases that present with the nephrotic syndrome disrupt the size and charge selective barriers that ordinarily prevent the ultrafiltration of macromolecules across the glomerular capillary wall. In general, these diseases disrupt the glomerular capillary wall without causing overt inflammation (FSGS, diabetic nephropathy, and amyloidosis), or they affect the epithelial cells without causing endovascular inflammation [membranous nephropathy and minimal change disease (MCD)].

D. Clinical assessment of glomerular disease

  1. The nephritic syndrome. In cases in which the nephritic syndrome is the predominant clinical presentation, a search for systemic diseases is warranted. The history and physical examination should particularly focus on the assessment of rashes, lung disease, neurologic abnormalities, evidence of viral or bacterial infections, and musculoskeletal and hematologic abnormalities. Laboratory assessment should be tailored to the clinical findings in the history and physical examination. A complete blood count (CBC), electrolyte panel, 24-hour urine collection for protein and creatinine clearance, and liver function tests should be obtained initially. Serum complement (C3) levels are often clinically helpful to assist in the diagnosis of a specific renal disease (Table 9-5). Further

TABLE 9-3	Systemic Diseases that Cause Glomerular Injury and a Nephrotic Clinical Presentation	

Disease state	Common etiologies	Laboratory findings
Infections	Hepatitis B (C less common)	Hepatitis B SAg, hepatitis B eAg
	HIV	HIV Ab
	Syphilis	RPR
Chronic diseases	Diabetes	Elevated HgbA$_{1c}$, blood glucose
	Amyloidosis	UPEP/IEP (when associated with light chains)
	Sickle cell disease	Hemoglobin electrophoresis
	Obesity	
Malignancies	Multiple myeloma	SPEP, UPEP
	Adenocarcinoma (lung, breast, colon most common)	Abnormal cancer screening studies (usually clinically evident tumor burden)
	Lymphoma	
Rheumatologic	Systemic lupus erythematosus	ANA, anti-dsDNA Ab
	Rheumatoid arthritis	Rheumatoid factor
	Mixed connective tissue disease	Anti-RNP (ribonuclear protein) Ab
Medications	NSAIDs	—
	Bucillamine	
	Penicillamine	
	Lithium	
	Ampicillin	
	Captopril	
	Probenecid	
	Gold	
	Mercury	

ANA, antinuclear antibody; HIV, human immunodeficiency virus; IEP, immunoelectrophoresis; NSAID, nonsteroidal anti-inflammatory drug; RPR, rapid plasma reagin; SPEP, serum protein electrophoresis; UPEP, urine protein electrophoresis; anti-dsDNA Ab, anti double-stranded DNA antibody.

laboratory assessment may be performed based on these findings, and may include an antistreptolysin (ASO) titer, antinuclear antibody (ANA), ANCA, cryoglobulins, and/or an anti-GBM antibody. These early assessments may provide a presumptive diagnosis and should lead the clinician to an appropriate therapeutic intervention while awaiting renal biopsy results. These laboratory assessments should not substitute for the renal biopsy; only with a tissue diagnosis that confirms the clinical findings and provides information regarding the acuity and chronicity of the disease process can a glomerular disease be properly managed.

2. **The nephrotic syndrome.** With the identification of significant proteinuria, with or without other features of the nephrotic syndrome, secondary causes of proteinuria should be considered (Table 9-3). History and physical examination should evaluate for the presence of viral and bacterial infections, malignancies (particularly lung, breast, and lymph node), and chronic diseases (such as diabetes), and medications should be reviewed for their potential to cause glomerular proteinuria. Laboratory assessment initially includes CBC, electrolyte panel, 24-hour urine collection for protein and creatinine clearance, liver function tests, and a cholesterol panel. Further assessment may include hepatitis and human immunodeficiency virus (HIV) serologies, ANA, rapid plasma reagin (RPR), and serum and urine electropheresis. Renal biopsy should be performed in all cases in which no cause is evident, or to determine the extent of renal disease to guide therapy or prognosis.

TABLE 9-4   Primary Glomerular Diseases, Defined by Histology

Nephritic	Histologic findings	Nephrotic	Histologic findings
Renal limited vasculitis/microscopic polyangiitis	Necrotizing capillary lesions, crescents; negative IF, EM	Minimal change disease	Normal light microscopy, effaced foot processes on EM
Antiglomerular basement membrane disease	Linear IgG staining along glomerular basement membrane	Membranous nephropathy	Thickened GBM on light, subepithelial "spikes" on light, IF, EM, granular IgG and C3
Essential cryoglobulinemia	Fibrils on electron microscopy	Membranoproliferative glomerulonephritis	Thickened mesangial matrix, splitting ("double contour") of the glomerular basement membrane, C3 granular staining on IF
		Focal segmental glomerulosclerosis	Sclerosis in portions of glomeruli, C3 in areas of sclerosis on IF
		IgA nephropathy	IgA in mesangium on IF
		Fibrillary glomerulonephritis	Fibrillar deposits in mesangium, negative Congo red staining on IF

EM, electron microscopy; GBM, glomerular basement membrane; IF, immunofluorescence; Ig, immunoglobulin.

TABLE 9-5 Clinical Approach to Glomerulonephritis Based upon Serum Complement Level

Low serum complement level	Normal serum complement level
Systemic diseases	*Systemic diseases*
SLE	Polyarteritis nodosa
Subacute bacterial endocarditis	Hypersensitivity vasculitis
"Shunt" nephritis	Wegener's granulomatosis
Cryoglobulinemia	Henoch-Schönlein purpura
	Goodpasture's syndrome
	Visceral abscess
Primary renal diseases	*Primary renal diseases*
Poststreptococcal glomerulonephritis	IgA nephropathy
Membranoproliferative glomerulonephritis (MPGN)	Idiopathic rapidly progressive glomerulonephritis (antiglomerular basement membrane disease, pauci-immune glomerulonephritis, immune complex disease)
Type 1	
Type 2	

Ig, immunoglobulin; SLE, systemic lupus erythematosus.
(Adapted from Madaio MP, Harrington JT. Current concepts. The diagnosis of acute glomerulonephritis. *N Engl J Med* 1983;309:1299, with permission.)

V. THERAPY FOR GLOMERULONEPHRITIS. The management of systemic diseases that cause secondary glomerular injury is rapidly changing (e.g., new antiviral therapies for HIV and hepatitis B and C, and clinical trials using chemotherapeutic regimens for malignancies and vasculidities); therefore the reader is encouraged to refer to recent disease-specific reviews of the literature for current management strategies for these systemic diseases. This chapter reviews the treatment of the most frequent systemic diseases that cause glomerular injury. The treatment of glomerular disorders can be approached by general management of the nephrotic syndrome and proteinuria and immunomodulating therapies for specific glomerular diseases and vasculidities.

A. General management of the nephrotic syndrome and proteinuria. Four general treatment strategies should be considered in the patient with nephrotic syndrome: management of edema, proteinuria, hyperlipidemia, and hypercoagulability. Management of edema should initially focus on sodium restriction and diuretics. Thiazides are a reasonable treatment choice for patients with mild edema and normal renal function; however, most patients will require a loop diuretic such as furosemide for adequate sodium balance. The cornerstone to management of proteinuria is the inhibition of the renin-angiotensin system using either angiotensin-converting enzyme inhibitors (ACEis) or angiotensin receptor blockers (ARBs). Using these medications, intraglomerular pressure is reduced due to efferent arteriolar vasodilation, thereby resulting in a reduced amount of protein filtration. In diabetes, ACEi have been shown to be critical in slowing the development of overt diabetic nephropathy in patients with type 1 diabetes and microalbuminuria (30 to 300 mg per day) and reducing the incidence of end-stage renal disease (ESRD) and overall mortality in patients with type 1 diabetes and overt diabetic nephropathy (urine protein excretion greater than 300 mg per day). ARBs have shown similar benefits in patients with type 2 diabetes with either microalbuminuria or overt nephropathy. In nondiabetic proteinuric renal disease, ACEi also significantly reduces the risk of developing ESRD. The maximal therapeutic dose of single agent and the role of a combination of ACEi and ARB for treatment of significant proteinuria and progression of renal disease are in need of further study. Proteinuria may also be reduced by lowering patients' mean arterial pressure (MAP) to levels lower than 92 mm Hg, independent of the class of antihypertensive agents used to achieve this target. Finally, dietary protein restriction in the range of 0.6 to 0.8 g per kg per day has been suggested, both to slow the rate of loss of renal function and as a further means of diminishing proteinuria. Long-term studies regarding nutritional safety are still necessary before this strategy should be advocated in patients, particularly those with heavy proteinuria (i.e., more than 10 g per day).

Control of hyperlipidemia often can be accomplished with the use of HMG-CoA reductase inhibitors or agents such as gemfibrozil. The issue of anticoagulation arises due to a hypercoagulable state induced by nephrotic proteinuria. Protein losses include the loss of antithrombotic factors such as antithrombin III, leading to an increased frequency of renal vein thrombosis and, less commonly, arterial thrombosis or pulmonary emboli. Long-term anticoagulation for the duration of the nephrotic syndrome is recommended for patients with documented thrombotic episodes. Debate still exists regarding prophylactic anticoagulation for all patients with nephrotic syndrome.

B. Therapies for specific glomerular diseases. The specific management of glomerular diseases requires the information obtained by renal biopsy, but is also influenced by the patient's clinical presentation. For example, more aggressive treatment may be undertaken in patients with a faster rate of progression or a greater degree of proteinuria. Specific histologic patterns will frequently present as either the nephritic or the nephrotic syndrome. Patients with IgA nephropathy, poststreptococcal glomerulonephritis, anti-GBM disease, or small vessel vasculitis of the kidney generally present with the nephritic syndrome. MCD, membranous nephropathy, and FSGS typically present with the nephrotic syndrome. However, there are exceptions to such generalizations. For example, patients with IgA nephropathy and MPGN may present with the nephrotic syndrome.

1. **Minimal change glomerulopathy.** Approximately 15% of cases of idiopathic nephrotic syndrome in adults, and 85% in children, are due to MCD. Light microscopy is normal, and on electron microscopy there is effacement of podocyte foot processes. IgM deposits may be seen in the mesangium on immunofluorescence, which may portend a poorer prognosis. In addition to the conservative management of nephrotic syndrome, high-dose prednisone (1 mg per kg, maximum, 80 mg) is used as primary therapy for at least 12 weeks. Whereas greater than 90% of children with MCD will have a complete remission of proteinuria within 2 months of starting steroid therapy, in adults this figure is approximately 50% to 60%. Extending the duration of high-dose prednisone to 5 to 6 months increases the rate of complete remission to 80%. Prednisone should then be slowly tapered over approximately 4 months. For relapsing cases and cases in which steroids cannot be tapered (steroid dependence), recycling of steroids with or without the addition of cytotoxic agents (e.g., cyclophosphamide or chlorambucil), cyclosporine A, or possibly mycophenolate mofetil, may be effective.

2. **Membranous nephropathy.** Approximately 30% to 40% of cases of idiopathic nephrotic syndrome in adults are due to membranous nephropathy. This disease is often slowly progressive and patients may have spontaneous remissions. Certain patients, however, are at high risk for progressive renal injury. Clinical risk factors associated with progression include heavy proteinuria greater than 8 g per day, hypertension, diminished GFR (creatinine greater than 1.2 for women, greater than 1.4 for men), male gender, and greater than 20% tubulointerstitial fibrosis on renal biopsy. For these patients, steroids combined with a cytotoxic agent (either chlorambucil or cyclophosphamide) alternating monthly for 6 months appears to be more effective than steroids alone in inducing a complete or partial remission. Preliminary data suggest that mycophenolate therapy also may be effective in the management of low- to moderate-risk patients.

3. **MPGN.** Idiopathic MPGN can be subcategorized to two types, type I (immune complex-mediated) and type II (thought to be complement-mediated). Both types, however, appear similar on light microscopy with hypercellularity, expansion of the mesangial matrix, and lobulation of the glomerular tuft. On electron microscopy, type II MPGN shows dense longitudinal deposits within the GBM versus the subendothelial immune deposits seen in type I MPGN. Together, these entities account for approximately 5% of glomerular disease in adults, and they tend to carry a poor renal prognosis. Of patients with type I MPGN and nephrotic proteinuria, 60% will progress to ESRD in 10 years. Unfortunately, no established therapy exists for MPGN. Despite conflicting data regarding its efficacy, long-term alternate-day prednisone is the current therapy of choice, particularly for children and teenagers. In any case of MPGN, secondary causes must be fully evaluated, because diseases such as chronic bacterial infection, hepatitis C infection, and cryoglobulinemia, as well as leukemias and lymphomas all have therapies that may lead to remission of the renal disease.

4. **Focal and segmental glomerulosclerosis.** Approximately 20% of cases of idiopathic nephrotic syndrome in adults is due to FSGS. Some consider FSGS and MCD to occur within the same spectrum of disease, but the prognosis is significantly worse in FSGS. Light microscopy in FSGS demonstrates focal areas of segmental glomerular sclerosis, and, as with MCD, electron microscopy demonstrates foot process effacement. Previously considered an untreatable renal lesion, recent evidence suggests that with prolonged courses (at least 6 months) of high-dose corticosteroid therapy approximately 30% of patients will achieve remission of the nephrotic syndrome. The remaining 70% who fail to respond to steroids may occasionally experience remission on cytotoxic agents such as cyclosporin, cyclophosphamide, or chlorambucil.

5. **IgA nephropathy (Berger's disease).** IgA nephropathy is the most common form of primary glomerular disease in the world. It is particularly prevalent in Asia and Australia (perhaps due to sampling bias resulting from a more

TABLE 9-6	Histologic Classification of Crescentic (or Rapidly Progressive) Glomerulonephritis		
Linear immunofluorescence	**Granular immunofluoroescence**		**Absent (pauci-immune) immunofluorescence**
Goodpasture's disease Anti-GBM disease	SLE Henoch-Schönlein purpura, IgA nephropathy Cryoglobulinemia		ANCA-associated vasculitis: Wegener's granulomatosis, Churg-Strauss syndrome, microscopic polyangiitis

ANCA, antineutrophil cytoplasmic antibody; Ig, immunoglobulin; SLE, systemic lupus erythematosus.

frequent biopsy rate in these regions), and it is rare in African-Americans. Although generally considered to be a slowly progressive renal disease, with ESRD occurring in 20% to 40% of patients by 20 years, a minority of patients may experience an RPGN with crescent formation on biopsy. Occasionally, reversible acute renal failure occurs, particularly in association with gross hematuria. Several clinical trials have demonstrated that corticosteroids are effective at slowing the progression of IgA nephropathy. Although further studies are needed, patients with proteinuria greater than 1 g per day may benefit from treatment with a 6-month course of corticosteroids (0.5 mg per kg on alternate days). Some studies advocate the use of fish oil in slowing the progression of renal insufficiency. For crescentic disease, short-term, high-dose prednisone may be of benefit. The use of cytotoxic agents such as cytoxan remains investigational at this time, but these agents are sometimes employed in patients with rapidly progressive disease (Table 9-6).

6. **Lupus nephritis.** Lupus nephritis is the paradigmatic immune complex disease of the kidney. In patients with lupus, immune complexes may be seen within the mesangium, the subendothelial space, and the subepithelial space, and the location of the immune deposits often correlates with the clinical presentation. Subepithelial deposits, for example, cause an injury similar to membranous nephropathy and can cause nephrotic syndrome. Mesangial and subendothelial deposits can cause glomerular inflammation and a nephritic syndrome. Immunofluorescence may demonstrate C3, IgG, IgM, IgA, and C1q all within the same kidney. These deposits appear as "lumps and bumps" and are distinguishable from the linear pattern seen in anti-GBM disease. In general, therapy for immune complex–mediated glomerulonephritis includes high-dose corticosteroids and cytoxan, particularly for the treatment of diffuse proliferative lupus nephritis. Recent studies have also demonstrated that mycophenolate mofetil is effective in proliferative lupus nephritis. Plasmapheresis has not been demonstrated to be of benefit.

7. **Anti-GBM disease and Goodpasture's syndrome.** When glomerulonephritis is accompanied by crescents and immunofluorescent staining for IgG demonstrates a linear pattern along glomerular capillaries on biopsy, the presence of an anti-GBM autoantibody is the most likely etiology. Clinically, this may present either as isolated renal dysfunction (anti-GBM disease) or as renal disease in conjunction with pulmonary involvement (Goodpasture's syndrome) with IgG staining of the pulmonary capillary basement membrane. Treatment of this disorder involves the combination of high-dose steroids, cytoxan therapy, and plasmapheresis to remove the anti-GBM antibody. Patients who present with oliguria have a poor renal prognosis, but occasionally may avoid chronic dialysis with aggressive and early therapy.

8. **Renal vasculitis.** When crescentic glomerulonephritis is accompanied by necrotizing capillary lesions, but no immunofluorescent staining of immune deposits is present on renal biopsy, the differential diagnosis of "pauci-immune"

diseases is considered. These diseases are generally considered to be secondary to antibodies to lysosomal enzymes of neutrophils (ANCA). Two ANCAs have been identified. Antibody to myeloperoxidase (MPO) results in perinuclear staining of neutrophils (p-ANCA), whereas antibody to proteinase-3 results in cytoplasmic staining of neutrophils (c-ANCA). Both systemic diseases (such as Wegener's granulomatosis, associated primarily with c-ANCA; Churg-Strauss syndrome, associated with either c- or p-ANCA; and polyarteritis nodosa) and primary renal disease (microscopic polyangiitis) can cause a pauci-immune necrotizing glomerulonephritis. Whether systemic or primary, these diseases are managed with high-dose steroids and cyclophosphamide as the therapy of choice. Oral cytoxan seems to be more effective than intravenous pulse cytoxan therapy. Eighty percent of patients respond to therapy, although patients with a serum creatinine of greater than 6 mg per dL at presentation are less likely to respond than patients with a lower serum creatinine at the time of presentation.

VI. THE THROMBOTIC MICROANGIOPATHIES: GLOMERULAR INJURY THAT MAS-QUERADES CLINICALLY AS GLOMERULONEPHRITIS. Systemic disorders that may produce a nephritic clinical presentation include a number of diseases that are not classical inflammatory diseases or vasculidities. Systemic diseases such as scleroderma, thrombotic thrombocytopenic purpura (TTP), hemolytic uremic syndrome (HUS), malignant hypertension, and antiphospholipid syndrome (APS) can present with hematuria, hypertension, and proteinuria (although usually less than 1 to 1.5 g per day), but all have renal histologic findings distinct from glomerulonephritis. Common histologic findings on renal biopsy in HUS, TTP, and APS include glomerular capillary thrombi and afferent arterioles, with fibrinoid necrosis from endothelial injury. Immunofluorescence is typically negative, with the exception of the presence of fibrinogen. Electron microscopy is also usually unremarkable, with no deposits noted. Additionally, malignant hypertension and scleroderma can cause subintimal proliferation within blood vessels, leading to an "onion-skin" appearance of arterioles. Microthrombi may be present as well.

The specific management of the thrombotic microangiopathies differs significantly from other disorders that lead to a nephritic clinical presentation; therefore, a correct diagnosis rather than empiric therapy is critical under circumstances of a nephritic presentation. For treatment of malignant hypertension and scleroderma renal crisis, blood pressure control is paramount. ACEi therapy is the first-line therapy in the setting of scleroderma, because data demonstrate improved patient survival and renal outcomes using this form of therapy. In HUS, the clinical picture is predominantly one of acute renal failure, thrombocytopenia, and hemolysis resulting either from verotoxin (from *Escherichia coli* 0157:H7 gastrointestinal infection) or from secondary causes such as idiosyncratic reactions to medications such as cyclosporin and mitomycin, or postpartum HUS. Therapy is supportive, with dialysis and correction of electrolytes and treatment of anemia providing reasonable short-term outcomes. Ninety percent of cases of diarrhea-associated HUS will completely recover, whereas 5% die within the acute phase and 5% remain with severe renal and extrarenal complications. Long-term follow-up demonstrates a diminished GFR in 40% of these patients at 10 years. Approximately half of the cases of HUS not associated with diarrhea (atypical HUS) occur in patients with mutations in complement regulatory proteins. These patients have a worse prognosis than those with diarrhea-associated HUS. Currently, therapy for atypical HUS involves plasma exchange and supportive care.

For TTP, the clinical picture is a pentad of neurologic signs, purpura, fever, thrombocytopenia, hemolysis, and renal failure that usually do not coexist but rather wax and wane. Secondary forms of TTP exist, and include pregnancy-, malignancy-, and HIV-associated causes. However, the most common cause of primary TTP is secondary to endothelial injury and the persistence of abnormally large von Willebrand factor (vWF) multimers into the microcirculation. This leads to platelet aggregation and thrombi formation. The failure to cleave large vWF multimers is usually caused by a functional deficiency of the metalloproteinase ADAMTS13, which, in most cases, is caused by an inhibitory autoantibody to the ADAMTS13. For this syndrome, fresh frozen plasma exchange or infusion is the most effective therapeutic intervention. It is felt that plasma exchange may remove autoantibody when it is present, and replace ADAMTS13 when there is a deficiency of this protein. Plasma exchange should be continued until the platelet count has normalized and the serum lactate dehydrogenase (LDH) enzyme level returns to normal range. This typically takes 7 to 16 exchanges to induce remission, followed by a slow taper of therapy. Additional therapies that have been described include high-dose prednisone therapy, vincristine, and other chemotherapeutic agents. The benefit of these therapies is not clear. In some patients in whom plasma exchange is only transiently effective, splenectomy may be necessary.

Suggested Readings

Agrawal N, Chiang LK, Rifkin IR. Lupus nephritis. *Semin Nephrol* 2006;26(2):95–104.

Appel GB, Waldman M, Radhakrishnan J. New approaches to the treatment of glomerular diseases. *Kidney Int* 2006;70:S45–S50.

Fakhouri F, Fremeaux-Bacchi V. Does hemolytic uremic syndrome differ from thrombotic thrombocytopenic purpura? *Nat Clin Pract Nephrol* 2007;3(12):679–687.

Falk RJ, Nachman PH, Hogan SL, et al. ANCA glomerulonephritis and vasculitis: a Chapel Hill perspective. *Semin Nephrol* 2000;20(3):244–255.

Kuhn K, Haas-Wohrle A, Lutz-Vorderburgge A, et al. Treatment of severe nephrotic syndrome. *Kidney Int* 1998;64(Suppl):S50–S53.

Madaio MP, Harrington JT. The diagnosis of glomerular diseases, acute glomerulonephritis and the nephrotic syndrome. *Arch Intern Med* 2001;161(1):25–34.

Schnaper HW. Idiopathic focal segmental glomerulosclerosis. *Semin Nephrol* 2003;23(2):183–193.

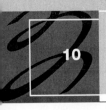

THE PATIENT WITH ACUTE RENAL FAILURE

*Sarah Faubel, Robert E. Cronin,
and Charles L. Edelstein*

10

I. **DEFINITION AND RECOGNITION OF ACUTE RENAL FAILURE (ARF).** ARF is a sudden and usually reversible decrease in the glomerular filtration rate (GFR) occurring over a period of hours to days. ARF may occur in patients with previously normal renal function or patients with chronic kidney disease (CKD); in either case, the clinical approach to find and treat the cause remains similar. The Acute Dialysis Quality Initiative (ADQI) has developed the *R*isk, *I*njury, *F*ailure, *L*oss, *E*nd-stage kidney disease (RIFLE) classification of ARF because of the lack of a universal definition of ARF (Fig. 10-1). The RIFLE classification conveys the concept that renal dysfunction is not only considered to be significant when it reaches the stage of failure but also it is a spectrum that ranges from early risk to long-term failure. **The term *acute kidney injury* (AKI) now replaces the term *ARF*; the term *ARF* should now be restricted to patients who have AKI and need renal replacement therapy.** Therefore, the RIFLE criteria have a high sensitivity for the early diagnosis of AKI and should allow detection of patients at risk to develop AKI as well as those patients with established AKI. The RIFLE criteria have been validated in multiple studies.

A. **Serum creatinine as a marker for AKI and GFR.** Normal serum creatinine is 0.6 to 1.2 mg per dL and is the most commonly used parameter to assess renal function. Unfortunately, the correlation between serum creatinine concentration and GFR may be confounded by several factors.

1. **Creatinine excretion is dependent on renal factors independent of function.** Certain medications such as trimethoprim or cimetidine interfere with proximal tubular creatinine secretion and may cause a rise in serum creatinine without a fall in GFR (Table 10-1). Once filtered, creatinine cannot be reabsorbed.

2. **Serum creatinine is dependent on nonrenal factors independent of kidney function.** For example, creatinine production is dependent on muscle mass. Muscle mass declines with age and illness. Therefore, a serum creatinine of 1.2 mg per dL in an elderly, 40-kg patient with cancer and wasted muscles may represent a severely impaired GFR, whereas a serum creatinine of 1.2 mg per dL in a 100-kg weightlifter with large muscle mass may represent a normal GFR. Serum creatinine is also dependent on other factors such as nutritional status, infection, volume of distribution, age, gender, race, body habitus, presence of amputations, malnutrition, and diet.

3. **Creatinine production and excretion must be in a steady state before creatinine may be used in any formula for the estimate of GFR.** The most commonly used formulae to estimate GFR are the Cockcroft-Gault, Modification of Diet in Renal Disease (MDRD), and the modified MDRD. In a steady state, the modified MDRD is as good as the MDRD for estimating renal function; both equations are superior to the Cockcroft-Gault formula. After an acute insult, it may take several days for creatinine excretion and production to reassume a steady state. For example, if a 60-kg, 30-year-old woman with a serum creatinine of 1.0 mg per dL suddenly loses all renal function, her serum creatinine may only rise to 2.0 mg per dL after 1 day. By the modified MDRD her GFR is 31 mL per minute; by Cockgroft-Gault it is 39 mL per minute, but it is actually zero.

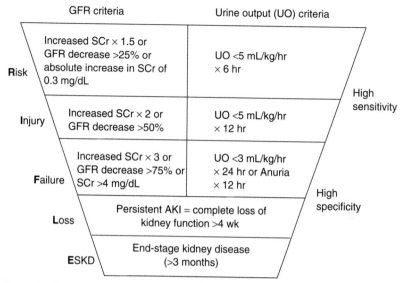

Figure 10-1. Risk, injury, failure, loss, end-stage kidney disease (RIFLE) definition/classification of acute kidney injury (AKI). Serum creatinine changes from baseline at 48 hours. (AKI, acute kidney injury; ESKD, end-stage kidney disease; GFR, glomerular filtration rate; Scr, serum creatinine.)

a. **Cockcroft-Gault formula**

$$GFR = [([140 - age\ (years)] \times lean\ body\ weight\ in\ kg)/(serum\ Cr \times 72)] \times (0.85\ if\ female)$$

b. **MDRD formula**

$$GFR,\ in\ mL\ per\ minute\ per\ 1.73\ m^2 = 170 \times (serum\ Cr^{-0.999})$$
$$\times (age^{-0.176}) \times (BUN^{-0.170})$$
$$\times (serum\ albumin^{+0.318})$$
$$\times (0.762\ if\ female)$$
$$\times (1.180\ if\ black)$$

Where serum Cr (creatinine) and blood urea nitrogen (BUN) are in mg per dL; serum albumin is in g per dL

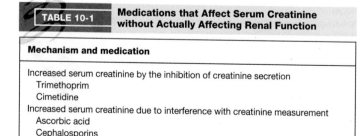

TABLE 10-1	Medications that Affect Serum Creatinine without Actually Affecting Renal Function

Mechanism and medication
Increased serum creatinine by the inhibition of creatinine secretion
Trimethoprim
Cimetidine
Increased serum creatinine due to interference with creatinine measurement
Ascorbic acid
Cephalosporins

c. Modified MDRD formula

$$\text{GFR, in mL per minute per } 1.73 \text{ m}^2 = 186.3 \times (\text{serum Cr}^{-1.154})$$
$$\times (\text{age}^{-0.203}) \times (0.742 \text{ if female})$$
$$\times (1.21 \text{ if black})$$

d. **Creatinine clearance** (CCr) gives a better estimate of GFR than the formulae listed earlier in the acute setting. This requires a 24-hour urine collection. Normal ranges for CCr are 120 ± 25 mL per minute for men and 95 ± 20 mL per minute for women.

$$\text{CCr} = [\text{urine creatinine (mg per dL)} \times \text{urine volume (mL per 24 hour)}]$$
$$/[\text{serum Cr (mg per dL)} \times 1,440 \text{ minute}]$$

B. **BUN as a marker for AKI and GFR.** Normal BUN is 8 to 18 mg per dL. An increase in BUN typically accompanies a rise in serum creatinine in the setting of AKI. Urea is filtered, but not secreted. Increased reabsorption of urea by the proximal tubule and arginine vasopressin (AVP)-sensitive urea transporters in the collecting duct occurs in states of volume depletion. In this setting, BUN can rise without a rise in creatinine, resulting in a BUN to serum creatinine ratio that is greater than 20 (see section IV.H.3).

BUN levels are affected by multiple factors not related to GFR. Because BUN production is related to protein metabolism, an increase in BUN without a decline in GFR may occur with hypercatabolic states, protein loading, upper gastrointestinal (GI) bleeding, and high-dose steroid administration, Conversely, a low BUN may be present in the setting of reduced GFR in patients who are on a low-protein diet, are severely malnourished, or have severe liver disease.

C. **Cystatin C as a marker for AKI and GFR.** Cystatin C is a protein produced by all nucleated cells. It is freely filtered by the glomerulus, completely reabsorbed by the proximal tubules, and is not secreted by the renal tubules. Therefore, some of the limitations of serum creatinine, for example, effect of muscle mass are not a problem with cystatin C. In AKI, changes in cystatin C occur sooner after changes in kidney function than serum creatinine. In studies, serum cystatin C correlated better with GFR than did serum creatinine and was diagnostically superior to creatinine especially in patients with liver cirrhosis. Cystatin C is best measured by an immunonephelometric assay, but is not yet routinely measured except in patients in whom serum creatinine is judged to be a poor marker of renal function, for example liver cirrhosis, and in patients with reduced muscle mass.

D. **Biomarkers of AKI.** A biomarker that is released into the blood or urine by the injured kidney and is analogous to the troponin release by injured myocardial cells after myocardial ischemia, is a more sensitive and specific marker of AKI than BUN and serum creatinine. Urinary interleukin-18 (IL-18), neutrophil gelatinase–associated lipocalin (NGAL), kidney injury molecule-1 (Kim-1), and tubular enzymes have been found to increase 1 to 2 days before serum creatinine in patients with ischemic AKI. Many studies are in progress to develop biomarkers of AKI that are superior to BUN and serum creatinine and will allow the early detection of AKI.

E. **Distinguishing ARF from chronic renal failure (CRF).** Distinguishing ARF from CRF may be challenging. Laboratory findings such as hyperphosphatemia, hypoalbuminemia, and hyperkalemia are unreliable factors to distinguish ARF from CRF and may be present in either case. Symptoms such as nausea, vomiting, and malaise may also occur in ARF or CRF. Potential methods to distinguish between the two include:
1. **Old records.** The most reliable way to distinguish ARF from CRF is an evaluation of old records. Increased BUN or serum creatinine documented months earlier and/or a history of kidney disease suggest that the renal failure is chronic.
2. **Small kidneys (less than 10 cm) on renal ultrasonography.** Although many patients with CKD do have a reduction in kidney size, if small kidneys are present it suggests that renal failure is chronic.

3. **Anemia.** Normochromic normocytic anemia is common in patients with CKD and a GFR less than 30 mL per minute; in patients with a GFR of 30 to 44 mL per minute, only approximately 20% of patients have anemia. Therefore, with a GFR of 30 mL or below, the absence of anemia suggests that the decline in renal function is acute. In some etiologies of CKD (e.g., autosomal dominant polycystic kidney disease), anemia may be absent. In some etiologies of AKI, anemia may be present, for example hemolytic uremic syndrome (HUS) or thrombotic thrombocytopenic purpura (TTP).

F. **Urine output in AKI.** AKI is typically described as either oliguric or nonoliguric. **Oliguria** is defined as a urine output of less than 400 mL per day; 400 mL is the minimum amount of urine that a person in a normal metabolic state must excrete to get rid of the daily solute production. For example, a person with a daily solute production of 500 mOsm who concentrates urine to a maximum of 1,200 mOsm per L would need to pass approximately 400 mL of urine per day to excrete the daily solute production (i.e., 500 mOsm/1,200 mOsm/L = 417 mL of urine per day).

      Anuria is defined as a lack of urine obtained from a bladder catheter; it has a short list of potential causes. It is most often caused by complete bilateral urinary tract obstruction, urinary tract obstruction in a solitary kidney, and shock. Less common causes are the HUS and rapidly progressive glomerulonephritis (RPGN), particularly anti-glomerular basement membrane (GBM) antibody disease; bilateral renal arterial or venous occlusion can also cause anuria.

II. **CLASSIFICATIONS OF AKI: DEFINITIONS AND CAUSES.** AKI is classified as either intrinsic renal or postrenal. Prerenal azotemia, in the absence of kidney injury, may also cause a decline in GFR which is reflected by increased serum creatinine and BUN.

A. **Prerenal azotemia** (Fig. 10-2). Prerenal azotemia is a fall in the GFR due to reduced renal perfusion in which minimal or no structural or cellular damage to the kidney has occurred. Urine sediment may be bland, but granular casts may be present.

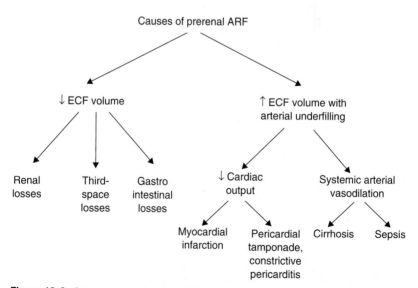

Figure 10-2. Causes of prerenal azotemia. Prerenal azotemia may be secondary to true intravascular volume depletion or arterial underfilling from a decrease in cardiac output or arterial vasodilatation. The extracellular fluid volume (ECF) comprises the intravascular and the interstitial body water compartments. (ARF, acute renal failure.)

Essential to this diagnosis is that renal function returns to normal within 24 to 72 hours of correction of the hypoperfused state. Prerenal azotemia occurs in the following situations:

1. **Total intravascular volume depletion.** This condition can occur in a number of settings where intravascular volume is reduced and may be secondary to
   a. Hemorrhage
   b. Renal fluid loss
      ■ Excessive diuresis (e.g., diuretics)
      ■ Osmotic diuresis (e.g., glucosuria)
      ■ Primary adrenal insufficiency (i.e., hypoaldosteronism)
      ■ Salt-wasting nephritis
      ■ Diabetes insipidus
   c. GI fluid loss
      ■ Vomiting
      ■ Diarrhea
      ■ Nasogastric tube drainage
   d. Skin fluid loss
      ■ Burns
      ■ Excessive sweating
      ■ Hyperthermia
   e. Third-space fluid loss
      ■ Peritonitis
      ■ Pancreatitis
      ■ Systemic inflammatory response syndrome (SIRS)
      ■ Profound hypoalbuminemia
2. **Effective volume depletion from arterial underfilling.** Arterial underfilling is a state in which intravascular volume is actually normal (or even increased) but circulatory factors are inadequate to maintain renal perfusion pressure. Underfilling may be due to either a decrease in cardiac output or arterial vasodilatation and may occur in a number of clinical settings:
   a. Reduced cardiac output
      ■ Congestive heart failure (CHF)
      ■ Cardiogenic shock (e.g., acute myocardial infarction)
      ■ Pericardial effusion with tamponade
      ■ Massive pulmonary embolism
   b. Peripheral vasodilation
      ■ Sepsis
      ■ Antihypertensive medications
      ■ Anaphylaxis
      ■ Anesthesia
      ■ Cirrhosis and other liver diseases
3. **Intrarenal hemodynamic changes**
   a. Glomerular afferent arteriole vasoconstriction (preglomerular effect)
      ■ Nonsteroidal anti-inflammatory drugs (NSAIDs) (prostaglandin inhibition)
      ■ Cyclo-oxygenase 2 (Cox-2) inhibitors (prostaglandin inhibition)
      ■ Cyclosporine
      ■ Tacrolimus
      ■ Radiocontrast dye
      ■ Hypercalcemia
   b. Glomerular efferent arteriole vasodilation (postglomerular effect)
      ■ Angiotensin-converting enzyme inhibitors (ACEIs)
      ■ Angiotensin II receptor blockers (ARBs)

B. **Postrenal AKI.** It is caused by the acute obstruction of the flow of urine. Urinary obstruction of both ureters, the bladder, or the urethra may cause postrenal AKI. Patients most at risk for postrenal AKI are elderly men, in whom prostatic hypertrophy or prostatic cancer may lead to complete or partial obstruction of urine flow. In women, complete urinary tract obstruction is relatively uncommon in the absence of pelvic surgery, pelvic malignancy, or previous pelvic irradiation. The causes of postrenal AKI include:

1. **Bilateral ureteral obstruction or unilateral obstruction in a solitary kidney (upper urinary tract obstruction)**
   a. Intraureteral
      - Stones
      - Blood clots
      - Pyogenic debris or sloughed papillae
      - Edema following retrograde pyelography
      - Transitional cell carcinoma
   b. Extraureteral
      - Pelvic or abdominal malignancy
      - Retroperitoneal fibrosis
      - Accidental ureteral ligation or trauma during pelvic surgery
   c. Bladder neck/urethral obstruction (lower urinary tract obstruction)
      - Prostatic hypertrophy
      - Prostatic and bladder carcinoma
      - Autonomic neuropathy or anticholinergic agents causing urinary retention
      - Urethral stricture
      - Bladder stones
      - Fungal infection (e.g., fungus balls)
      - Blood clots

C. **Intrarenal or intrinsic AKI.** In contrast to prerenal azotemia and postrenal AKI, the disorders listed here represent problems which originate within the kidney itself. These problems may be vascular, glomerular, interstitial, or tubular. The diseases may be primary renal or part of a systemic disease. The course of AKI in these situations cannot be changed by manipulating factors outside the kidney (e.g., performing volume repletion, improving cardiac function, correcting hypotension, or removing obstruction).

1. **Vascular.** Vascular disorders causing AKI are classified based on the size of the vessels involved.
   a. Large- and medium-sized vessels
      - Renal artery thrombosis or embolism
      - Operative arterial cross-clamping
      - Bilateral renal vein thrombosis
      - Polyarteritis nodosa
   b. Small vessels
      - Atheroembolic disease
      - Thrombotic microangiopathies
      - HUS
      - TTP
      - Scleroderma renal crisis
      - Malignant hypertension
      - Thrombotic microangiopathies of pregnancy
      - Hemolysis, Elevated Liver enzymes, and Low Platelets (HELLP) syndrome
      - Postpartum AKI

2. **Glomerular.** Glomerular diseases are typically categorized based on urine findings as either nephrotic or nephritic.
   a. **Nephrotic** glomerular disorders are characterized by large proteinuria (greater than 3 g in 24 hours) and minimal hematuria. Nephrotic glomerular disorders are uncommonly associated with AKI, but may occur in minimal-change disease, due to volume depletion, or focal segmental glomerulosclerosis (FSGS), particularly collapsing FSGS.
   b. **Nephritic** glomerular disorders (glomerulonephritis) are characterized by hematuria and proteinuria (typically 1 to 2 g in 24 hours). Patients with known glomerulonephritis may develop AKI; alternatively, glomerulonephritis may commonly present as AKI. Rapidly progressive glomerulonephritis (RPGN), also called *crescentic nephritis*, should be suspected in a patient with

glomerulonephritis who has a doubling of serum creatinine within a 3-month period. RPGN is caused by injury to the glomerular capillary wall, which results in subsequent inflammation, fibrosis, and crescent formation. Urgency is required to make the diagnosis of RPGN, because crescent formation can rapidly destroy the glomeruli; response to therapy is directly correlated with the percentage of glomeruli having crescents. Because the diagnosis is typically made by renal biopsy, the causes of glomerulonephritis and RPGN are classified according to immunofluorescence staining on renal biopsy.

    i. Diseases with linear (anti-GBM) immune complex deposition
- Goodpasture's syndrome (renal and pulmonary complications are present)
- Renal-limited Goodpasture's syndrome

    ii. Diseases with granular immune complex deposition
- Acute postinfectious glomerulonephritis
- Lupus nephritis
- Infective endocarditis
- Immunoglobulin (Ig) A glomerulonephritis
- Henoch-Schönlein purpura
- Membranoproliferative glomerulonephritis
- Cryoglobulinemia

    iii. Diseases with no immune deposits (pauci-immune)
- Wegener's granulomatosis
- Microscopic polyangiitis
- Churg-Strauss syndrome (CSS)
- Idiopathic crescentic glomerulonephritis

3. Interstitium. AKI from an interstitial cause is known as *acute interstitial nephritis (AIN)*. The primary histologic lesion of AIN is marked edema of the interstitial space with a focal or diffuse infiltration of the renal interstitium with inflammatory cells (lymphocytes and/or eosinophils). AIN (also called *acute tubulointerstitial nephritis*) is most commonly due to drug hypersensitivity, but may also be a consequence of infections or systemic disease [e.g., systemic lupus erythematosus (SLE)].

    a. Drug-induced AIN. More than 100 drugs have been implicated in drug-induced AIN. Some of the drugs most commonly associated with AIN are:
- **Antibiotics** (e.g., methicillin, cephalosporins, rifampicin, sulfonamides, erythromycin, and ciprofloxacin)
- **Diuretics** (e.g., furosemide, thiazides, chlorthalidone)
- **NSAIDs**
- **Anticonvulsant drugs** (e.g., phenytoin, carbamazepine)
- **Allopurinol**

    b. Infection-associated AIN
- **Bacterial** (e.g., *Staphylococcus, Streptococcus*)
- **Viral** (e.g., cytomegalovirus, Epstein-Barr virus)
- **Tuberculosis**

4. Tubular. Acute tubular necrosis (ATN), which may be termed *AKI*, is characterized by an abrupt decrease in the GFR due to proximal tubular dysfunction caused by ischemia (50% of cases) and nephrotoxins (35% of cases). Although this type of renal injury has long been designated ATN, in many cases little true necrosis of tubular cells is present on histologic examination. Most of the renal biopsies are, however, late and therefore could miss early tubular necrosis. The tubules may demonstrate morphologic changes of sublethal injury (e.g., swelling, vacuolization, loss of brush border, apical blebbing, and loss of basolateral infoldings). Loss of viable and nonviable tubular epithelial cells into the urine also occurs. The continued presence of renal blood flow and reversibility of tubular dysfunction is compatible with the recovery of renal function that is seen in some patients with ATN.

Ischemic ATN is a consequence of reduced blood flow to the kidneys, which results from a decreased total blood volume or arterial underfilling with a redistribution of blood away from the kidney. Ischemic ATN is seen most commonly after septic or hemorrhagic shock. **Nephrotoxic ATN** is most commonly caused by aminoglycoside antibiotics and radiocontrast dye. In most cases the insults are multifactorial.

Causes of ATN include:

a. Renal ischemia
- Shock
- Hemorrhage
- Trauma
- Gram-negative sepsis
- Pancreatitis
- Hypotension from any cause

b. Nephrotoxic drugs
- Aminoglycoside antibiotics
- Amphotericin B
- Pentamidine
- Foscarnet
- Acyclovir
- Indinavir
- Antineoplastic agents (e.g., cisplatin)
- Radiocontrast dye
- Organic solvents (e.g., carbon tetrachloride)
- Ethylene glycol (antifreeze)
- Anesthetics (enflurane)
- Oral sodium phosphosoda used for bowel preparation for colonoscopy can cause acute phosphate nephropathy resulting in acute nephrocalcinosis

c. Endogenous toxins
- Myoglobin (e.g., rhabdomyolysis)
- Hemoglobin (e.g., incompatible blood transfusion, acute falciparum malaria)
- Uric acid (e.g., acute uric acid nephropathy)

III. EPIDEMIOLOGY OF AKI (Table 10-2).

A. Community-acquired AKI. AKI is present on admission in approximately 1% of hospitalized patients. Half of the cases occur in patients with CKD. The most common causes of community-acquired AKI include prerenal (70%) and postrenal (17%). The overall mortality of patients presenting with community-acquired AKI is 15%.

B. Hospital-acquired AKI. The development of AKI in hospitalized patients is common and carries with it a significant independent risk of mortality. Using the RIFLE criteria, up to 20% of hospitalized patients may develop AKI. The most common causes of AKI in hospitalized patients include ischemia, sepsis, medications, and radiocontrast dye. Prerenal azotemia a common cause of an increase in creatinine in ward patients, however, ATN accounts for the majority of causes of acute renal failure in ICU patients. ATN in the ICU is typically multifactorial and is frequently part of multisystem organ failure syndrome.

C. Prevention of AKI. Numerous factors predispose hospitalized patients to the development of AKI: volume depletion, drugs which affect renal blood flow (e.g., NSAIDs and Cox-2 inhibitors), and the use of nephrotoxic medications and contrast dye.

Although data are limited on treatments to prevent AKI, it is prudent to carefully follow volume status and maintain adequate hydration; discontinue (when possible) medications that are potentially nephrotoxic; choose alternate nonradiocontrast imaging techniques [e.g., magnetic resonance imaging (MRI) without gadolinium]; and use non-nephrotoxic antibiotics.

TABLE 10-2	Characteristics of Acute Kidney Injury (AKI) in Regard to the Location of its Development

Community-acquired AKI		
History/symptoms	Predisposing factor(s)	Type of AKI
Acute systemic illness (e.g., viral influenza, gastroenteritis)	Volume depletion	Prerenal azotemia or ATN
Streptococcal pharyngitis or pyoderma (vesicular skin lesions, typically located on the extremities, which become pustular and then crust)	Immune complex deposition in the glomeruli	Acute poststreptococcal glomerulonephritis
Trauma, crush injury, prolonged immobilization, "found down"	Extensive muscle damage and tissue breakdown	Rhabdomyolysis
Urinary tract symptoms such as difficulty voiding, incontinence, dribbling	Obstruction to urine flow or neurogenic bladder	Postrenal
Fever and/or rash in a patient recently prescribed a new medication	NSAIDS, antibiotics, and diuretics are frequently prescribed on an outpatient basis	Allergic interstitial nephritis
Accidental or intentional overdose of a nephrotoxin (altered mental status may be a frequent accompaniment)	Heavy metal compounds, solvents, ethylene glycol, salicylates, and acetaminophen	ATN

Acute renal failure occurring inside the hospital		
History/symptoms	Predisposing factor(s)	Type of AKI
Excessive fluid loss from aggressive diuresis, nasogastric suction, surgical drains, diarrhea, etc.	Volume depletion	Prerenal azotemia or ATN
Surgery with or without concomitant volume depletion	Anesthesia causes renal vasoconstriction, which reduces renal blood flow	Prerenal azotemia or ATN
Radiologic (contrast CT) or other procedures (e.g., coronary angiography)	Intravenous contrast dye	ATN
Sepsis	Infection, volume depletion, hypotension, nephrotoxic antibiotics (e.g., aminoglycosides)	ATN

ATN, acute tubular necrosis; CT, computed tomography; NSAID, nonsteroidal anti-inflammatory drug.

D. Morbidity and mortality associated with AKI. It is commonly thought that AKI from ATN is a completely reversible disorder. Recent data suggest that of patients who develop AKI in the ICU and require dialysis, 10% to 30% may require maintenance dialysis after discharge from the hospital.

Another widely held belief is that patients die with AKI, not from AKI. Numerous well-controlled studies have challenged this notion and found that after adjusting for comorbidities, the development of AKI in hospitalized

TABLE 10-3	Mortality of Acute Kidney Injury (AKI)

Type of AKI	Mortality
AKI in the ICU associated with respiratory failure and the requirement of dialysis	>90%
AKI in the ICU	72%
AKI in hospitalized patients, not in the ICU	32%
AKI following intravenous contrast	34% (compared to 7% in controls) Adjusted odds ratio of death: 5.5
AKI following cardiac surgery	64% (compared to 4.3% in controls) Adjusted odds ratio of death: 7.9
AKI following administration of amphotericin B	Adjusted odds ratio of death: 6.6

ICU, intensive care unit.

patients is an independent and significant predictor of in-hospital mortality (Table 10-3).

IV. **EVALUATION OF THE PATIENT WITH AKI.** A stepwise evaluation approach to the patient with AKI is recommended. A comprehensive **history** and thorough **physical examination** suggest the diagnosis in most patients.

Whether the patient is seen for the first time in the office, emergency room, hospital, or ICU, careful tabulation and recording of data are the first steps in determining the diagnosis. Vital signs, daily weights, records of intake and output, past and current laboratory data, and the fluid and medication list should be recorded on a flow sheet and included in the patient's chart. When the patient has been hospitalized for several days or weeks with a complicated course before developing AKI, a carefully prepared flow sheet may often be the only way to comprehend the problem and guide the selection of proper therapy.

Urinalysis by dipstick and the evaluation of **urine sediment** by microscopy should always be performed in patients with AKI. **Urine chemistries** that may be helpful in the diagnosis of AKI include sodium, creatinine, urea, osmolality, and protein content.

Clinical features of the common causes of AKI are described in the following sections.

A. **Prerenal azotemia.** This may occur in patients who are clinically hypovolemic (total intravascular volume depletion) or hypervolemic (arterial underfilling).

1. **History.** The following history is suggestive of prerenal azotemia from true volume depletion or hypovolemia: thirst, decreased fluid intake, fever, nausea, vomiting, diarrhea, burns, peritonitis, and pancreatitis. Prerenal azotemia from arterial underfilling occurs most commonly in patients with CHF or liver disease. Features of the history that are suggestive of CHF include recent myocardial infarction, orthopnea, paroxysmal nocturnal dyspnea, or dyspnea on exertion. Features suggesting liver disease and cirrhosis include a history of alcohol abuse or hepatitis. A complete documentation of medications (prescribed and over-the-counter) is important in the evaluation of prerenal azotemia. Medications that affect intrarenal hemodynamics include cyclosporine, tacrolimus, NSAIDs, Cox-2 inhibitors, ACEIs, and ARBs.

2. **Physical examination.** Assessment of volume status and the adequacy of the extracellular fluid (ECF) volume are critical to the diagnosis of prerenal azotemia.

   a. **Physical findings that suggest a reduction in intravascular volume** include:
   - Absence of axillary sweat
   - A recent reduction in body weight

- Orthostatic hypotension. Defined as a fall in systolic blood pressure of more than 20 mm Hg or a rise in pulse rate of more than 10 beats per minute after standing
- Tachycardia
- Dry mucous membranes
- "Tenting" of upper thorax skin when pinched between the fingers
- Jugular venous pressure not visible when supine

b. Physical examination findings generally found in arterial underfilling states with an excess of ECF include:
- Elevated jugular venous pressure
- Ascites
- Lower extremity pitting edema
- Anasarca
   CHF in particular may be identified by:
- Pulmonary crackles
- S3 gallop
   Liver failure may be identified by:
- Jaundice
- Decreased liver size
- Palmar erythema
- Spider angiomas

3. Urinary findings. Regardless of the cause of prerenal azotemia (hypovolemic, arterial underfilling, or medication induced) the urine dipstick, sediment, and chemistries will be the same (Table 10-4 for a comparison of urinary findings in various types of AKI).

a. The urine **dipstick** should be normal with negative protein, heme, leukocyte esterase, and nitrate. The specific gravity is increased (greater than 1.020).

b. The **urine sediment** may be bland but granular casts may be present.

c. Urine chemistry and indices. Frequently it is difficult to distinguish between prerenal azotemia and AKI, particularly ATN. Laboratory tests and indices characteristic of prerenal azotemia versus other causes of AKI are summarized in Table 10-5. The pathophysiologic basis of these tests is discussed in section IV.G.3.

4. Specific disorders of prerenal azotemia

a. Hepatorenal syndrome (HRS) occurs in patients with severe liver failure. It is characterized by peripheral vasodilatation (low systemic vascular resistance) accompanied by intense renal vasoconstriction that causes renal insufficiency. Two forms of HRS are recognized. **Type I HRS** is the more severe form and is characterized by an abrupt (within 2 weeks) decline of renal function, defined as a doubling of serum creatinine to greater than 2.5 mg per dL or a 50% reduction in creatinine clearance to less than 20 mL per minute. Without liver transplantation, the mortality of this condition is greater than 90% at 3 months. **Type II HRS** is characterized by slowly progressing renal insufficiency (serum creatinine greater than 1.5 mg per dL and CCr less than 40 mL per minute) in a patient with refractory ascites; it has a much better prognosis. Patients with type II HRS may convert to type I in the setting of certain insults such as the development of infections (e.g., spontaneous bacterial peritonitis) or the use of NSAIDs. HRS is typical of other forms of prerenal azotemia, and the kidney functions normally if transplanted into a person with a normal liver. The only permanent cure for HRS is liver transplantation unless there is substantial recovery of an acute liver insult.

The **diagnostic criteria for HRS** have recently been revised. CCr has been excluded. Renal failure in the setting of ongoing bacterial infection, but in the absence of septic shock, does not explain HRS. This implies that treatment of HRS can be initiated without waiting for recovery from infection. Minor diagnostic criteria have been removed. To diagnose HRS, each of the criteria must be present.

TABLE 10-4   Urinary Findings in Various Causes of Acute Kidney Injury (AKI)

Dipstick	Prerenal azotemia[a]	Postrenal[b]	Small vessel vascular	Nephrotic glomerular	Nephritic glomerular	AIN	ATN[c]
Leukocyte esterase	(−)	(−)	(−)	(−)	(−)	(++)	(−)
Heme	(−)	(−)	(±)	(−) or trace	(±)	(±)	(−)
Protein	(−)	(−)	(±)	(+)	(±)	(±)	(−) or trace
Specific gravity	>1.020	1.010	Variable	Variable	Variable	1.010	1.010
Microscopy							
RBCs	(−)	(−)	(+)	(−) or few	(+)	(±)	(−)
WBCs	(−)	(−)	(±)	(−)	(±)	(±)	(−)
RBC casts	(−)	(−)	(±)	(−)	(±)	(±)	(−)
WBC casts	(−)	(−)	(−)	(−)	(−)	(−)	(−)
Granular casts	(−)	(−)	(−)	(−)	(−)	(−)	(±)
Renal tubular epithelial cells	(−)	(−)	(−)	(−)	(−)	(−)	(±)
Tests							
Osmolality (mOsm/L)	>500	≤350	Variable	Variable	Variable	≤350	≤350
Protein (g/d)	(−)	(−)	1–2	>3	1–2	1–2	≤1

AIN, acute interstitial nephritis; ATN, acute tubular necrosis; RBCs, red blood cells; WBCs, white blood cells.
[a] Although classically associated with a bland urinary sediment, a few granular casts may occasionally be present.
[b] If a superimposed infection is present due to urine stasis, the leukocyte esterase, heme, protein, RBCs, and WBCs may be positive.
[c] If ATN is secondary to rhabdomyolysis, heme will be positive on dipstick and RBCs will be absent on microscopy.

Index	Prerenal azotemia	Acute tubular necrosis
Urine sodium (Una), mEq/L	<20	>40
Urine osmolality, mOsm/kg H$_2$O	>500	<350
Urine creatinine (UCr) to plasma creatinine (PCr)	>40	<20
Serum BUN/serum creatinine	>20	≤10
Fractional excretion of sodium (FENa):		
FENa = [(Una/Pna)/(Ucr/Pcr)] × 100	<1	>1
Fractional excretion of urea (FEUN):		
FEUN = [(Uun/Pun)/(Ucr/Pcr)] × 100	<35	>50

BUN, blood urea nitrogen (mg/dL); Pcr, plasma creatinine (mg/dL); Pna, plasma sodium (mEq/L); Pun, plasma urea nitrogen (mg/dL); Uun, urine urea nitrogen (mg/dL).

Diagnostic criteria for HRS
- Cirrhosis with ascites
- Serum creatinine greater than 1.5 mg per dL
- Absence of another cause of renal failure [e.g., proteinuria greater than 500 mg per dL; hematuria (greater than 50 red blood cells (RBCs) per high-power field); abnormal renal ultrasonography]
- Absence of ongoing fluid loss
- Absence of shock
- Absence of a sustained improvement in renal function following at least 2 days of diuretic withdrawal and volume expansion with albumin. Recommended dose of albumin is 1 g per kg per day up to a maximum of 100 g per day.

b. Vasomotor prerenal azotemia due to NSAIDs. A history of NSAID use in all patients with prerenal azotemia or AKI should be aggressively sought. Under euvolemic conditions with normal kidney, liver, and cardiac function, the administration of NSAIDs does not cause an increase in serum creatinine. In the presence of clinical conditions with increased renal vasoconstrictor activity (e.g., CHF, cirrhosis, nephrotic syndrome, hypertension, sepsis, volume depletion, anesthesia), NSAIDs can cause prerenal azotemia. Patients with chronic renal insufficiency (e.g., diabetic nephropathy) are also at risk of acute vasomotor decline in renal function with NSAIDs. Typical clinical features include the presence of risk factors, decreased urinary output, usually bland urine sediment, low (less than 1%) fractional excretion of sodium (FENa), and prompt improvement in renal function after discontinuation of NSAIDs. NSAIDs may predispose AIN and ATN.

c. Cyclosporine and tacrolimus may cause a dose-dependent, hemodynamically mediated prerenal azotemia in patients who have undergone solid-organ and bone marrow transplantation. A large increase in renal vascular resistance occurs. The loss of renal function is generally reversible when the dosage of the drug is reduced. The urine sediment is bland, and ATN is not typically present.

d. ACEIs and ARBs are widely used for the treatment of hypertension, CHF, and diabetic nephropathy. Prerenal azotemia may occur in conditions where angiotensin plays a crucial protective role in maintaining GFR by constricting the glomerular efferent arteriole, such as volume depletion, bilateral renal artery stenosis, autosomal dominant polycystic kidney disease, cardiac failure, cirrhosis, and diabetic nephropathy. Diuretic-induced sodium depletion and underlying chronic renal insufficiency are other major predisposing factors.

The decline in renal function is usually asymptomatic, nonoliguric, and associated with hyperkalemia; renal function returns to baseline in most cases after discontinuation of the ACEI or ARB. Prerenal azotemia from ACEI/ARB can usually be managed in the outpatient setting by discontinuation of the ACEI/ARB and discontinuation of diuretics if present. An increase in BUN and serum creatinine in a patient on an ACEI or ARB should raise the possibility of renal artery stenosis.

B. Postrenal AKI

1. History. Symptoms that suggest urinary tract obstruction are anuria or intermittent anuria and polyuria, prostatic symptoms (urinary frequency and urgency, dysuria, straining upon urination), pelvic malignancy on previous radiotherapy, and recurrent renal stones. Patients may complain of pain over a distended bladder; severe pain (renal colic) may be present if obstruction is due to renal calculi. Patients with diabetes mellitus, sickle cell anemia, analgesic nephropathy, and benign prostatic hypertrophy are predisposed to papillary necrosis that causes obstruction.

2. Physical examination. The physical examination is important in diagnosing postrenal AKI, especially in the unconscious patient or in the confused patient in whom otherwise unexplained agitation may be the only clue to acute urinary retention. Careful abdominal examination may uncover a distended, tender bladder or bilaterally hydronephrotic kidneys. A digital examination of the prostate should be performed routinely in any male patient with AKI, and pelvic masses should be sought in female patients through a bimanual pelvic examination. In any patient in whom lower tract obstruction is suspected as the cause of acute AKI, a sterile in-and-out diagnostic postvoid bladder catheterization should be performed as a routine part of the physical examination. The postvoid residual urine volume should be less than 50 mL. The urine volume should be recorded and the specimen saved for studies.

3. Urine findings. The typical urinalysis and sediment finding in postrenal AKI compared to other causes of AKI is presented in Table 10-4.

  a. Urinalysis. The urine dipstick should be normal with negative protein, heme, leukocyte esterase, and nitrite. The specific gravity is typically isosmotic (1.010). Heme test for RBCs may be positive if obstruction is due to renal calculi. A secondary infection may be present due to urine stasis; in this setting the dipstick may be positive for leukocyte esterase, nitrite, heme, and trace protein.

  b. Urine sediment is typically bland without cells or casts. As noted, hematuria may be present if obstruction is due to renal calculi. Prostatitis and some cases of benign prostatic hypertrophy may also be associated with hematuria. In the setting of a secondary urinary tract infection (UTI), the sediment may contain white blood cells (WBCs), RBCs, and/or bacteria.

4. Radiologic tests. Renal ultrasonography is sufficient to diagnose urinary obstruction in most patients. Because of the risk of intravenous contrast dye, intravenous pyelogram (IVP) should be avoided.

  a. Renal ultrasonography is the radiologic test of choice to evaluate for obstruction, characterized by dilatation of the urinary tract (hydronephrosis). The absence of hydronephrosis virtually excludes important urinary tract obstruction; hydronephrosis may be absent, however, in the following settings: early obstruction (before the urinary tract has been able to dilate) and obstruction due to the encasement of the urinary system by retroperitoneal fibrosis or tumor.

    Hydronephrosis that is not functionally significant may occur in pregnancy and in people with anatomic variants of the collecting system. If the functional importance of hydronephrosis is in doubt, a furosemide isotope renogram can evaluate the functional significance of the obstruction.

  b. Isotope renography is performed by the intravenous injection of a radionucleotide and furosemide. Furosemide increases urinary flow and normally causes a rapid washout of the radionucleotide. Persistence of the isotope in the renal parenchyma suggests obstruction. Poor renal function limits the usefulness of this test because the diuretic response may be blunted, thereby making interpretation of the test difficult.

    c. Noncontrast computed tomography (CT) of the kidneys, ureters, and abdomen is often done following renal ultrasonography to identify the cause and location of urinary obstruction.

    d. Cystoscopy and retrograde pyelography. In instances of AKI with a high clinical suspicion of urinary tract obstruction (e.g., calculi, pyogenic debris, blood clots, bladder cancer), cystoscopy and retrograde or anterograde pyelography should be performed, even if ultrasonographic finding is negative for obstruction.

C. Intrinsic renal disease — large vessel disease

    1. History. Renal artery thrombosis or embolism, or bilateral renal vein thrombosis may present with flank pain. Predisposing disorders such as membranous nephropathy or antiphospholipid antibody syndrome may be present.

    2. Urine findings

        a. Urinalysis. The urine dipstick is positive for heme.

        b. Urine sediment. RBCs.

    3. Laboratory findings and radiology. An elevated serum lactic dehydrogenase (LDH) may be present. Doppler ultrasonography may be used to assess renal blood flow and to evaluate for renal vein thrombosis. CT or magnetic resonance (MR) angiography are useful for detecting clots in the renal vein or inferior vena cava. Angiography may be required in emergent cases (e.g., acute anuria due to acute renal embolization).

D. Intrinsic renal disease — small vessel disease. Intrinsic renal disease due to small vessel disease is caused by either atheroembolic disease or thrombotic microangiopathy. The clinical and laboratory features of these disorders are as follows:

    1. Atheroembolic disease is caused by the detachment of atheromatous plaques from the intimal surface of large vessels. These plaques travel distally and occlude small arteries or large arterioles of the kidney. Showers of cholesterol crystals or microemboli from the surface of ulcerated plaques may also occur, traveling distally to occlude small arterioles throughout the body (e.g., kidney, gut, or skin). The presentation and clinical findings of atheroembolic disease can be confused with those of polyarteritis nodosa, allergic vasculitis, subacute bacterial endocarditis, or left atrial myxoma.

        The usual course is progressive renal insufficiency. However, milder forms of renal failure with some recovery of function have been described. No treatment is known. Prevention of the disease involves avoiding unnecessary invasive procedures (e.g., renal arteriogram in patients with clinical evidence of widespread atherosclerosis).

        a. History. A history of AKI occurring after cardiovascular surgery, angiography, or administration of intravenous thrombolytics should raise a suspicion of atheroembolic disease as the cause of AKI, particularly in a patient with known atherosclerosis. Occasionally, the disease occurs spontaneously.

        b. Physical examination. Skin manifestations of cholesterol emboli include discrete peripheral necrotic areas, blue toe syndrome, and livido reticularis. Small cholesterol emboli to the gut and pancreas may cause abdominal pain.

        c. Laboratory investigation may reveal an increased erythrocyte sedimentation rate, eosinophilia, and hypocomplementemia (C3 is reduced whereas C4 remains normal). Biopsy of the skin, muscle, or kidney reveals intravascular cholesterol crystals.

        d. Urinary evaluation

            i. Urinalysis. Dipstick is frequently negative although heme and protein or both may be positive. Specific gravity is variable.

            ii. Urine sediment. Sediment is often bland, although RBCs, granular casts, RBC casts, or all may be present.

            iii. Urine tests. Proteinuria is typically less than 1 g in 24 hours.

2. **Thrombotic microangiopathies** are characterized by a microangiopathic hemolytic anemia, thrombocytopenia, and variable renal and neurologic manifestations. These disorders begin with endothelial injury followed by secondary platelet thrombi formation in renal arterioles; renal cortical necrosis may result from the arterial lesions. The primary site of injury is the glomerulus or the vascular supply of the glomerulus; the proximal tubule and interstitium are relatively uninvolved.

   a. **History and physical examination.** HUS-TTP should be suspected in patients with anemia, AKI, thrombocytopenia, and neurologic signs such as confusion and seizures. Malignant hypertension causing a thrombotic microangiopathy is characterized by high blood pressure associated with papilledema and/or retinal hemorrhages; other organ involvement may manifest as chest pain, shortness of breath from pulmonary edema, and confusion from brain involvement. Scleroderma renal crisis should be considered in patients with scleroderma and an abrupt rise in serum creatinine associated with hypertension.

   b. **Laboratory findings.** Peripheral blood smear demonstrates increased RBC fragmentation (schistocytes) and thrombocytopenia. Indices of hemolysis (e.g., LDH) are elevated.

   c. **Urine findings**

      i. **On dipstick.** Variable specific gravity; heme positive, protein positive, or both.

      ii. **Urine sediment** is characterized by granular casts, RBC casts, or both.

E. **Intrinsic renal disease–glomerular disease from a nephrotic cause.** Nephrotic glomerular disorders are characterized by a urine protein excretion of greater than 3 g in 24 hours. Nephrotic glomerular disorders are uncommonly associated with AKI, but it may occur in patients with minimal-change disease (especially in the elderly) and FSGS (especially from collapsing FSGS). This generally occurs when the serum albumin concentration is less than 2.0 g per dL.

   1. **History and physical examination.** Clinical symptoms and signs characteristic of a nephrotic disorder include pitting peripheral edema, hypertension, periorbital edema, and anasarca.

   2. **Laboratory findings.** Typically hypoalbuminemia and hypercholesterolemia are present.

   3. **Urine findings.** In cases of minimal change–induced AKI, urine dipstick and sediment may also include features of ATN.

      a. **Dipstick** is strongly positive for protein. Heme is negative or trace.

      b. **Urine sediment** is typically bland; possibly with few RBCs. Oval fat bodies reflecting lipiduria may be present.

      c. **Urine tests** show proteinuria greater than 3 g in 24 hours.

F. **Intrinsic renal disease – glomerular disease from a nephritic cause.** Nephritic glomerular disorders (glomerulonephritis) frequently cause AKI. Nephritic glomerular disorders are characterized by hematuria and proteinuria (typically 1 to 2 g in 24 hours). RPGN should be suspected in a patient with glomerulonephritis who has a doubling of serum creatinine within a 3-month period.

   1. **History and physical examination.** Clinical symptoms and signs that suggest that the glomerulonephritis is part of a systemic disease include palpable purpura, skin rash, arthralgias, arthritis, fever, cardiac murmurs, sinusitis, hemoptysis, abdominal pain, and acute neuropathy. Hemoptysis is an ominous symptom in a patient with AKI and may indicate a life-threatening vasculitis, such as Goodpasture's syndrome or Wegener's granulomatosis.

   2. **Urine findings.** Glomerulonephritis is characterized by hematuria and proteinuria. The identification of RBC casts confirms the presence of glomerular disease.

   3. **Laboratory findings.** ANCAs are helpful in determining the cause of glomerulonephritis. ANCA staining by immunofluorescence is either cytoplasmic (c-ANCA) or perinuclear (p-ANCA). Although c-ANCA and p-ANCA are sensitive screening tests, numerous conditions other than vasculitis and

glomerulonephritis may result in c-ANCA or p-ANCA positivity. Therefore, all positive results must be confirmed with enzyme-linked immunosorbent assay (ELISA) tests for the more specific antigen targets proteinase 3 (PR3) and myeloperoxidase (MPO). The PR3-ANCA antibody is typically responsible for c-ANCA staining and the MPO-ANCA antibody for the p-ANCA staining.

Of patients with active Wegener's disease, 90% are ANCA positive (the majority are PR3-ANCA positive). Of patients with microscopic polyangiitis, 70% are ANCA positive (the majority are MPO-ANCA positive). Of patients with CSS, 50% are ANCA positive (PR3- and MPO-ANCA detected with about equal frequency). More than 90% of patients with renal limited, idiopathic pauci-immune vasculitis are ANCA positive (the majority are MPO-ANCA positive).

4. **Anti-GBM antibodies** are useful for the diagnosis of Goodpasture's disease, although false-negative results may occur.

5. Evaluation of **serum complement** (C3 and C4) may be helpful in the evaluation of patients with AKI and glomerulonephritis. Hypocomplementemia is common in postinfectious glomerulonephritis, lupus nephritis, membranoproliferative glomerulonephritis, and mixed cryoglobulinemia. Another cause of AKI associated with hypocomplementemia includes atheroembolic renal disease. It is important to recognize that other nonrenal conditions may lower serum complement levels (e.g., sepsis, acute pancreatitis, and advanced liver disease).

G. **Intrinsic renal disease — AIN.** Intrinsic renal disease due to AIN may be secondary to medications, infections, or a systemic illness such as lupus. Drug-induced AIN may be divided into three categories: AIN from methicillin, AIN from a medication other than methicillin, and NSAID-induced AIN. Interstitial nephritis from methicillin is no longer seen because this drug is no longer clinically available; however, methicillin-induced AIN remains the prototype for the classification of AIN. The clinical presentation and findings of these three major forms of drug-induced AIN are described in Table 10-6. Renal insufficiency typically persists for a mean of 1.5 months; however, complete recovery of renal function occurs in most patients.

1. **History.** In NSAID-induced AIN, symptoms and findings do not occur until several months after initiation of drug therapy (average 6 months); fenoprofen is the culprit in half of cases. AIN from other medications typically occurs within a few weeks of drug therapy. Patients may complain of fever, rash, or flank pain.

2. **Physical examination.** Physical findings with acute drug-induced interstitial nephritis may be lacking, although fever and a maculopapular or petechial skin eruption may occur with any of the agents, particularly the penicillin derivatives and allopurinol.

3. **Laboratory findings.** Eosinophilia was common in methicillin-induced AIN, but is present in less than 50% of cases of AIN from NSAIDs and other drugs.

4. **Urine findings.** When AIN is caused by methicillin and other drugs, RBCs and WBCs are present in most cases; also present are WBC casts, the urine is typically

TABLE 10-6		Three Types of Drug-Induced Interstitial Nephritis					
Drug group	Age	Duration of therapy	Fever	Rash	Hematuria and pyuria	Eosinophilia	Nephrotic syndrome
Methicillin	Any age	2 wk	80%	25%	90%	80%	No
Nonmethicillin	Any age	3 wk	<50%	<50%	50%	<50%	No
NSAIDs	>50 yr	Mo	10%	10%	<50%	20%	70%

NSAIDs, nonsteroidal anti-inflammatory drugs.

isotonic, and 20% of cases are oliguric. In NSAID-induced AIN, nephrotic-range proteinuria is present in 80% of cases (greater than 3 g in 24 hours); WBCs, RBCs, and eosinophils are present in less than 50% of cases.

The evaluation for urinary eosinophils should be performed with Hansel's secretion stain (methylene blue and eosin Y in methanol), which is superior to Wright's stain, because urinary eosinophils are readily identified by their brilliant red-pink granules. In contrast to Wright's stain, Hansel's stain is not influenced by urinary pH. In a recent review of four series of drug-induced AIN, the positive predictive value for eosinophils in the urine was only 50%; however, the negative predictive value was 90%.

H. Intrinsic renal disease — ATN. ATN typically occurs in hospitalized patients as a consequence of ischemia or nephrotoxins.

   1. History. The evaluation of a patient with suspected ATN must focus on identifying a predisposing cause. The chart should be reviewed for a history of hypotensive episodes, fluid losses, aminoglycoside use, NSAID administration, or radiologic procedures associated with contrast administration.

   2. Physical examination. Signs of sepsis or ongoing infection should be evaluated. Volume status should be determined (see section IV.A.2.a.).

   3. Laboratory findings and urinalysis. Distinguishing ATN from prerenal azotemia is often very difficult; this is an important clinical problem because a decline in GFR in hospitalized patients is most commonly due to either ATN or prerenal azotemia. In addition, prolonged prerenal azotemia often predisposes to the development of ATN. Because the causative factors for prerenal azotemia and ATN overlap, distinguishing between the two may become possible only by the outcome of therapy (e.g., if volume repletion improves renal function, then prerenal azotemia was present).

   In general, a urine sediment with muddy brown granular casts is characteristic of ATN. However, this finding may be lacking, and other clinical clues will be necessary to make the diagnosis. To distinguish between the two, numerous diagnostic indices and formulae have been developed based on their pathophysiologic differences.

   Prerenal azotemia is a hemodynamic condition in which tubular function is normal, whereas ATN is characterized by tubular dysfunction. This distinction is the basis for the following tests (Table 10-5):
   - Urine specific gravity
   - Urine osmolality
   - Urine creatinine/plasma creatinine
   - Urine sodium concentration
   - FENa
   - Serum BUN to creatinine ratio

   Prerenal azotemia is characterized by the increased reabsorption of water and sodium by the nephron. The increased reabsorption of water increases urine specific gravity and osmolality. Tubular reabsorption of urea increases, thereby increasing the serum BUN to creatinine ratio; creatinine, however, is not reabsorbed, and its concentration increases in the urine and increases the urine to plasma creatinine ratio. Sodium reabsorption increases, resulting in a low urine sodium concentration and FENa. In ATN, these processes typically cannot occur. Therefore, urine specific gravity and osmolality are isotonic, the urine creatinine to plasma creatinine ratio does not increase above a 20:1 ratio, the serum BUN to creatinine ratio does not increase, and urine sodium and FENa are higher than in prerenal azotemia. FENa is not always increased in ATN; the causes of ATN that are associated with a low urine sodium concentration and low FENa include radiocontrast nephropathy and rhabdomyolysis.

   The use of loop diuretics in AKI is a confounding factor in the use of FENa to distinguish prerenal azotemia and ATN. Distal acting diuretics (e.g., furosemide) increase urinary sodium excretion and increase FENa even if the patient is prerenal. A recent study evaluated the use of the fractional excretion of urea nitrogen (FEUN) to distinguish prerenal azotemia in the setting of diuretic use from ATN (both of which are typically associated with a FENa of greater than 2%). The basis of this test is that urea absorption increases in the proximal tubule in prerenal azotemia and would not be affected by the use of diuretics, which act on the distal tubule. In the setting of loop diuretic use, FEUN was an excellent test to distinguish between these conditions. In prerenal azotemia, the FEUN is less than 35% and in ATN it is greater than 50%. The use of FEUN in cases of ATN associated with a low FENa could not be assessed in this study because of the lack of patients with this condition. Keep in mind that FEUN cannot be used in the setting of osmotic diuretic use (e.g., mannitol), because these agents affect proximal tubular absorption. A recent study, however, has indicated that the specificity of FEUN to distinguish between prerenal azotemia and ATN is poor.

4. **Specific causes of ATN**
   a. **Aminoglycoside nephrotoxicity.** AKI occurs in up to 20% of patients on aminoglycosides, even with careful dosing and therapeutic plasma levels. The incidence of nephrotoxicity correlates better with total cumulative dose than with plasma levels. Predisposing factors are old age, preexisting renal disease, volume depletion, and combination with other agents (e.g., diuretics, cephalosporins, vancomycin). Nephrotoxicity is usually clinically apparent after 5 to 10 days of therapy; early findings are isosthenuria caused by nephrogenic diabetes insipidus, and magnesium and potassium wasting. Later findings include azotemia, which may not develop for the first time until after the drug has been discontinued; conversely, recovery of renal function after discontinuation of the nephrotoxic aminoglycoside is often delayed and may require weeks or months to be complete. AKI from aminoglycosides is typically nonoliguric.

   In Table 10-7, a comparison of the clinical characteristics of aminoglycoside and radiocontrast nephropathy are shown.
   b. **Radiographic contrast nephropathy.** Radiocontrast agents cause AKI through a direct nephrotoxic effect and by causing renal vasoconstriction. Risk factors include old age, high contrast dose, preexisting renal disease, (especially diabetes mellitus), volume depletion, and recent exposure to other agents, such as NSAIDs. Renal failure develops 1 to 2 days after exposure and is typically nonoliguric and associated with a high urine specific gravity, bland urine sediment, and low FENa. Serum creatinine typically peaks at 3 to 4 days and returns to baseline after about a week.
      i. **Prevention.** Nonionic contrast agents are less nephrotoxic and should be used in high-risk patients, especially patients with preexisting renal dysfunction. Drugs that affect renal hemodynamics (e.g., NSAIDs) and diuretics should be discontinued before the procedure if possible.

      Although numerous agents have been studied to prevent contrast nephropathy, the only therapies that have been shown to be beneficial are intravenous hydration with either isotonic saline or isotonic sodium bicarbonate before and after the contrast load. Reports are conflicting whether isotonic saline or bicarbonate is superior, but one of these forms of hydration should be utilized in patients who receive intravenous contrast.

      N-acetylcysteine (NAC) may be beneficial in the prevention of contrast nephropathy, and its administration before contrast is reasonable. In a frequently cited prospective trial, patients treated with NAC had a significantly lower serum creatinine 48 hours after contrast administration. The benefit of NAC in the prevention of contrast nephropathy, however, remains uncertain. Some studies have confirmed the benefit of NAC in the prevention of contrast nephropathy, others have not. The weight of the evidence of meta-analysis and other studies suggest that administration of NAC at either 600 or 1,200 mg doses is beneficial. Given the potential benefit, and the minimal risk, the authors recommend that 1,200 mg of NAC be given orally twice a day on the day of the procedure and the day

TABLE 10-7   A Comparison between Aminoglycoside Nephrotoxicity and Contrast Nephropathy

	Pathophysiology	Risk factors	Onset of renal failure	Urine output	Prevention
Aminoglycoside	Direct tubular toxin	Older age Volume depletion Diuretics Cephalosporins Vancomycin	5–10 d	Nonoliguric	Avoidance Correct drug dosing
Contrast	Vasoconstriction	Older age Diabetes Multiple myeloma ACE inhibitors NSAIDs	1–2 d	Nonoliguric	Nonionic, iso-osmotic contrast NAC Isotonic saline or isotonic bicarbonate

ACE, angiotensin-converting enzyme; NAC, N-acetylcysteine; NSAIDs, nonsteroidal anti-inflammatory drugs.

after. It was previously thought that NAC may artificially lower serum creatinine measurement; however, the very small lowering of serum creatinine seen with NAC administration does not explain the magnitude of the protective benefit seen in clinical trials.

Studies are ongoing to address whether prophylactic hemofiltration or hemodialysis (HD) may be of benefit to patients who receive intravenous contrast. Currently, insufficient data exists for hemofiltration or dialysis to be recommended as a standard approach.

The clinical significance of contrast nephropathy should not be underestimated. It has been demonstrated that the development of AKI after contrast administration is associated with an adjusted odds ratio of death of 5.5 versus patients who do not develop AKI (see Table 10-3, mortality associated with AKI).

Agents tested and demonstrated to be ineffective in the prevention of contrast nephropathy include furosemide, mannitol, theophylline, dopamine, fenoldopam, and atrial natriuretic peptide.

c. Rhabdomyolysis is caused by muscle injury (traumatic or atraumatic) that leads to the systemic release of muscle contents including myoglobin. Myoglobin is a heme pigment that is directly nephrotoxic; the intratubular precipitation of myoglobin causes obstruction and also contributes to the development of renal failure. Rhabdomyolysis should be considered in patients with trauma, muscle pain, and dark brown urine. However, rhabdomyolysis is frequently atraumatic, and up to 50% of patients have no muscular complaints. In Table 10-8 predisposing factors for rhabdomyolysis are listed.

The characteristic **urine finding** is a heme-positive urine with absence of RBCs. Pigmented granular casts are typically present on urine sediment. Laboratory clues to the diagnosis include a rapid rise of serum creatinine, massively increased creatine phosphokinase, hyperphosphatemia, hyperuricemia, hypocalcemia, increased anion gap, and disproportionate hyperkalemia. Serum calcium is reduced due to the sequestration of calcium into injured muscle; this calcium is released from the tissue during the recovery phase and may cause hypercalcemia. Therefore, replacement of serum calcium should be avoided unless symptoms of hypocalcemia are present.

The only proven **therapy** in the treatment of rhabdomyolysis is early and vigorous infusion of intravenous isotonic saline. In crush injury, it is recommended that intravenous saline be administered even before extrication. Mannitol administration and urinary alkalinization are often attempted in the treatment of rhabdomyolysis, although their efficacy may not be superior to vigorous hydration with saline alone. Theoretically, forced diuresis with mannitol may aid in the washout of obstructing myoglobin pigment. Mannitol administration may be attempted only after the correction of volume deficits; saline and mannitol should be administered together with a goal urine output

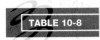

TABLE 10-8	Causes of Rhabdomyolysis

Direct muscle damage (e.g., crush injuries, polymyositis, prolonged immobilization associated with unconsciousness)
Muscle ischemia (e.g., arterial occlusion or embolism)
Excess energy consumption (e.g., seizures, hyperthermia, delirium tremens)
Decreased energy production (e.g., severe hypophosphatemia, hypokalemia, myxedema, genetic defect)
Drugs and toxins (e.g., alcohol, heroin, cocaine, amphetamines, poisonous insect, and snake bites)
Severe infections (e.g., tetanus, Legionnaire's disease, influenza)

of 300 mL per hour. Urinary alkalinization may inhibit myoglobin precipitation; however, urinary alkalinization is difficult to achieve in practice and requires the administration of a large quantity of bicarbonate. Bicarbonate administration in rhabdomyolysis carries the risk of worsening hypocalcemia due to increased calcium and phosphorus precipitation into injured muscle.

d. **Acute uric acid nephropathy** causes AKI due to the intratubular deposition of uric acid crystals. A very high serum uric acid concentration is present (e.g., greater than or equal to 15 mg per dL). The condition typically occurs during induction chemotherapy for malignancies with high cell turnover (e.g., leukemias and lymphoproliferative malignancies). Acute uric acid nephropathy and AKI occur in the tumor lysis syndrome, but may occur spontaneously in patients with high tumor burden. Clinical features of acute uric acid nephropathy are hyperuricemia, hyperkalemia, hyperphosphatemia, and a urine urate to creatinine ratio higher than 1. Preventive measures include allopurinol administration (300 to 600 mg per day) and vigorous hydration and forced diuresis with mannitol. Alkalinization of the urine has been traditionally recommended, but has not been proved more beneficial than saline administration alone; additionally, bicarbonate therapy carries the risk of increased calcium precipitation. Rasburicase, a recombinant urate oxidase, can lower uric acid levels rapidly allowing earlier institution of chemotherapy, and may reduce the risk of acute uric acid nephropathy.

V. AKI IN SPECIAL CLINICAL CIRCUMSTANCES

A. **Crystal-associated AKI.** A number of important causes of AKI may be due to the formation of urinary crystals. In Table 10-9 the causes of AKI associated with crystal formation are listed.

B. **Acute phosphate nephropathy.** A number of case reports and case series have described a potential association between use of oral sodium phosphosoda (used as a bowel preparation for colonoscopy) resulting in hyperphosphatemia, hypocalcemia, and the development of acute nephrocalcinosis, AKI, and CKD. Oral or enema sodium phosphosoda therefore is contraindicated in patients with kidney disease.

C. **AKI in patients with AIDS** (Table 10-10). The approach to the causes of AKI in AIDS patients is the same as that for other patients (i.e., classification into prerenal, intrinsic renal, and postrenal causes). AKI may develop in up to 20% of hospitalized

| **TABLE 10-9** | Urinary Crystals Associated with Acute Kidney Injury (AKI) |

Type of AKI	Crystal	Shape/appearance
ATN from ethylene glycol	Calcium oxalate monohydrate or	Needle shaped
	Calcium oxalate dihydrate	Envelope shaped
ATN from uric acid nephropathy	Uric acid	Diamond shaped, yellow or brown
AKI from sulfadiazine (intratubular obstruction)	Sulfadiazine	Needle shaped or shocks of wheat
AKI from acyclovir (intratubular obstruction)	Acyclovir	Needle shaped, birefringent
AKI from indinavir (intratubular obstruction)	Indinavir sulfate	Needle shaped, occasionally forming rosettes

ATN, acute tubular necrosis.

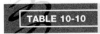

TABLE 10-10	Acute Kidney Injury (AKI) in Acquired Immunodeficiency Syndrome (AIDS) Patients

Prerenal azotemia
Hypovolemia (diarrhea)
Hypotension (sepsis, bleeding)
Decreased effective arterial blood volume (hypoalbuminemia, cachexia, HIV nephropathy)
Vasoconstriction (radiocontrast agents)
Postrenal AKI
Tubular obstruction due to crystalluria (intravenous acyclovir, sulfadiazine, indinavir, saquinavir, ritonavir)
Extrinsic ureteral compression (lymph nodes, tumors)
Intrinsic ureteral obstruction (fungus balls)
Bladder obstruction (tumors, fungus balls)
Renal AKI
Hemolytic uremic syndrome and thrombotic thrombocytopenic purpura
Postinfectious glomerulonephritis
Collapsing focal segmental glomerular sclerosis
Acute allergic interstitial nephritis (penicillins, sulfonamides)
Plasmacytic interstitial nephritis
Acute tubular necrosis (shock, sepsis, aminoglycosides, amphotericin)
Rhabdomyolysis (pentamidine, zidovudine)

HIV, human immunodeficiency virus.

patients with AIDS and is in most cases multifactorial. ATN is seen in AIDS because the patients are often acutely ill with multiple infections or malignancies. Their clinical course is often complicated by hypovolemia, multiorgan failure, compromised cardiovascular status, invasive diagnostic procedures complicated by bleeding, and the administration of multiple nephrotoxic drugs and radiocontrast agents. Although ATN is a major cause of morbidity and mortality in AIDS patients, it is also potentially reversible and treatable. All supportive measures, including dialysis, should be used as warranted by the clinical situation. Importantly, ATN is avoidable in some cases when preventative measures are used (e.g., maintaining adequate hydration before use of radiocontrast agents and during use of antibiotics and antiretroviral therapy that precipitates crystalluria).

D. **AKI in bone marrow transplant patients.** AKI is a common complication of bone marrow transplant. [This procedure is now referred to as *hematopoietic cell transplant* (HCT), because other cells, such as stem cells, are transplanted as well as bone marrow.] Approximately 90% of patients have a doubling of serum creatinine after allogeneic HCT. This incidence is higher in patients who receive allogeneic as opposed to autologous transplantation. AKI also occurs in nonmyeloablative HCT, also known as *mini-allo* transplants. The incidence of AKI is high in HCT because of the life-threatening nature of the underlying diseases and the toxicity of the cancer drugs, immunosuppressive regimens, and antibiotics. Patients who have undergone autologous HCT do not receive immunosuppressive drugs and have less AKI than allogeneic HCT. Patients with AKI after HCT who require dialysis have a greater than 90% incidence of mortality.

Factors that predispose to ATN are vomiting and diarrhea due to radio-chemotherapy or acute graft-versus-host disease; nephrotoxic drugs such as aminoglycosides and amphotericin B; and hemorrhagic and septic shock. Hepatic veno-occlusive disease, which is more common in allogeneic than autologous bone marrow transplants, is a syndrome that may resemble the HRS. A sodium retention state occurs and leads to weight gain, edema, and a low FENa of less than 1%, despite the use of diuretics. Progressive hyperbilirubinemia and nonoliguric AKI occur.

By far, the most common time for development of AKI is 7 to 21 days after the transplant. The renal syndromes unique to bone marrow transplant recipients are classified according to the time of presentation:

■ **Immediate (first few days)**
   Tumor lysis syndrome
   Stored marrow toxicity
■ **Early (7 to 21 days)**
   Hepatic veno-occlusive disease
   Sepsis
   ATN
   Cyclosporin or FK506 toxicity
■ **Late (6 weeks to 1 year)**
   Bone marrow transplant–associated HUS
   Chronic cyclosporine nephrotoxicity

E. AKI in the setting of liver disease. In addition to HRS, AKI in patients with liver disease may also occur in other clinical settings. Jaundice and AKI may be due to HUS, leptospirosis, mismatched blood transfusion, acute hemorrhage, or falciparum malaria. Simultaneous AKI and acute liver failure suggests acetaminophen overdose, bacteremia, or carbon tetrachloride exposure. Glomerulonephritis and liver cirrhosis are associated with cryoglobulinemia, IgA nephropathy, membranous glomerulonephritis (associated with hepatitis B), and membranoproliferative glomerulonephritis (associated with hepatitis C).

F. Indications for renal biopsy. Renal biopsy is not performed in patients with prerenal azotemia or the typical features of ATN. However, important indications for a renal biopsy in a patient with AKI exist.

1. AKI of unknown etiology. In most cases, a stepwise approach reveals a cause of the AKI. However, in some patients with AKI, the diagnosis is not clear.

2. Suspicion of **glomerulonephritis,** systemic disease (e.g., vasculitis), or **AIN** as the cause of AKI. A renal biopsy in such circumstances may provide the basis and justification for aggressive and life-saving therapy (e.g., high-dose steroids, cytotoxic agents, plasmapheresis, cessation of causative agent for AIN).

3. ATN not recovering after 4 to 6 weeks of dialysis with no more recurrent insults. A renal biopsy may determine that a less favorable condition, such as diffuse cortical necrosis, has developed and that chronic HD may need to be instituted.

VI. MANAGEMENT

A. Prerenal azotemia

1. True volume depletion or hypovolemia. Therapy in this setting is directed toward correcting volume deficits. If volume depletion is due to hemorrhage, then the administration of packed RBCs is indicated; otherwise, the administration of 0.9% normal saline (NS) is appropriate. When 1 L of 0.9 NS is given, approximately 250 mL remain in the plasma compartment, whereas 750 mL enter the interstitial compartment.

The amount of intravenous fluid (IVF) and the rapidity of administration depend on the clinical situation. In a young, stable patient, IVF should be given in one-time boluses (e.g., 500 to 1,000 mL over 1 hour). Smaller boluses (e.g., 250 mL over 1 hour) may be prudent in elderly patients in whom cardiac status is unknown. After a bolus, the patient should be evaluated clinically for signs of hypovolemia or volume overload. Bedside evaluation includes monitoring of orthostatic changes in blood pressure and pulse and jugular venous pulsation (JVP). JVP is a gross indicator of pressure in the central venous area of the right heart. In a normovolemic patient, JVPs are visible when the patient is supine but disappear when the patient assumes the sitting position. JVPs are not visible in the volume-depleted patient; therefore, their reappearance following fluid administration suggests that the central venous pressure (CVP) has returned to normal. The presence of basilar crackles or a third heart sound implies too vigorous fluid replacement, with resultant cardiopulmonary congestion. Intravenous boluses of fluid should continue until euvolemia is achieved. Electrolyte deficits (e.g., potassium) should be monitored and replaced if necessary.

In patients in whom vigorous resuscitation efforts are required, and cardiovascular tolerance to sudden fluid challenges is in doubt, some form of indwelling monitoring system is desirable. Hemodynamic monitoring may be achieved through the use of a central venous catheter or Swan-Ganz catheter.

   a. Central venous catheter. When rapid fluid administration is required, and severe heart or lung disease (or both) is absent, a catheter positioned in the central venous area of the right heart is a satisfactory guide to the speed of fluid administration. The CVP normally ranges between 2 and 12 cm of water. In volume-depleted states, values of zero or below can be expected. Before vigorous volume repletion is begun, a fluid challenge of 200 to 300 mL of NS should be attempted over a 10- to 20-minute period. In an otherwise uncomplicated volume-depleted patient, this amount of saline has little effect on the CVP reading. A CVP rise of more than 5 cm of water suggests cardiac failure, and the infusion should be immediately discontinued.

   b. Swan-Ganz catheter. When a volume deficit must be repaired in the presence of tricuspid stenosis, acute or chronic pulmonary disease, or an unstable cardiovascular system, the CVP does not give a reliable index of left ventricular performance. In this situation, a balloon-tipped Swan-Ganz catheter can be wedged in a pulmonary artery. This gives a measurement of pulmonary artery wedge pressure (PAWP), an indirect measurement of left ventricular end-diastolic pressure. The PAWP is a good guide to the adequacy and speed of fluid replacement. Because of the complications of infection, pulmonary infarction, and hemopneumothorax, this device should be inserted and placed only by trained professionals and should be removed as early as possible. In patients with liver encephalopathy and AKI, a clinical judgment of fluid balance may be difficult because of massive edema and ascites. The measurement of PAWP gives critical information about fluid balance: AKI in the presence of a low PAWP may respond to fluid administration.

2. **Arterial underfilling with an ECF excess.** Prerenal azotemia in this setting is usually a secondary problem overshadowed by primary cardiac or liver disease. The management goal, therefore, is to treat the underlying cause; if the primary disease cannot be treated, then conservative management of symptoms is desirable.

   a. Heart failure. Numerous medications may be employed to improve cardiac output in patients with cardiac disease. In the outpatient setting of a patient with CHF, diuretic agents in combination with digitalis therapy may increase the cardiac output and improve renal perfusion, and thereby lessen the azotemia. Cardiac unloading agents such as ACEIs, ARBs, nitrates, and hydralazine may also improve cardiac function. However, with advanced heart failure that is refractory or only partially responsive to these agents, the physician may be forced to accept mild to moderate prerenal azotemia as a tradeoff. Such azotemia rarely leads to symptomatic uremia.

   In hospitalized patients with CHF who are diuretic resistant, fluid may be removed with continuous venovenous hemofiltration (CVVH), slow continuous ultrafiltration (SCUF), or intermittent ultrafiltration, without dialysis.

   b. Liver disease. Prerenal azotemia associated with advanced hepatic cirrhosis and patients with type II HRS are often refractory to attempts to improve intravascular volume. Ordinarily, however, the management goal is to reduce symptoms and treat ascites and edema with a sodium-restricted diet (1 to 2 g of salt per day), an aldosterone antagonist (e.g., spironolactone 200 to 400 mg per day), and a loop diuretic (e.g., furosemide) while the usually mild prerenal state may persist. Diuretic-resistant patients can be treated with intermittent large volume paracentesis, transjugular intrahepatic portosystemic stent shunt (TIPS), or liver transplantation. Treatment of hospitalized patients with type I HRS may include vasopressin analogs with albumin, somatostatin, or TIPS (see Chapter 2) in an attempt to improve renal blood flow. These therapies have yet to be proved to impact mortality, which is greater than 90% in type I HRS. In reports from Europe, the antidiuretic hormone (ADH) analogs, specifically terlipressin, with albumin infusion, have shown some promise in the treatment of HRS; however, these agents may have significant ischemic side effects. It remains to be determined if the benefits of these agents will outweigh the risk of use (terlipressin is currently available in the United States, but AVP can be used). TIPS may be an option for some patients; improved mortality was demonstrated in one study. However, further studies have not confirmed this benefit. To date, liver transplant is the only definitive cure for HRS.

B. Postrenal failure. Foley catheter drainage is usually successful for acute obstruction secondary to prostatic hypertrophy. The decision regarding further therapy must be made in consultation with a urologist. Medical therapy with finasteride or an α-blocker, or surgical removal of prostatic tissue may be recommended.

With ureteral obstruction, cystoscopy and the placement of ureteral drainage catheters or stents may allow passage of obstructing stones, sludge, or pus, but if this fails, surgical intervention is required.

C. Primary renal disease: vasculitis and glomerulonephritis. When renal failure develops in the course of a systemic or vascular disorder, it is usually a grave sign. A comprehensive discussion of the treatment of these systemic and vascular disorders is beyond the scope of this chapter. Obtaining a renal biopsy early after presentation is essential to make the diagnosis and to guide appropriate therapy. Therapeutic options include immunosuppressive therapy with steroids and/or cyclophosphamide. A subset of patients may benefit from plasmapheresis (e.g., Goodpasture's syndrome).

D. AIN. When a therapeutic agent is identified as the cause of AIN, removal of the agent is the obvious first step in therapy. Bacterial infectious etiologies should be treated with the appropriate antibiotics. When renal impairment is minor, nothing more need be done. If renal impairment has been present for weeks, or if renal involvement is severe, high-dose, short-term prednisone therapy (60 mg per day for 3 to 4 weeks) may speed recovery of renal function. Before initiating prednisone therapy, it is important to confirm the diagnosis with a renal biopsy.

E. Intrinsic renal disease, ATN. No specific therapy exists for the treatment of AKI due to ATN, although this is a widely investigated area of interest.

  1. What to avoid in ATN

    a. High-dose diuretics. No data support the use of high-dose diuretic therapy in established ATN. Furosemide and other loop diuretics are frequently used in oliguric AKI in an effort to convert it to nonoliguric AKI. Although the conversion of oliguric to nonoliguric renal failure may simplify fluid management, clinical trials have failed to demonstrate that the use of diuretics is associated with improved outcome in patients with AKI.

    b. Renal dose dopamine. Dopamine is a selective renal vasodilator. It elicits profound natriuresis and increases urine output in patients with normal kidney function. The renal selective dose is 1 to 3 μg per kg per minute. No evidence suggests that renal dose dopamine is beneficial in AKI. In fact, several studies have identified deleterious effects, such as bowel ischemia and arrhythmias. Unless dopamine is required for circulatory support, it should not be used for AKI.

    c. Nephrotoxic drugs. Potentially nephrotoxic drugs and agents should be avoided in AKI, because they may perpetuate the renal injury. These agents and drugs include NSAIDs, ACEIs, ARBs, cyclosporine, tacrolimus, aminoglycosides, radiocontrast agents, and amphotericin B.

    d. Gadolinium-based contrast agents (GBCAs). Nephrogenic systemic fibrosis (NSF) is a rare but devastating disorder that can occur in patients with kidney failure who are given GBCA. NSF is characterized by sclerosis of the skin, muscle, and internal organs and can be debilitating or even fatal. Most cases have been identified in patients with end-stage kidney disease on dialysis; however, cases in patients with chronic renal failure (stage IV), not requiring dialysis, have been reported. The latest boxed warning from the U.S. Food and Drug Administration (FDA) states that exposure to GBCA increases the risk of NSF in patients with acute or chronic renal insufficiency (GFR less than 30 mL per minute per 1.73 m^2) or acute renal insuffiency of any severity due to the HRS or in the perioperative liver transplantation. Because of the risk of NSF, GBCA should be avoided in AKI. Although the risk of NSF appears to be greatest with a low GFR (less than 30 mL per minute), accurate assessment of GFR in patients with AKI is very difficult because serum creatinine is typically not in a steady state. Current recommendations are that if GBCA are to be used in a patient at risk, informed consent needs to be provided.

    e. Volume overload. The amount of IVF necessary for critically ill patients is unknown, and IVFs must be given judiciously in the setting of ATN, especially if the patient is oliguric. In patients with acute lung injury, conservative fluid management improves outcomes without increasing the development of nonpulmonary organ failures such as the kidney. In general, IVFs should not contain potassium.

2. Supportive therapy in ATN

    a. Drug dosages. Drug dosages should be adjusted based on the measured or best estimate of CCr, not merely on the serum creatinine. Certain medication doses also must be adjusted if the patient with AKI is receiving dialysis [intermittent hemodialysis (IHD) or continuous renal replacement therapy (CRRT)].

    b. Nutritional support. AKI is a hypercatabolic state associated with increased protein breakdown. Nitrogen balance is extremely negative, especially in AKI associated with sepsis, postsurgery, and multiorgan dysfunction syndrome. Renal factors contributing to the negative nitrogen balance include uremia, acidosis, parathyroid hormone abnormalities, inadequate protein intake, and protein losses. In critically ill patients, supplemental nutritional support with enteral versus parenteral nutrition may improve nutritional status, a reduction in infections and sepsis, and better survival. Therefore, enteral feeding is the preferred method of nutritional support, although it is not always possible. The use of parenteral nutrition remains controversial, and randomized controlled clinical trials have yet to demonstrate a benefit in acutely ill patients with AKI. Opinion papers in AKI have suggested that protein intake not exceed 1.5 g of protein per kg of body weight, that early nutritional supplementation may not be beneficial, and that supplementation after 2 to 3 weeks of not eating is likely to be beneficial.

    c. Dialysis therapy. In general, the indications to start dialysis in ATN and AKI are not specific and should be individualized by nephrology consultation. Although not yet proved in clinical trials, some studies do suggest that early dialysis is associated with improved outcome, and therefore a trend in clinical practice is to initiate dialysis early to avoid the potential consequences of uremia. Uremia that results in altered mental status or pericarditis is an absolute indication for dialysis. The initiation of dialysis depends on the entire clinical picture, not just the presence or absence of certain factors.

        The main modalities of dialysis are IHD and CRRT.

    i. IHD is the same form of dialysis used in patients with end-stage renal disease (ESRD). IHD is typically used in otherwise stable patients who can tolerate rapid fluid removal (e.g., 1 L per hour). IHD is mandatory in ambulatory patients.

        In this form of dialysis, the patient is connected to a dialysis machine for 4 hours at a time, daily or every second day. Fluid removal and urea clearance for the day is achieved during the period of a few hours. Rapid removal of solutes and fluids may cause hemodynamic instability. The technique requires a double-lumen catheter, tubing, an HD machine (blood pump, dialysate generation system, dialysate pump, and alarms and safety monitoring devices), a dialysis membrane, and a dialysis nurse. Daily treatment for 4 hours, with a blood urea clearance of 200 mL per minute, can achieve a weekly urea clearance of 350 L.

The frequency of IHD and delivered dose of dialysis required in AKI is a matter of debate. In patients with chronic ESRD, IHD is typically performed on alternate days (3 days per week) for approximately 4 hours at a time. The dose and frequency of dialysis for AKI may need to be much higher than in the chronic setting, because patients with AKI are typically hypercatabolic and most temporary catheters have a high recirculation rate. A number of recent studies demonstrate that intensive dialysis achieved by daily HD or CVVH, with increased ultrafiltration (35 mL per hour per kg), are associated with a lower mortality rate as compared to conventional dialysis, that is HD three times a week or CVVH with 20 mL per hour per kg ultrafiltration. The Acute Renal Failure Trial Network (ATN) study is a large multicenter study though sought to determine the mortality benefit of intensive idalysis in patients with AKI. In their recently published report, no martality benefit was observed for intensive dialysis [IHD hemodialysis or sustained low-efficiency dialysis six days a week, or continuous venovenous hemodiafiltration (CVVHDF) at 35 mL per kg per hour] versus less intensive dialysis (IHD thrice weekly or CVVHDF at 20 mL per kg per hour). Achieved target clearance goals for IHD were 1.2 to 1.4 Kt/V_{urea} per treatment, suggesting that this level of clearance be maintained in patients receiving IHD.

ii. **CRRT.** Currently, four main types of **CRRT** are used: SCUF, CVVH, continuous venovenous hemodialysis (CVVHD), and continuous venovenous hemodiafiltration (CVVHDF). In Table 10-11 the different characteristics of each CRRT are summarized. The type of CRRT is individualized. A common approach is to start with CVVH and then add dialysate (CVVHDF), if clearance rates are too low. A single center, prospective randomized study demonstrated improved mortality in patients on CVVH who had an ultrafiltrate formation of 45 mL per kg per hour or 35 mL per kg per hour compared with 20 mL per kg per hour. Notably, however, in a multicenter ATN study, discussed above, found no mortality benefit of CVVHDF performed at 35 mL per hour versus 20 mL per hour.

In CRRT, the goal is for the patient to undergo continuous dialysis for 24 hours a day. In practice, interruptions in dialysis for patient procedures, radiologic testing, and dialysis membrane clotting are frequent and reduce the amount of time the patient is actually receiving dialysis. CRRT is the mandatory form of dialysis for patients who are hemodynamically unstable. Because the removal of solutes and fluid is slow and continuous, hemodynamic instability and hypotensive episodes are reduced. Minimization of hypotension theoretically avoids the perpetuation of renal injury. CRRT requires a double-lumen catheter (the same catheter that is used for IHD), tubing, a simple blood pump with safety devices, sterile replacement fluid, volumetric pumps to control replacement and ultrafiltration rate, continuous anticoagulation, and a high-flux dialysis membrane. ICU nurses typically monitor therapy.

iii. **Intermittent versus continuous dialysis.** Many nonrandomized studies have compared IHD and CRRT. Prospective randomized studies are difficult to carry out, because patients who are hemodynamically unstable and cannot tolerate IHD are almost always started on CRRT. Alternatively, confining a mobile patient to bed to receive CRRT may be unethical. Therefore, any randomization may be biased. CRRT is believed to be the modality of choice in very ill patients, and IHD is used in less ill patients. At present, IHD and CRRT are regarded as equivalent methods for the treatment of AKI. The choice of IHD or CRRT should be made in consultation with a nephrologist and tailored for the individual

TABLE 10-11 Comparison of Intermittent Hemodialysis (IHD) and Various Types of Continuous Renal Replacement Therapy (CRRT)

Type of renal replacement	Amount of ultrafiltrate formed/hour (mL)[a]	Use of replacement fluid[b]	Use of dialysate	Urea clearance (L/d)
Intermittent hemodialysis (IHD)	500–1,000	No	Yes	40–60
Slow continuous ultrafiltration (SCUF)	50–100	No	No	2–5
Continuous venovenous hemofiltration (CVVH)	1,000–2,000	Yes	No	20–50
Continuous venovenous hemodialysis (CVVHD)	50–100	No	Yes	20–55
Continuous venovenous hemodiafiltration (CVVHDF)	1,000–2,000	Yes	Yes	25–75

[a]The ultrafiltrate formed has the same electrolyte composition as plasma; therefore, with high ultrafiltrate formation, increased losses of potassium, phosphorous, calcium, and magnesium may occur. These electrolytes may need to be replaced intravenously.
[b]Replacement fluid typically contains sodium, chloride, and calcium and replaces fluid lost in the ultrafiltrate and other sources (GI, etc.) to achieve the desired hourly net fluid loss. In IHD, net fluid loss is typically 500 to 1,000 mL per hour, whereas in CRRT net fluid loss is typically 50 to 100 mL per hour.

patient. The decision may also depend on facility-specific issues, such as experience, nursing resources, and technical proficiency. The cost of CRRT is greater than that of IHD. At present, indications for CRRT in AKI include hemodynamic instability, cerebral edema, hypercatabolism, and severe fluid overload. In Table 10-12 a comparison of IHD and CRRT is listed. CRRT is similar in solute clearance to a GFR of 15 to 20 mL per minute. A day of CRRT is roughly equivalent to one HD treatment. Therefore, drug-dosing adjustments must be made in CRRT.

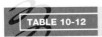

TABLE 10-12 Analysis of Continuous Renal Replacement Therapy (CRRT) versus Intermittent Hemodialysis

Advantages
Hemodynamic stability (may relate in part to decreased body temperature)
Unlimited alimentation
Avoidance of rapid fluid and electrolyte shifts
Aggressive correction of acid–base status
Massive fluid removal
Potential elimination of mediators (e.g., cytokines) by membrane absorbance
Disadvantages
Immobilization
Lactate load[a]
Continuous anticoagulation[b]

[a]Lactate should be avoided in patients with severe liver disease who cannot metabolize lactate. The lactate load may be avoided by making a custom dialysate that contains bicarbonate instead.
[b]CRRT may be performed without anticoagulation; however, frequent clotting of the membrane may occur.

iv. Type of dialysis membrane. Some studies have demonstrated that the dialysis of patients with AKI having biocompatible membranes is associated with improved mortality; therefore, biocompatible membranes are used for dialysis in AKI. Biocompatible membranes are made of synthetic polymers and include polyamides, polycarbonate, and polysulfone. The adverse effects of bioincompatible cellulosic membranes (e.g., cellulose, cuprophane, hemophane, cellulose acetate) include activation of complement, increased production of cytokines, and hypotension.

v. Temporary vascular access. The primary vascular sites used for insertion of temporary dialysis catheters are the internal jugular or femoral vein. The internal jugular access is required in patients who are mobile. Femoral access is indicated when the cardiopulmonary condition of the patient limits attempts at thoracic catheterization; it is useful in bedridden patients. The subclavian vein may be used if other access sites are unavailable; however, use of subclavian catheters entails a major risk of stenosis or thrombosis of the subclavian vein or its branches.

vi. Peritoneal dialysis is uncommonly used as a mode of dialysis therapy in AKI in the United States despite the fact that it is not technically difficult and can be used with minimally trained staff. It may be an option in locations where IHD or CRRT is not available. It can be used in patients with minimally increased catabolism without an immediate or life-threatening indication for dialysis. It is ideal for patients who are hemodynamically unstable. For short-term dialysis, a rigid dialysis catheter is inserted into the peritoneum, through the anterior abdominal wall, 5 to 10 cm below the umbilicus. Exchanges of 1.5 to 2.0 L of standard peritoneal dialysis solutions are infused into the peritoneum. The major risks are bowel perforation during insertion of the catheter and peritonitis. Acute peritoneal dialysis offers the same potential advantages to the pediatric patient that CRRT offers to the adult with AKI.

Suggested Readings

Carvounis CP, Nisar S, Guro-Razman S. Significance of the fractional excretion of urea in the differential diagnosis of acute renal failure. *Kidney Int* 2002;62:2223–2229.

Choudhury D, Ahmed Z. Drug-associated renal dysfunction and injury. *Nat Clin Pract Nephrol* 2006;2:80–91.

Dursun B, Edelstein CL. Acute renal failure – core curriculum. *Am J Kidney Dis* 2005;45:614–618.

Edelstein CL, Schrier RW. Pathophysiology of ischemic acute renal injury. In: Schrier, RW, ed. *Diseases of the kidney and urinary tract*. Philadelphia: Lippincott Williams & Wilkins, 2007:930–961.

Lameire N, Van Biesen W, Vanholder R. The changing epidemiology of acute renal failure. *Nat Clin Pract Nephrol* 2006;2:364–377.

Langford CA, Balow JE. New insights into the immunopathogenesis and treatment of small vessel vasculitis of the kidney. *Curr Opin Nephrol Hypertens* 2003;12:267–272.

Molitoris BA, Levin A, Warnock DG, et al. Improving outcomes of acute kidney injury:report of an initiative. *Nat Clin Pract Nephrol* 2007;3:439–442.

Parikh C, Cantley L, Devarajan P, et al. Biomarkers of acute kidney injury – early diagnosis, pathogenesis and recovery. *J Investig Med* 2007;55(7):333–340.

Pepin M-N, Bouchard J, Legault L, et al. Diagnostic performance of fractional excretion of fractional excretion of urea and fractional excretion of sodium in the evaluations of patients with acute kidney injury with or without diuretic treatment. *Am J Kidney Dis* 2007;50(4):566–573.

Ronco C. Continuous dialysis is superior to intermittent dialysis in acute kidney injury of the critically ill patient. *Nat Clin Pract Nephrol* 2007;3:118–119.

Schrier RW, Wang W. Acute renal failure and sepsis. *N Engl J Med* 2004;351:159–169.

Schrier RW, Wang W, Poole B, et al. Acute renal failure: definitions, diagnosis, mechanisms, and therapy: historical perspective and definitions. *J Clin Invest Sci Med Ser* 2004;114(1):5–14.

Van Biesen W, Vanholdert R, Lameire N. Defining acute renal failure: RIFLE and beyond. *Clin J Am Soc Nephrol* 2006;1:1314–1319.

Yalavarthy R, Edelstein CL, Teitelbaum I. Acute renal failure and chronic kidney disease following liver transplantation. *Hemodial Int* 2007;11(Suppl 3):S7–S12.

THE PATIENT WITH CHRONIC KIDNEY DISEASE

Michel Chonchol and David M. Spiegel

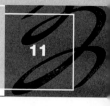

11

*P*atients with end-stage renal disease (ESRD) have decreased quality of life, high morbidity, and an annual mortality of approximately 22%. The number of persons with kidney failure who are treated with dialysis and transplantation is projected to increase from 340,000 in 1999 to 651,000 in 2010. The high morbidity and mortality seen in chronic dialysis patients may decrease significantly if patients were healthier at the time of initiating renal replacement therapy.

This chapter presents an overview of the current recommendations designed to retard the progression of chronic kidney disease (CKD); to optimize the medical management of comorbid medical conditions, such as cardiovascular disease (CVD), diabetes, and lipid disorders; and to decrease the complications secondary to progression of kidney disease including hypertension, anemia, secondary hyperparathyroidism, and malnutrition. These recommendations are derived from the clinical practice guidelines published by the Kidney Disease Outcomes Quality Initiative (K/DOQI) of the National Kidney Foundation (NKF).

I. DEFINITION AND STAGING OF CKD. The definition of CKD is:
   A. Kidney damage for 3 months or longer, as defined by structural or functional abnormalities of the kidney, with or without decreased glomerular filtration rate (GFR), manifest by either:
      1. Pathological abnormalities; or
      2. Markers of kidney damage, including abnormalities in the composition of the blood or urine, or abnormalities in imaging tests
   B. GFR of less than 60 mL per minute per 1.73 m^2 for 3 months or longer, with or without kidney damage.

   In a recent NKF report, CKD was divided into stages of severity (Table 11-1). Importantly, the staging system is based on estimated GFR and not on the measurement of serum creatinine. Stage 1 CKD is recognized by the presence of kidney damage at a time when GFR is conserved; this includes patients with albuminuria or abnormal imaging studies. For example, a patient with type 2 diabetes and normal GFR, but with microalbuminuria, is classified as stage 1 CKD. The definition for microalbuminuria is 30 to 300 mg per day (24-hour excretion) and for clinical proteinuria: more than 300 mg per day (24-hour excretion). Stage 2 CKD takes into account patients with evidence of kidney damage with decreased GFR (60 to 89 mL per minute per 1.73 m^2). Lastly, all patients with a GFR of less than 60 mL per minute per 1.73 m^2 are classified as having CKD irrespective of whether kidney damage is present.

   The staging of CKD is useful because it endorses a model in which primary physicians and specialists share responsibility for the care of patients with CKD. This classification also offers a common language for patients and the practitioners involved in the treatment of CKD. For each stage of CKD, K/DOQI provides recommendations for a clinical action plan (Table 11-1).

   An essential requirement for the classification and monitoring of CKD is the measurement or estimation of GFR. Serum creatinine is not an ideal marker of GFR, because it is both filtered at the glomerulus and secreted by the proximal tubule. Creatinine clearance (CrCl) is known to overestimate GFR by as much as 20% in healthy individuals and by even more in patients with CKD. Estimates of GFR based on 24-hour CrCL require timed urine collections, which are difficult to obtain and often involve errors in collection. Classic methods for measurements

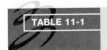

TABLE 11-1	National Kidney Foundation Kidney Disease Outcomes Quality Initiative Classification, Prevalence, and Action Plan for Stages of Chronic Kidney Disease

Stage	Description	GFR, mL per min per 1.73 m^3	Prevalence, n (%)	Action
—	At increased risk	≥60 (with chronic kidney disease risk factors)	—	Screening: chronic kidney disease risk reduction
1	Kidney damage with normal or increased GFR	≥90	5,900,000 (3.3)	Diagnosis and treatment; treatment of comorbid conditions; slowing progression; CVD risk reduction
2	Kidney damage with slightly decreased GFR	60–89	5,300,000 (3.0)	Estimating progression
3	Moderately decreased GFR	30–59	7,600,000 (4.3)	Evaluating and treating complications
4	Severely decreased GFR	15–29	400,000 (0.2)	Preparation for kidney replacement therapy
5	Kidney failure	<15 (or dialysis)	300,000 (0.1)	Kidney replacement (if uremia present)

CVD, cardiovascular disease; GFR, glomerular filtration rate.
(National Kidney Foundation-K/DOQI. Clinical practice guidelines for chronic kidney disease: evaluation, classification, and stratification: *Am J Kidney Dis* 2002;39(Suppl 1):S1–S266.)

of GFR, including the gold standard inulin clearance, are cumbersome, require an intravenous infusion and timed urine collections, and are not clinically feasible. In adults, the normal GFR based on inulin clearance and adjusted to a standard body surface area of 1.73 m^2 is 127 mL per minute per 1.73 m^2 for men and 118 mL per minute per 1.73 m^2 for women, with a standard deviation of approximately 20 mL per minute per 1.73 m^2. After age 30, the average decrease in GFR is 1 mL per minute per 1.73 m^2 per year.

Equations based on serum creatinine but factored for gender, age, and ethnicity are the best alternative for estimation of GFR. The most commonly used formula is the Cockcroft-Gault equation. This equation was developed to predict CrCl, but has been used to estimate GFR:

$$\text{CrCl} = \frac{(140 - \text{age})(\text{weight in kg})}{(\text{Serum creatinine})(72)} \times 0.85 \text{ if female} \quad (11.1)$$

The Modification of Diet in Renal Disease (MDRD) study equation was derived on the basis of data from more than 500 patients with a wide variety of kidney diseases and GFRs up to 90 mL per minute per 1.73 m^2. Therefore, the abbreviated MDRD equation is recommended for routine use and requires only serum creatinine, age, gender, and race:

$$\text{GFR (mL per minute per 1.73 m}^2) = 186 \times (\text{SCR})^{-1.154} \times (\text{age})^{-0.203}$$
$$\times (0.742 \text{ if female})$$
$$\times (1.210 \text{ if African-American}) \quad (11.2)$$

The calculations can be made using available web-based and downloadable medical calculators (www.kidney.org/professionals/KDOQI/gfr_calculator.cfm).

The MDRD study equation has many advantages. It is more accurate and precise than the Cockcroft-Gault equation for persons with a GFR of less than approximately 90 mL per minute per 1.73 m². This equation predicts GFR as measured by using an accepted method [urinary clearance of iodine 125 (^{125}I)-iothalamate]. It does not require height or weight and has been validated in kidney transplant recipients and African-Americans with nephrosclerosis. It has not been validated in diabetic kidney disease, in patients with serious comorbid conditions, in healthy persons, or in individuals older than 70 years.

II. **PREVALENCE OF CKD.** The Third National Health and Nutrition Examination Survey (NHANES III) included 15,625 participants aged 20 years or older and was conducted, between 1988 to 1994, by the National Center for Health Statistics (NCHS) of the Centers for Disease Control and Prevention. The goal of this survey was to provide nationally representative data on the health and nutritional status of the civilian, noninstitutionalized U.S. population. The results, when extrapolated to the U.S. population of adults older than 20 years ($n = 177$ million), revealed the following findings relevant to CKD:

   A. A total of 6.2 million individuals had a serum creatinine equal to or greater than 1.5 mg per dL, which is a 30-fold higher prevalence of reduced kidney function compared with the prevalence of treated ESRD during the same time interval.

   B. A total of 2.5 million individuals had a serum creatinine equal to or greater than 1.7 mg per dL.

   C. A total of 800,000 individuals had a serum creatinine equal to or greater than 2.0 mg per dL.

   D. Of individuals with elevated serum creatinine, 70% have hypertension.

   E. Only 75% of patients with hypertension and elevated serum creatinine received treatment, with only 27% having a blood pressure (BP) reading lower than 140/90 mm Hg and 11% having their BP reduced to lower than 130/85 mm Hg.

   In a further analysis of NHANES III data, estimated GFR was calculated from the serum creatinine using the MDRD study equation (2). The prevalence of the different stages of CKD clearly shows that the CKD population is several times larger than the ESRD population. The challenge for the medical community is to identify earlier stages of CKD and institute correct treatment strategies to decrease complications and slow the progression to ESRD.

   More recently it was noticed that the prevalence of CKD stages 1 to 4 increased from 10.0% in 1988 to 1994 to 13.1% in 1999 to 2004 in the U.S. population. This increase was partly explained by the increasing prevalence of diabetes and hypertension.

III. **MECHANISM OF KIDNEY DISEASE PROGRESSION.** Diabetes and hypertension are responsible for the largest proportion of ESRD. Glomerulonephritis represents the third most common cause of ESRD. Despite the many diseases that can initiate kidney injury, a limited number of common pathways are available for kidney disease progression. A general theme of many of these pathways is that adaptive changes in the nephron lead to maladaptive consequences. One of the best developed of these themes is the hyperfiltration that occurs in remaining nephrons after loss of renal mass. Elevated glomerular pressures drive this hyperfiltration. Glomerular hyperfiltration has initial adaptive effects by maintaining GFR, but later may lead to glomerular injury. Abnormal glomerular permeability is common in glomerular disorders, with proteinuria being the clinical consequence. Evidence has accumulated that this proteinuria might be a factor inciting tubulointerstitial disease. The extent of tubulointerstitial damage is a prime risk factor for subsequent renal disease progression in all forms of glomerular diseases studied. In experimental models and in human trials, an association has been consistently demonstrated between the reduction of proteinuria and renoprotection.

IV. **RISK FACTORS FOR PROGRESSION TO ESRD.** The quantity of protein excreted in the urine is one of the strongest predictors of kidney disease progression and response to antihypertensive therapy in almost all studies of CKD. Therefore, the greater the proteinuria the higher the risk for progression.

As described in the previous section, an important risk factor for most glomerular diseases is the extent of tubulointerstitial disease on renal biopsy.

A. Ethnicity is a risk factor for many kidney diseases. For example, African-American patients with diabetes have a twofold to threefold higher risk for developing ESRD compared with white patients. Some of this increased risk is attributable to such modifiable factors as suboptimal health behaviors, suboptimal glucose and BP control, and lower socioeconomic status. Human immunodeficiency virus (HIV)-associated nephropathy is also more common in African-American patients compared with white patients.

B. Gender is an additional risk factor for the development and progression of certain types of kidney disease. Overall, the incidence of ESRD is greater in males than females.

C. Smoking has been associated with proteinuria and kidney disease progression in both type 1 and 2 diabetes, as well as in immunoglobulin (Ig) A nephropathy, lupus nephritis, and polycystic kidney disease. Smoking cessation has been associated with a slower rate of progression of kidney disease in type 1 diabetic patients.

D. Finally, heavy consumption of nonnarcotic analgesics, particularly phenacetin, has been associated with an increased risk of CKD.

V. RETARDING PROGRESSION TO ESRD

A. Antihypertensive therapy. Hypertension is a risk factor for the progression of kidney disease, and it is the second most common cause of ESRD. The opinion of the seventh report of the Joint National Committee (JNC VII) recommended that BP be lowered to levels below 130/80 mm Hg in patients with diabetes or CKD.

An increasing amount of evidence has demonstrated that the inhibition of the renin-angiotensin system by either inhibiting angiotensin II generation with angiotensin converting enzyme (ACE) inhibitors or blocking the angiotensin type 1 A receptor with angiotensin receptor blockers (ARBs) has renoprotective effects above and beyond the effects of these therapies on reducing BP.

1. Studies in patients with diabetic kidney disease with established nephropathy

   a. Type 1 diabetic patients with established nephropathy

    A pronounced benefit of ACE inhibitors in type 1 diabetic patients who already had overt nephropathy has been demonstrated in the largest study to date. Four hundred and nine patients with overt proteinuria and a plasma creatinine concentration equal to or greater than 2.5 mg per dL were randomized to therapy with either captopril or placebo. Further antihypertensive drugs were then added as necessary, although calcium channel blockers and other ACE inhibitors were excluded. At approximately 4 years of nearly equivalent BP control, patients treated with captopril had a slower rate of increase in the plasma creatinine concentration and a lesser likelihood of progressing to ESRD or death.

   b. Type 2 diabetic patients with established nephropathy

    i. The Reduction of Endpoints in type 2 diabetes with the Angiotensin II Antagonist Losartan (RENAAL) study examined the effects of losartan versus non-ACE inhibitors or ARB antihypertensive therapy in 1,513 patients with type 2 diabetes and nephropathy, followed for a mean of 3.4 years. The results of this study demonstrated a beneficial effect of losartan, beyond its effects on lowering BP, on the time to doubling of serum creatinine concentration and onset of ESRD.

    ii. In the Irbesartan Diabetic Nephropathy Trial (IDNT), 1,715 patients with nephropathy secondary to type 2 diabetes were randomly assigned to receive irbesartan, amlodipine, or placebo. The mean duration of follow-up was 2.6 years. This study revealed that patients assigned to irbesartan had a 33% reduction of risk for the doubling of serum creatinine compared with placebo and a 37% decrease compared with patients on amlodipine.

c. **Studies in patients with diabetic kidney disease with microalbuminuria**
   i. **Meta-analysis of published trials.** Diabetic nephropathy trialists have examined 12 selected studies involving 698 patients to compare the effects of ACE inhibitors versus placebo in type 1 diabetic patients with microalbuminuria and normal BP. Results showed that ACE inhibitors were more likely associated with regression of microalbuminuria. This effect persisted despite adjustment for any changes in BP.
   ii. **The United Kingdom Prospective Diabetes Study (UKPDS)** examined the efficacy of atenolol and captopril in reducing the risk of both macrovascular and microvascular complications in type 2 diabetic patients with hypertension. This study found that both captopril and atenolol were equivalent in reducing the renal endpoints of progression of albuminuria, overt nephropathy, a twofold increase in serum creatinine, and the development of ESRD.
   iii. The Appropriate Blood Pressure Control in Diabetics **(ABCD)** trial was a prospective randomized trial of 950 type 2 diabetic patients examining whether intensive versus moderate BP control affected the incidence of progression of type 2 diabetic complications. The hypertensive patients ($n = 470$) were randomized to intensive BP control [diastolic blood pressure (DBP) goal of 75 mm Hg] versus moderate BP control (DBP goal of 80 to 89 mm Hg) and to either nisoldipine or enalapril as the initial antihypertensive medication. BP control of 138/86 or 132/78 mm Hg with either nisoldipine or enalapril as the initial antihypertensive medication appeared to stabilize kidney function in hypertensive type 2 diabetic patients without overt albuminuria over a 5-year period. The enalapril-treated patients had significantly fewer heart attacks than the nisoldipine-treated patients. The more intensive BP control decreased all-cause mortality. The effects of intensive versus moderate DBP control were also studied in 480 normotensive type 2 diabetic patients. Over a 5-year follow-up period, intensive (approximately 128/75 mm Hg) BP control in normotensive type 2 diabetic patients: (a) slowed the progression to incipient and overt diabetic nephropathy, (b) decreased the progression of diabetic retinopathy, and (c) diminished the incidence of stroke. Cardiovascular events occurred more commonly in the nisoldipine group.
   iv. The **Heart Outcomes Prevention Evaluation (HOPE)** study included 3,577 people with diabetes. Of the patients recruited in the study, 1,120 had microalbuminuria. Patients were randomized to the ACE inhibitor ramipril or placebo. Patients treated with ramipril had a 25% reduction in myocardial infarction, stroke, or cardiovascular death. In the ramipril group, the risk of developing overt nephropathy decreased by 24%.
   v. **Irbesartan Microalbuminuria Study.** The effects of the ARB irbesartan were examined in 590 hypertensive patients with type 2 diabetes and microalbuminuria. The primary endpoint was time from baseline visit to the first detection of overt nephropathy. This study revealed that irbesartan had a renoprotective effect independent of its BP lowering effect.

d. **Studies in patients with nondiabetic kidney disease**
   i. **The African-American Study of Kidney Disease and Hypertension (AASK)** was designed to study the effect on progression of hypertensive kidney disease of (a) two different mean arterial pressure (MAP) goals—usual (MAP: 102 to 107 mm Hg) and lower (MAP: equal to below 92 mm Hg)—and (b) treatment with three different antihypertensive drug classes: an ACE inhibitor (ramipril), a dihydropyridine calcium channel blocker (amlodipine), and a β-blocker (metoprolol). This study concluded that lowering BP below the achieved 141/85 mm Hg was not associated with added beneficial effects and that ACE inhibitors are more

effective antihypertensives in slowing the progression of hypertensive nephrosclerosis.

ii. In the **Ramipril Efficacy in Nephropathy (REIN)** study, patients were stratified before randomization by the level of 24-hour urinary protein, with stratum 1 having less than 3 g per 24-hour proteinuria, and stratum 2 having 3 or more g per 24-hour proteinuria. The patients were then randomized to receive ramipril or placebo, with other medications added to achieve a target DBP of lower than 90 mm Hg. An analysis of the results of this study demonstrated a beneficial effect of ramipril on slowing GFR decline that was more than expected from the reduction in BP.

The care of diabetic and nondiabetic kidney disease has been significantly advanced by this series of controlled trials. The results of these studies clearly demonstrate the renoprotective effects of ACE inhibitors and ARBs in both reducing proteinuria and slowing the progression of kidney disease. The effects of these medications may be related to decreases in glomerular capillary pressure or other effects of angiotensin II on fibrosis and growth. These agents should be considered the drugs of first choice in patients with CKD, and the BP goal should be lower than 130/80 mm Hg.

e. **Combined therapy with ACE inhibitors and ARBs in nondiabetic renal disease**

i. **COOPERATE study.** This study was a randomized, double-blind study designed to test the efficacy and safety of combination therapy with an ACE inhibitor (trandolapril) and an ARB (losartan), compared with monotherapy with each drug in 263 patients with nondiabetic kidney disease. Combination therapy was associated with a marked antiproteinuric effect, and fewer patients reached the combined primary endpoint of time to doubling of serum creatinine or ESRD compared with either of the monotherapy groups.

f. **Combined therapy with ACE inhibitors and ARBs in diabetic renal disease**

i. In the **Candesartan and Lisinopril Microalbuminuria (CALM)** study, the effects of candesartan or lisinopril or both on BP or urinary albumin excretion was examined in patients with microalbuminuria, hypertension, and type 2 diabetes.

Combination therapy reduced BP and albumin excretion more than either agent alone.

In summary, these studies provide some evidence that combining an ACE inhibitor with an ARB may be more effective than either agent alone in reducing proteinuria and improving kidney survival. An increase in adverse events does not appear to exist with combination therapy. However, at present, it is not clear in some studies whether maximizing the dose of either agent is better than the combination or whether the effect of combination therapy is independent of BP reduction.

VI. MANAGING COMPLICATIONS OF CKD

A. **Anemia.** The anemia secondary to kidney disease develops during the course of CKD. The degree of anemia is better evaluated using hemoglobin values rather than hematocrit. A direct correlation exists between the level of hemoglobin and GFR. In the NHANES III data, this association exists at GFR levels of less than 90 mL per minute per 1.73 m^2, but was most marked when the GFR was less than 60 mL per minute per 1.73 m^2. The etiology of the anemia of CKD is multifactorial, with the major factor being a decline in erythropoietin synthesis by the kidneys. Anemia is a common complication of CKD and recently there has been considerable interest in the relationship between hemoglobin targets and major cardiovascular outcomes in patients with stage 3 and 4 CKD. The publication of two large randomized control trials of recombinant human erythropoietin in CKD patients—Cardiovascular Risk Reduction by Early Anemia Treatment with Epoetin Beta (CREATE) and Correction of Hemoglobin and Outcomes in Renal Insufficiency (CHOIR)—have received intense attention and discussion by the nephrology community. Both studies tested the hypothesis that early and complete correction of anemia with the use of recombinant human erythropoietin would result in improvements of major cardiovascular outcomes; however, both studies resulted in negative findings. K/DOQI guidelines recommend that patients with CKD be evaluated for anemia when the GFR is less than 60 mL per minute per 1.73 m^2. Erythropoietin levels are not helpful in assessing the anemia of kidney disease. The iron status of patients should be assessed, including measurements of serum ferritin, iron, and transferrin saturation. Transferrin saturations and ferritin levels should exceed 20% and 100 ng per mL, respectively, to optimize erythropoiesis. The ideal hemoglobin level for CKD patients has not been definitively determined. NKF-DOQI guidelines recommend a target hemoglobin level of 11 to 12 g per dL.

B. Phosphate control. Phosphate control in CKD is important to preserve the bone mineral content and avoid hyperparathyroidism. Phosphate binders can be instituted when the GFR falls below 30 to 50 mL per minute. Vitamin D analogs can clearly help suppress parathyroid gland overactivity, but often at the expense of higher serum phosphate levels and the risk of hypercalcemia, both of which can worsen extraskeletal calcifications. Recommendations for patients with CKD include:

1. Maintain serum phosphorus between 3.0 and 4.6 mg per dL.
2. Restrict dietary phosphorus to 800 to 1,000 mg per day when serum phosphorus is greater than 4.6 mg per dL.
3. Restrict dietary phosphorus to 800 to 1,000 mg per day when serum levels of intact parathyroid hormone (PTH) are greater than 65 pg per mL.
4. Monitor serum phosphorus every 3 months if patients are on a phosphorus-restricted diet.
5. The target range for corrected serum calcium (for every 1 g decrease in serum albumin, the serum calcium should be corrected by 0.8 mg) is 8.8 to 9.5 mg per dL.
6. If serum calcium is greater than 10.2 mg per dL, reduce or discontinue vitamin D analogs, and/or switch to a noncalcium-based phosphate binder.
7. Serum calcium-phosphorus product should be less than 55 mg^2 per dL^2.

C. Acid–base control. Acidosis is common in almost all forms of CKD. The main mechanism responsible for the acidosis is a decrease in total ammonia excretion, leading to a decrease in net hydrogen secretion and a fall in serum bicarbonate. This net positive acid balance results in dissolution of bone, ultimately worsening uremic osteodystrophy. Other adverse consequences of metabolic acidosis include protein malnutrition and the suppression of albumin synthesis. Early treatment of acidosis with oral bicarbonate therapy may help prevent some of the bone disease of chronic uremia. K/DOQI recommends maintaining a serum bicarbonate level of greater than 22 mEq per L. Care must be taken, however, not to precipitate or worsen hypertension with the added sodium intake.

VII. MANAGING CARDIOVASCULAR COMORBIDITY. CVD remains the most common cause of death in patients with ESRD, and CKD patients are more likely to die from CVD than are expected to progress to ESRD. The CKD population has a higher incidence of traditional cardiovascular risk factors, including diabetes, hypertension, and dyslipidemias. In addition, overwhelming scientific evidence has shown that decreased GFR and proteinuria are independent risk factors for cardiovascular disease. Consensus exists in the nephrology community that the CKD population should undergo aggressive risk factor management. This includes strict control of BP and lipids, as well as smoking cessation. K/DOQI clinical practice guidelines on the management of dyslipidemias in CKD have recommended drug therapy for patients with a low-density lipoprotein (LDL) cholesterol level equal to or greater than 100 mg per dL after 3 months of therapeutic lifestyle changes. Statins are recommended as initial drug therapy for high LDL, and fibrates (e.g., gemfibrozil) are recommended for an elevated fasting triglyceride.

VIII. WHEN TO REFER TO A NEPHROLOGIST. Several studies have shown that delayed referral to a nephrologist is common and is associated with adverse consequences, including greater morbidity and mortality, more severe uremia, increased use of percutaneous vascular access with associated morbidity, reduced use of the preferred arteriovenous fistula for vascular access, restricted patient choice of treatment modality, prolonged and more costly hospitalization at initiation of dialysis, and higher rates of emotional and socioeconomic problems. An early referral allows the patient to develop an effective relationship with a multidisciplinary team consisting of a nephrologist, vascular surgeon, nurse, dietitian, social worker, and mental health professional. This relationship allows for a more informed consideration by patients of renal replacement options including transplantation, initiation of renal replacement therapy to maintain optimal patient health, timely placement of a dialysis access, supervision of dietary modification, and support services regarding unmet psychological, social, and financial needs. A nephrologist should participate in the care of patients with a GFR of less than 30 mL per minute per 1.73 m^2.

Suggested Readings

Brenner BM, Cooper ME, De Zeeuw D, et al. Effects of losartan on renal and cardiovascular outcomes in patients with type 2 diabetes and nephropathy. *N Engl J Med* 2001;345:861–869.

Cockcroft DW, Gault MH. Prediction of creatinine clearance from serum creatinine. *Nephron* 1976;16:31–41.

Coresh J, Selvin E, Stevens LA, et al. Prevalence of chronic kidney disease in the United States. *JAMA* 2007;298:2038–2047.

Estacio R, Jeffers B, Gifford N, et al. Effect of blood pressure control on diabetic microvascular complications in patients with hypertension and type 2 diabetes. *Diabetes Care* 2000;23(Suppl 2):B54–B64.

Estacio R, Jeffers B, Gifford N, et al. Effect of blood pressure control on diabetic microvascular complications in patients with hypertension and type 2 diabetes. *N Engl J Med* 1998;338:645–652.

Keane W. Proteinuria: its clinical importance and role in progressive renal disease. *Am J Kidney Dis* 2000;35:S97–S105.

Krop J, Coresh J, Chambless L, et al. A community-based study of explanatory factors for the excess risk for early renal function decline in blacks versus whites with diabetes. *Arch Intern Med* 1999;159:1777–1783.

Kshirsagar AV, Joy MS, Hogan SL, et al. Effect of ACE inhibitors in diabetic and nondiabetic chronic renal disease: a systematic overview of randomized placebo-controlled trials. *Am J Kidney Dis* 2000;35:695–707.

Levin A. Understanding recent haemoglobin trials in CKD: methods and lesson learned from CREATE and CHOIR. *Nephrol Dial Transplant* 2007;22:309–312.

Lewis EJ, Hunsicker LG, Clarke WR, et al. Effect of ACE inhibition on nephropathy in type 1 diabetes. *N Engl J Med* 1993;329:1456–1462.

Lewis EJ, Hunsiker LG, Clarke WR, et al. Renoprotective effect of the angiotensin receptor antagonist irbesartan in patients with nephropathy due to type 2 diabetes. *N Engl J Med* 2001;345:851–860.

Mann JF, Gestein H, Pogue J, et al. Renal insufficiency as a predictor of cardiovascular outcomes and the impact of ramipril: the HOPE randomized trial. *Ann Droit Int Med* 2001;134:629–636.

Mogensen CE, Neldam S, Tikkanen I, et al. Randomized controlled trial of dual blockade of renin-angiotensin system in patients with hypertension, microalbuminuria, and non-insulin dependent diabetes: the candesatan and lisinopril microalbuminuria (CALM) study. *Br Med J* 2000;321:1440–1444.

Nakao N, Yoshimura A, Morita H, et al. Combination treatment of angiotensin II receptor blocker and angiotensin-converting enzyme inhibitor in non-diabetic renal disease (COOPERATE): a randomized controlled trial. *Lancet* 2003;361:117–124.

Nath K. The tubulointerstitium in progressive renal disease. *Kidney Int* 1998;54:992–994.

National Kidney Foundation-K/DOQI. Clinical practice guidelines for chronic kidney disease: evaluation, classification, and stratification. *Am J Kidney Dis* 2002;39(Suppl 1):S1–S266.

Orth SR, Ritz E, Schrier RW. The renal risks of smoking. *Kidney Int* 2003;51:1669–1677.

Parving HH, Lehnert H, Brochner-Mortensen J, et al. The effect of irbesartan on the development of diabetic nephropathy in patients with type 2 diabetes. *N Engl J Med* 2001;345:870–878.

Remuzzi G, Bertani T. Pathophysiology of progressive nephropathies. *N Engl J Med* 1998;339:1448–1456.

Schrier RW, Estacio R, Esler A, et al. Effect of aggressive blood pressure control in normotensive type 2 diabetic patients on albuminuria, retinopathy and strokes. *Kidney Int* 2002;61:1086–1097.

Shemesh O, Golbetz H, Kriss JP, et al. Limitations of creatinine as a filtration marker in glomerulopathic patients. *Kidney Int* 1985;28:830–838.

The GISEN Group. The GISEN Group: randomized placebo-controlled trial of effect of ramipril on decline in glomerular filtration rate and risk of terminal renal failure in proteinuric, non-diabetic nephropathy. *Lancet* 1997;349:1857–1863.

The JNC 7 Report. *JAMA* 2003;289:2560–2572.

UK Prospective Diabetes Study Group. Efficacy of atenolol and captopril in reducing risk of macrovascular and microvascular complications in type 2 diabetes: UKPDS 39. *Br Med J* 1998;317:713–720.

United States Renal Data System. Excerpts from the 2000 U.S. Renal Data System annual data report: atlas of end stage renal disease in the united states. *Am J Kidney Dis* 2000;36:S1–S279.

Wright JT, Bakris G, Greene T, et al. Effect of blood pressure lowering and anti-hypertensive drug class on progression of hypertensive kidney disease. Results from the AASK Trial. *JAMA* 2002;288:2421–2431.

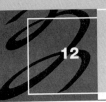

THE PATIENT RECEIVING CHRONIC RENAL REPLACEMENT WITH DIALYSIS

David M. Spiegel and Rebecca Moore

*T*he number of individuals kept alive by dialysis therapy in the United States continues to increase each year. Currently approximately 350,000 patients receive chronic dialysis treatments. Approximately 7% to 8% of these patients are on peritoneal dialysis (PD), whereas the large majority are treated with hemodialysis (HD). This life-prolonging therapy continues to make end-stage kidney failure the only major organ system failure that does not result in certain death without organ transplantation. However, the morbidity and mortality associated with end-stage renal disease (ESRD) remains high. Increased understanding of the disease process, new insights into pathogenic mechanisms, and new therapeutic options are emerging that may improve survival rates and quality of life for patients with ESRD.

   I. **THE NEED FOR RENAL REPLACEMENT THERAPY (RRT).** RRT is required when kidney function deteriorates to the point where the accumulation of waste products begins to interfere with life functions. As kidney function deteriorates, a number of physiologic alterations occur, many of which are ultimately detrimental. RRT is indicated when these changes can no longer be controlled by medications and diet. The progressive deterioration of kidney function has been defined as chronic kidney disease (CKD). Appropriate care designed to slow the progression of CKD, control factors known to contribute to the morbidity and mortality of kidney failure, and appropriate preparation for RRT during the stages of CKD ensure that patients are in the best overall condition at the time they start dialysis.

  II. **PREPARING FOR RRT**
   A. **Access creation.** Preparation for dialysis therapy is critical for the smooth transition from CKD care to RRT. Poor planning for RRT is a major cause of increased morbidity and mortality at the initiation of dialysis therapy. The use of temporary or tunneled dialysis catheters contributes to dialysis mortality by increasing the incidence of sepsis, acting as a stimulus for chronic inflammation, and damaging the central veins, thereby preventing or shortening the survival of more permanent vascular access once created.
      1. **HD.** Permanent access for HD requires either a native arterial venous fistula (AVF) or an artificial arteriovenous (AV) graft. Both types of accesses are placed surgically. Native AVFs are always preferable to artificial grafts, because they have a significantly lower incidence of infection and a longer event-free survival. Vein mapping by ultrasonography or venography may increase the likelihood of successful AVF placement by identifying suitable veins for access creation. In ideal candidates, an AVF may mature in as little as 4 weeks. However, in patients with less than ideal veins, AVFs can take 6 months or longer to mature. Therefore, access planning should start 6 to 12 months before dialysis is anticipated. As a general rule, the longer an AVF matures before first use the better the chance for long-term success. For artificial grafts, surgery should be performed 4 to 6 weeks before the anticipated start of dialysis. Usually the access is placed in the nondominant arm, in the most distal position available.
      2. **PD.** PD catheters are surgically inserted into the peritoneal cavity. Several types of catheters are now available and the time from placement to first use may vary greatly. Most nephrologists allow 7 to 10 days before using a catheter that is externalized at the time of implantation. Many PD catheters are left in a subcutaneous tunnel for several months before being externalized. This option

may allow better ingrowth of the catheter in a sterile environment and allows for externalization at the time of training.

III. **MODALITY SELECTION.** Current evidence suggests that both PD and HD provide equal RRT for most patients. Modality selection should be based on patient preference, which is largely related to lifestyle decisions. Proper education, starting early in the course of CKD, is the best means of ensuring that patients are able to make rational and educated decisions.

A. **Hemodialysis**

1. **In-center HD.** The largest percentages of patients on dialysis in the United States are dialyzed using this modality. As a general rule, patients dialyze three times per week for approximate 4 hours each session. At the beginning and throughout the treatment, vital signs are measured. Two needles are placed in the AVF or graft so that blood can be circulated through the artificial kidney at a rate of 300 to 500 mL per minute. Excess fluid is removed by a transmembrane pressure gradient, whereas toxins are removed by diffusion down their concentration gradient. At the end of the treatment, the needles are removed and bleeding stopped by the application of local pressure. Some facilities promote "self-care," wherein patients actively participate in their care by setting up dialysis machines, monitoring their blood pressure (BP), responding to machine alarms, and cannulating their access by placing the dialysis needles.

2. **Home HD.** Traditionally, home HD was performed similar to in-center HD three times per week utilizing essentially the same machines. The introduction of new technologies has greatly simplified home HD and dramatically changed the way it is performed in the United States. As a result, the number of patients performing home HD has increased dramatically in the last few years. Many patients are now performing daily home HD, a technique that provides between 2 and 3 hours of dialysis 6 days a week. However, newer machines are making it possible for some patients without partners to receive the benefits of home HD. Traditionally, the average training time before patients were able to perform HD at home was approximately 6 weeks. Now, some patients are able to train in 3 weeks on the newer machines. Once trained, patients generally do quite well, having the lowest mortality rate of any group of patients on dialysis in the United States. Part of this low mortality may be related to patient selection, because traditionally the healthiest and most motivated patients select home HD.

3. **New HD therapies.** Emerging HD therapies offer some advantages over current treatment and may ultimately improve the quality of life of patients on dialysis, along with increasing survival. These therapies include daily home HD, nocturnal HD which can be performed at home or in-center, and daily in-center HD. In both daily home and daily in-center HD, patients dialyze 2 to 3 hours, 6 days per week. Nocturnal dialysis is typically 6 to 8 hours, 6 days per week, although fewer treatments per week are being evaluated. In addition to providing overall more toxin removal, these therapies also have the advantage of better control of fluid volume and BP. A number of studies suggest that patients feel better, experience a higher quality of life, and are more socially adjusted. Some studies have found a reduced requirement for erythropoietin (EPO), although this has not been universal. Patients on nocturnal HD generally have greatly reduced need for phosphate binders. Although these therapies are more expensive than traditional HD, emerging evidence suggests that the total cost of patient care may be decreased, because patients on these more frequent therapies have a decreased need for supplemental medications and experience fewer hospitalizations.

B. **Peritoneal dialysis**

1. **Continuous ambulatory peritoneal dialysis (CAPD)**, along with automated peritoneal dialysis (APD) accounts for less than 15% of all patients on dialysis in the United States. With this dialysis modality, the semipermeable lining of the peritoneal cavity serves as the dialysis membrane and toxins diffuse out of the blood into a sterile dialysate fluid that has been instilled into the abdominal cavity. The process of draining out the old PD dialysate and instilling fresh dialysate into the peritoneal cavity is referred to as an *exchange*. As patients

perform the PD exchanges at home, PD allows patients a more flexible schedule than traditional in-center HD, because the exchanges can be done around most schedules. Another advantage of PD is that patients in remote areas do not have to travel to a dialysis center.

2. **APD** uses a machine to perform the dialysis exchanges, usually overnight, thereby allowing patients greater daytime flexibility. This is especially useful for people in school or young children. The technology behind the PD machines continues to improve, and these machines are now about the size of a large DVD player.

IV. **RRT.** The appropriate time to initiate dialysis for a patient cannot be clearly defined. Most nephrologists base their decision on clinical laboratory data and a subjective patient assessment. By the time the glomerular filtration rate (GFR) falls below 10 mL per minute, most patients require dialytic intervention. However, many patients appear to function quite well until the GFR approaches 5 mL per minute. As a general rule, patients with diabetes require earlier intervention (GFR less than 15 mL per minute) than do those with other etiologies for their kidney failure. Clearly, dialysis must be initiated before the uremic symptoms of peripheral neuropathy, encephalopathy, malnutrition, or serositis (including pericarditis) become evident. Although many of these complications resolve with adequate dialysis, peripheral neuropathy and malnutrition may be exceedingly difficult to reverse. Some nephrologists believe that early initiation with dialysis may improve long-term outcome, although this has not been shown to be true.

A. **Hemodialysis**

1. **Technical aspects.** Although the basic principles of HD (diffusion-based mass transfer of solute and pressure gradient–driven water removal) have not changed a great deal in the last 20 years, the technology has dramatically improved. Most patients dialyze three times per week. For each treatment, two large-bore needles (15 to 17 gauge) are inserted into the vascular access for removal and return of blood. The patient must remain confined to the dialysis machine for the duration of the treatment. Currently, most dialysis units use volumetric machines designed to remove a precise amount of fluid. These volumetric machines permit the use of larger, highly porous dialyzers with high water and solute permeability. This new design not only allows for significantly more removal of larger molecules than older dialyzers but also increases the efficiency of urea removal.

2. **Adequacy.** What constitutes optimal HD remains controversial. Urea kinetic modeling is a useful tool to quantify dialysis and thereby prevent underdialysis. Care must be taken to ensure that the modeling is based on the delivered dose of dialysis, as treatments are often shorter than prescribed and prescribed blood flow rates are sometimes not achieved. Additionally, as dialysis treatment times are shortened, plasma urea rebound increases, due to delayed intercompartmental shifts of urea, making the delivered dose of dialysis less than the measured dose. Currently, a delivered dialysis dose, as measured by a urea removal rate (URR), of less than 65% or a K_t per V (where K equals the dialyzer clearance of urea, t is the treatment time, and V is the urea volume of distribution) of less than 1.2 is considered inadequate. To ensure adequate dialysis, the recommended targets have been set at a URR of greater than or equal to 70% [URR = $100 \times (1 - C_t/C_0)$, where C_t is the postdialysis blood urea nitrogen (BUN) and C_0 is the predialysis BUN] or a K_t per V of greater than or equal to 1.4 (determined by single pool urea kinetic modeling).

3. **BP control.** Cardiovascular mortality remains the leading cause of death in patients with ESRD. Whereas the condition of patients at the time they start dialysis clearly plays a role in their long-term outcome, optimal BP control remains important in patients receiving dialysis. Unfortunately, there are no prospective trials in patients on dialysis that define optimal BP control. In addition, many patients with CKD lose the normal diurnal variation in BP. The management of BP control in patients on HD is further complicated by the fact that most patients experience a fall in BP during the dialysis treatment, often correlated with the amount of fluid removed. Therefore, what might be considered optimal BP control in the general population may result in significant

intradialytic hypotension. The optimal time to measure BP in patients on HD is also controversial. Predialysis BPs are felt to overestimate the patient's average BP, whereas postdialysis BP may underestimate mean BP. In the few studies that have closely evaluated BP in patients on dialysis, it is clear that within 8 to 12 hours postdialysis, BP has returned to predialysis levels. It is therefore generally recommended that of the two, the predialysis BP better reflects overall hypertensive risk. However, a few studies utilizing 24-hour BP monitoring have suggested that neither measurement is adequate for BP management. In practice, it is generally accepted that a slightly higher than normal BP may be acceptable for patients if measured at the start of the dialysis treatment. Although there are no definitive studies, and the topic remains controversial, many nephrologists aim for a predialysis target of less than 140 to 160/95 mm Hg.

In the United States, 50% to 80% of patients on dialysis are receiving anti-hypertensive therapy. Some evidence suggests that many of these patients could have their BP adequately controlled without or with significantly less antihyper-tensive medications if adequate dialysis was provided along with vigilant control of fluid volume. Although all antihypertensive medications except diuretics are available to treat patients on dialysis, the use of both angiotensin-converting enzyme (ACE) inhibitors and β-blockers are increasing due to their cardiopro-tective advantage. Carvedilol has recently been shown to decrease mortality in a small prospective study of patients on dialysis with congestive heart failure measured by echocardiogram.

4. **Anemia.** Anemia occurs in most patients on dialysis and almost certainly con-tributes to cardiac hypertrophy. Studies have shown that the anemia of ESRD is primarily due to a deficiency of EPO and can be corrected by administration of exogenous EPO. Adequate iron stores are also required. The optimal man-agement of anemia in patients on dialysis is controversial. Partial correction of anemia improves patients' quality of life and exercise physiology. There are lim-ited data that some measures of quality of life continue to improve as hemoglobin is corrected toward normal. However, the only large outcome study showed a trend toward worsening outcomes as hemoglobin was increased toward the normal range. Therefore, the optimal level of hemoglobin for patients on dialysis remains to be determined. The current targets recommended by the package insert, the Center for Medicare Services, and the Veterans Administration is a hemoglobin of 10 to 12 g per dL. The most recent Kidney Disease Outcomes Quality Initiative (K/DOQI) guidelines recommend the narrower targets of 11 to 12 g per dL.

5. **Rehabilitation and psychosocial adjustment.** When compared to the normal U.S. population, patients on HD have a much lower employment rate and a much higher percentage of disability recipients. Efforts to improve these figures through vocational rehabilitation have been only marginally successful. However, on quality of life questionnaires, most patients on HD rate their quality of life only slightly below the general population. Despite their overall high self-rating on quality of life questionnaires, many patients on dialysis have depression and anxiety disorders. A social worker is a critical member of all dialysis facility teams and can play a vital role in helping patients adjust to dialysis and deal with feelings of depression and anxiety.

6. **Complications.** Despite its lifesaving nature, HD remains a poor substitute for normal renal function and is fraught with a number of complications, both technical and secondary to kidney failure itself.

   a. **Technical complications**
      i. **Vascular access.** Despite recent advances, vascular access remains the Achilles heel of HD. Although some AV fistulas last 5 to 20 years, many patients have poor native vessels and therefore have shortened AVF survival rates. These patients often must rely on artificial grafts, which are predisposed to thrombosis, pseudoaneurysm formation, and infection. The average survival of new grafts is approximately 2 years. Early intervention for failing grafts, along with new radiologic techniques, may

improve the average survival rate. Intervention can take several forms, including the measurement of static or dynamic venous pressures or indirect measures of access blood flow rate.

ii. **Hypotension.** Despite improvements in dialysis equipment, hypotension remains a common problem during HD. Use of bicarbonate dialysate, higher dialysate sodium concentrations, and volumetric machines have helped to decrease its frequency. However, hypotension continues to occur for a number of reasons including autonomic insufficiency, rapid ultrafiltration (fluid removal) that exceeds the rate of vascular refilling, or myocardial dysfunction.

iii. **Allergic reactions.** These can occur secondary to exposure to the dialyzer material or the sterilant. They can range from mild itching to anaphylaxis.

iv. **Other.** Air embolism, ruptured dialyzer, improper dialysate mixture, or failures of the water purification system are causes of rare but often life-threatening complications. Care and proper maintenance of dialysis machines and water treatment facilities, with special attention to the dialysis technique and to the safety and alarm mechanisms, help prevent these complications.

b. **Complications associated with inadequate dialysis**
   i. **Uremic pericarditis.** Although often thought of as a predialysis problem, occasionally patients on HD develop pericarditis. This often occurs in the setting of an acute illness, catabolic states, or at a time of vascular access difficulty, resulting in inadequate dialysis.
   ii. **Uremic neuropathy.** This complication is often overlooked by many nephrologists, because it is generally a peripheral neuropathy starting in the feet or hands. It must be differentiated from diabetic neuropathy, which is common in the dialysis population. Because the two conditions can coexist, chronic inadequate dialysis must be considered as a possible cause for any peripheral neuropathy.

c. **Long-term complications**
   i. **Cardiovascular.** Cardiovascular death remains the major cause of mortality in patients with ESRD. Many factors contribute, including hypertension, anemia, smoking, hypercholesterolemia, and the presence of an AV shunt. Most of these factors are present long before the development of ESRD. Although the aggressive treatment of these risk factors seems prudent, good clinical studies in patients with ESRD are lacking. In one of the few large prospective randomized trials in patients on dialysis, treatment of hypercholesterolemia failed to show a survival benefit. Increasing evidence suggests that disorders of mineral metabolism, that accompanies ESRD, may result in accelerated deposition of calcium in the intima and media of blood vessels. This calcium deposition appears to be an active process, much like the calcium deposition in bone. This vascular calcification has been associated with increased mortality presumably due to alterations in normal vascular physiology. Typical findings in patients with excessive vascular calcification are a widened pulse pressure and linear calcium deposition on plain films. In patients on dialysis, evidence of cardiac dysfunction and vascular calcification predict poor outcome.
   ii. **Infectious disease.** Infections remain a common cause of morbidity and mortality in patients on HD. Infection of temporary catheters and tunneled catheters is common. Infection of tunneled catheters is often classified as exit site infections, tunnel infections, or bacteremia. Exit site infections can often be treated without removal of the catheter. Tunnel infections generally require catheter removal. When bacteremia occurs tunneled catheter are often removed, although evidence suggests that changing the catheter over a guidewire, along with antibiotic therapy, may allow for resolution of the infection. Staphylococcal organisms

remain the most common, followed by other gram-positive bacteria. Endocarditis and spinal abscesses are not infrequent complications of catheter-related bacteremia. Native vein fistulas have a significantly lower infection rate than all forms of temporary catheters or artificial graft material and are the access of first choice. In addition to the vascular access as a route of infection, improper reprocessing of dialyzers can lead to sepsis, often from waterborne organisms.

iii. Bone disease. Bone disease starts before patients begin dialysis. Typically, high turnover bone disease is present in most patients with CKD. With increasing time on dialysis this bone disease often worsens although there has been some changes in the histologic patterns over the last 10 years. Hyperparathyroid bone disease (i.e., osteitis fibrosa) remains the most common. It results from overactivity of the parathyroid glands, occurring secondary to alteration in the serum calcium, hyperphosphatemia, and low 1,25-vitamin D_3 levels. Rapid bone turnover, increased osteoclastic activity, and ultimately fibrosis of the marrow space characterize this bone disease. It can range from mild to severe, pure or mixed with aluminum (Al) bone disease. Symptoms generally include bone pain and proximal muscle weakness and consequences include spontaneous tendon rupture and fractures. Aluminum is directly toxic to bone. Patients on dialysis can acquire Al either through oral Al-containing phosphate binders, other dietary sources, or through a contaminated water supply. It accumulates due to lack of renal excretion and deposits at the mineralization front of growing or remodeling bone. Al deposition produces a form of low turnover bone disease characterized by the accumulation of unmineralized matrix or osteoid (osteomalacia). A histologic pattern of low turnover bone disease without the presence of Al is increasingly reported in bone biopsies and has been termed *adynamic bone*. This bone is characterized by very low bone turnover with few osteoblasts or osteoclasts. Low turnover bone disease has been associated with increased vascular calcification. Both severe hyperparathyroidism and low turnover bone disease can predispose patients to hypercalcemia. Treatment for the abnormalities of mineral metabolism in ESRD involves control of the serum phosphorus, calcium, and parathyroid hormone. The traditional approach was limited to oral phosphate binders, often calcium containing, and intravenous or oral vitamin D preparations. Emerging evidence has raised concerns about calcium loading patients on dialysis and a number of new noncalcium phosphate binders are available and a great many more in development. The recent cloning of the calcium-sensing receptor has allowed for a new class of therapeutic agents called *calcimimetics*. These small organic compounds bind to the calcium-sensing receptor and amplify the calcium signal sent through a second intracellular messenger. The net effect is a reduction in parathyroid hormone production and release. Work is ongoing in an attempt to determine the link between abnormalities in bone mineral metabolism, abnormal vascular calcification, and the increased rate of cardiovascular mortality seen in patients on dialysis. It remains to be determined whether the move away from calcium-based phosphate binders, the more judicious use of vitamin D analogs, and the greater use of calcimimetic agents will improve bone health and help reduce the cardiovascular death rate. A final form of bone and osteoarticular disease seen in long-term patients on dialysis is β_2-microglobulin (β_2M) amyloidosis. β_2M is a small protein that accumulates in the blood of patients on dialysis and precipitates at osteoarticular surfaces to form amyloid. Symptoms include pain, swelling, bone cysts, and fractures. Recent data suggest that highly permeable dialysis membranes may delay the onset of disease symptoms.

iv. Malnutrition inflammation syndrome. Large-scale studies have demonstrated that the nutritional state of a patient on dialysis, as measured by the serum albumin, has a major impact on the long-term survival. Traditionally, it was believed that a low serum albumin reflected inadequate protein and calorie intake to maintain lean body mass. Whereas many patients do suffer from some degree of malnutrition, it is now recognized that albumin is an important inverse acute phase reactant, and the utility of a low serum albumin as a marker of mortality probably reflects in large part the presence of an active inflammatory process rather than specific nutritional deficiencies. Other inflammatory makers such as C-reactive protein and interleukin 6 (IL-6) have also been shown to be predictors of mortality in patients on dialysis. The finding of a low serum albumin and elevated levels of inflammatory markers has been termed the *malnutrition inflammation syndrome*. Identifying and correcting reversible causes of both inflammation and malnutrition are essential to maintaining optimal health in patients with ESRD.

   v. Skin disorders. Pruritus remains one of the most troubling complaints of patients on dialysis. Causes include an elevated calcium-phosphorus product, dry skin, and hyperparathyroidism. Some relief may be achieved with antihistamines and phosphate control. In severe cases, treatment with ultraviolet (UV) light has been effective. Other skin conditions in patients on dialysis include bullous dermatitis and porphyria cutanea tarda.

   vi. Acquired renal cystic disease. Many patients undergoing maintenance dialysis develop cysts in their native kidneys that tend to increase in size and number over time. Although these cysts are generally an incidental finding, complications have been reported including polycythemia, spontaneous rupture, and retroperitoneal bleeding. Patients on dialysis with acquired renal cystic disease appear to have a 100-fold increase in the incidence of renal cell carcinoma. However, deaths from renal cancer remains uncommon in the ESRD population, and routine screening has not been advocated due to the high rate of false-positive studies that might lead to unnecessary surgery in this high-risk population. Patients with hematuria, flank pain, or abnormal weight loss should be evaluated.

B. Peritoneal dialysis
   1. Technical aspects. Technically, PD is much less complex than HD. A sterile electrolyte and dextrose solution (dialysate) is allowed to flow into the peritoneal cavity through a previously implanted catheter using gravity or through a low-pressure pump. Following a specified period (dwell time), the fluid is drained out of the peritoneal cavity and fresh fluid is again infused. The peritoneal lining acts as the semipermeable membrane across which diffusion occurs. The process of fluid infusion and drainage (exchanges) can be performed manually (CAPD) or by a machine (APD). A new, nondextrose dialysate solution is now available. Its advantages include a long duration of osmotic activity due to its poor peritoneal transport and the lack of a glucose load to the patient that occurs when the dextrose in traditional PD fluid is absorbed across the peritoneal membrane.

   2. Adequacy. Because the quantity of PD that can be delivered is limited by the fixed peritoneal membrane kinetics and the amount of dialysate that can be comfortably infused and carried, it seems prudent to deliver as much dialysis as is reasonably possible. For many patients on PD, residual kidney function plays a vital role in their ability to achieve adequate clearance. The currently recommended minimum dose of delivered dialysis for patients on PD is 1.7 Kt/V.

   3. BP control. As in HD, BP control is important for the long-term well-being of patients on PD. Many patients on PD are able to discontinue their antihypertensives and maintain a normal BP. This may be attributable to the steady-state volume control achieved by this continuous dialysis modality.

   4. Anemia. The controversy regarding optimal anemia management in PD is identical to that in HD. EPO is generally administered subcutaneously in patients on PD, and erythropoiesis stimulating agents (ESAs) with longer duration of action are often used in patients on PD to minimize the frequency of injections.

A lower overall dose of ESA is needed to correct the anemia in patients on PD compared with patients on HD. This partly reflects the difference in routes of administration (subcutaneous is more effective than intravenous) and the small ongoing blood losses that occur with HD.

5. **Nutritional aspects.** Nutrition is critically important in patients on PD. Protein requirements for patients on PD are considered to be slightly higher than for patients on HD due to the ongoing loss of protein in the spent dialysate. Many patients on PD gain weight over the first 12 to 18 months. This phenomenon probably results from an increase in fat mass due to excess calorie intake, part of which comes from the high glucose content of the peritoneal dialysate solution. However, patients on long-term PD, like patients on HD, tend to lose lean body mass. It is unclear how this relates to the adequacy of PD or to underlying inflammatory processes.

6. **Rehabilitation and psychosocial adjustment.** Although PD allows individual patients more control over their health care and a more flexible dialysis schedule, the percentage of patients on PD in the workforce and the percentage on disability are no different from those on HD. On quality of life questionnaires, patients on PD as a group rate their quality of life about the same as patients on HD. Unfortunately, no prospective studies are available, and the variability in patient selection is certainly a major factor in these findings.

7. **Complications.** As in HD, PD has a number of associated complications. They can be divided into infectious and long-term complications. However, unlike HD, inadequate PD tends to result in malnutrition and technique failure, with pericarditis and peripheral neuropathy being less common, although they do occur.

   a. **Infectious disease.** Peritonitis remains the most frequent complication of PD. Technical improvements, including disconnect "flush before fill" systems, have reduced the peritonitis rates in most centers. Most episodes of peritonitis are treatable in the outpatient setting; however, severe infections require hospitalization and occasionally catheter removal. This is particularly true when peritonitis is caused by a fungal infection or *Pseudomonas aeruginosa*. Exit site infections are also common in PD and usually result from gram-positive organisms. These infections can generally be treated with antibiotics and increased exit site care. However, some infections, particularly those secondary to *Staphylococcus aureus* may require catheter removal. Although no consensus on proper exit site care has emerged, most experts agree that the catheter should exit the skin in a downward direction. Tunnel infections usually result from exit site infections and are frequently caused by *S. aureus*. Early diagnosis is often difficult. An episode of peritonitis, with the same organism causing an exit site infection, may be the presenting symptoms. In some centers, ultrasonography has been useful in detecting the fluid around the subcutaneous tunnel that indicates a tunnel infection. Tunnel infections usually necessitate catheter removal.

   b. **Long-term complications.** Although acute hemodynamic complications are less frequent with PD due to the continuous nature of the technique, cardiovascular disease remains the most common cause of death. Aggressive treatment of lipid abnormalities seems warranted, although no outcome studies are available. Disorders of mineral and bone disease also occur in patients on PD. The morphology is similar to that seen in patients on HD, with a slightly higher incidence of low turnover bone disease. β_2M amyloid can also occur in patients on PD. Acquired renal cystic disease and renal cell cancer appear to have the same increased incidence in PD as in HD. A number of long-term complications are unique to PD. These include a leak of PD fluid from the peritoneal space into either the pleural space or into the subcutaneous tissues, resulting in either pleural effusions or hernias, respectively. Sclerosing peritonitis resulting in ultrafiltration failure is an uncommon complication of PD; when it occurs, it is usually in the setting of repeated episodes of peritonitis. A much more common cause of failure of patients on PD is a gradual loss of residual renal function that results in a fall in total clearance, often leading to inadequate dialysis.

V. MORTALITY. Despite major advances in renal transplantation and the technology of HD and PD, the diagnosis of ESRD carries an increased mortality compared to age-matched controls. Patients starting dialysis typically have multiple comorbidities. More than 70% of patients have hypertension, 50% have diabetes, 45% have peripheral vascular disease, and 20% have congestive heart failure. Anemia remains common, despite more attention to treatment during the time period before dialysis. Although much of the increased mortality can be related to these underlying medical conditions, some can be directly attributable to the current practice of dialysis and transplantation. Dialysis in any form provides only a very small percentage of the clearance achieved by the normal kidneys. Although the hormones produced by the normal kidney, such as EPO and 1,25-dihydroxy vitamin D_3, have been available for some time, their optimal use remains to be determined. The optimal target hemoglobin remains unknown, as does the optimal use of vitamin D analogs and the new calcimimetic agent. Recently, it has become clear that most patients on dialysis are deficient in 25 vitamin D. Although this is the precursor vitamin for the circulating hormone 1,25 dihydroxy vitamin D, it is now apparent that many cells of the body contain the 1 hydroxylase enzyme, and can produce the active hormone for use in an autocrine manner. With increased recognition that 25 vitamin D plays an important role in cardiovascular health and immune function, interest is now focused on the potential benefit of vitamin D repletion in patients on dialysis.

A. HD versus PD. In the United States, the gross annual mortality among patients on dialysis is approximately 20% to 22%. This figure is 25% to 50% higher than that reported in much of Europe and Japan, and has raised questions about the delivery of dialysis in this country. However, differences in case mix remain a large confounding variable. The risk of death is higher for patients with diabetes as well as those with increasing age. For all race and age-groups, the life expectancy on dialysis is significantly shorter than that of the general population. As an example, a white man in the United States, at age 45, has a life expectancy of 32 years compared to white male patients on dialysis, whose life expectancy is approximately 7.4 years. For a black woman, the numbers are similar: normal population 33 years versus patient on dialysis 8.4 years. However, most studies comparing survival on HD versus PD have found little difference in overall mortality.

B. Dialysis versus transplantation. There is no doubt that a successful renal transplant improves an individual's quality of life and rehabilitation potential. For diabetic patients and the young, renal transplantation also significantly increases the average life expectancy of those with ESRD.

Suggested Readings

Besarab A, Bolton WK, Browne JK, et al. The effects of normal as compared with low hematocrit values in patients with cardiac disease who are receiving hemodialysis and epoetin. *N Engl J Med* 1998;339:584–590.

Blacher J, Guerin AP, Pannier B, et al. Arterial calcifications, arterial stiffness, and cardiovascular risk in end stage renal disease. *Hypertension* 2001;38:938–942.

Cice G, Ferrara L, D'Andrea A, et al. Carvedilol increases two-year survival in dialysis patients with dilated cardiomyopathy: a prospective, placebo-controlled trial. *J Am Coll Cardiol* 2003;41(9):1438–1444.

Collins AJ, Kasiske B, Herzog C, et al. Excerpts from the United States renal data system 2007 annual data report. *Am J Kidney Dis* 2008;51(Suppl 1):S1–S320; The data reported here have been supplied by the USRDS. The interpretation and reporting of these data are the responsibility of the authors and in no way should be seen as an official policy or interpretation of the US government.

Davies SJ, Woodrow G, Donovan K, et al. Icodextrin improves the fluid status of peritoneal dialysis patients: results of a double-blind randomized controlled trial. *J Am Soc Nephrol* 2003;14(9):2338–2344.

Foley RN, Parfrey PS, Harnett JD. Left ventricular hypertrophy in dialysis patients. *Semin Dial* 1992;5:34–41.

Lindberg JL, Moe SM, Goodman WG, et al. The calcimimetic AMG 073 reduces parathyroid hormone and calcium X phosphorus in secondary hyperparathyroidism. *Kidney Int* 2003;63:248–254.

NKF-K/DOQI. Clinical practice guidelines and clinical practice recommendations. *Am J Kidney Dis* 2006;48:S98–S127.

NKF-K/DOQI. Clinical practice guidelines and clinical practice recommendations. *Am J Kidney Dis* 2006;48:S132–S146.

Schwab SJ, Raymond JR, Saeed M, et al. Prevention of hemodialysis fistula thrombosis. Early detection of venous stenoses. *Kidney Int* 1989;36:707–711.

U.S. Renal Data System. *USRDS 2003 annual data report: atlas of end-stage renal disease in the united states.* Bethesda.: National Institutes of Health, National Institute of Diabetes and Digestive and Kidney Diseases, 2003.

Wanner C, Krane V, Marz W, et al. Atorvastatin in patients with type 2 diabetes mellitus undergoing hemodialysis. *N Engl J Med* 2005;353:238–248.

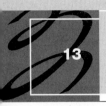

THE PATIENT WITH A KIDNEY TRANSPLANT

Eric Gibney, Chirag Parikh, and Alkesh Jani

I. INTRODUCTION AND EPIDEMIOLOGY

The prevalence of end-stage renal disease (ESRD) in the United States and developed nations is alarmingly high. In 2004, there were 104,000 new ESRD patients and more than 472,000 total patients with ESRD in the United States. These are dramatic increases from previous decades. Currently, hemodialysis, peritoneal dialysis, and kidney transplantation are the only available therapies for ESRD.

Comparisons of kidney transplant recipients to patients on dialysis awaiting transplantation have shown that kidney transplantation, in most cases, is the ideal treatment of ESRD. Advantages include longer patient survival, less morbidity, cost savings, and improved quality of life compared with dialysis. Living kidney donation remains the most effective therapy, with average graft survival of approximately 12 to 15 years, with longer survival for well-matched sibling transplants. This good news is tempered by the reality that demand for transplant kidneys far exceeds the supply of available organs. Although modest increases in deceased donor transplants have occurred owing to efforts to improve recovery from expanded donors, donors with cardiac death, and donors with brain death, these increases have not kept pace with demands. With more than 74,000 patients on the kidney waiting list in January 2008, the unfortunate result is that many patients will die on the waiting list before receiving a transplant.

II. PATIENT SELECTION

There are few contraindications to receiving a kidney transplant. However, patients should not receive a transplant if they have an active infection, ongoing active immunologic disease which led to kidney failure, metastatic malignancy, inability to follow a medical regimen due to medical or psychological reasons, or are at high operative risk due to other conditions. Although there is no definite age limit to receive a kidney transplant, elderly patients with comorbid conditions have less demonstrable survival benefit compared to dialysis and should be screened thoroughly and counseled regarding risks of transplantation. Human immunodeficiency virus (HIV) infection was historically a contraindication to transplantation, but successful kidney transplantation is now more common in patients free of opportunistic infections with undetectable viral replication and sustained CD4 counts greater than 200.

A. Recipient evaluation

The goals of evaluating a potential recipient should be to identify potential barriers to transplantation, identify treatable conditions that would attenuate the risk of the surgery or immunosuppression, and to explain benefits and risks. Attention is given to the cause of ESRD and its tendency to recur in kidney transplants. Comorbid conditions and the effects of immunosuppression on these conditions are considered. Patient age older than 50 years, diabetes, abnormal electrocardiogram, angina, or congestive heart failure have been demonstrated as predictors of cardiac death and nonfatal cardiac events with kidney transplantation. Noninvasive strategies such as thallium perfusion imaging and dobutamine stress echo have demonstrated the ability to predict cardiac events and may prevent high-risk patients from requiring angiography. Screening for malignancy should follow age-appropriate guidelines. In patients with malignancies, a 2- to 5-year remission may be required before transplantation depending on tumor type and invasiveness. Although obesity is a risk for wound-related complications, long-term outcomes are similar to nonobese patients unless cardiovascular disease exists. Psychosocial screening is usually performed. Testing generally includes evaluation for HIV and hepatitis B and C. Imaging or functional evaluation of the kidneys and lower urinary tract may be necessary in certain patients. After a patient has been accepted as a candidate, ABO and human leukocyte antigen (HLA) typing is performed, along with determination of serologic status for cytomegalovirus (CMV) and varicella. The candidate's blood is also screened with a panel reactive antibody (PRA) test for antibodies against common HLA antigens. A patient on the waiting list for more than 1 year should be seen periodically to update his or her condition.

B. Organ donors

1. Living donors. Although the risks of donation are small, these risks need to be carefully explained to a potential **living donor**. Mortality is uncommon, but has occurred in 0.02% of donors (2 per 10,000). Infection, bleeding, and other postoperative complications occur in up to 15% of patients. Progression to ESRD has occurred but does not appear to be more common than in the general population. Mild blood pressure elevation and proteinuria may occur after donation but the long-term consequences are currently unclear. After ABO compatibility and a negative cross match are assured, the donor evaluation process can begin. If there are multiple candidates, the donor with fewer HLA mismatches is usually selected. Donors are carefully screened for kidney disease to prevent the possibility of loss of function in the remaining kidney. Hypertension, proteinuria, obesity, kidney stones, and structural or functional kidney disease all are relative contraindications to donation depending on severity. Testing for latent diabetes mellitus with a glucose tolerance test may be performed if there is a family history or perceived risk for future diabetes. When recipients are affected by hereditary disorders such as polycystic kidney disease (PKD) or hereditary nephritis, the condition must be ruled out in related donors either clinically or with genetic testing. If a donor is thought to be acceptable, imaging of the kidneys is performed with computed tomographic angiography (CTA) or other modalities, allowing the team to assess for structural or vascular anomalies and suitability for laparoscopic donation.

2. Deceased donors

A deceased donor also must be evaluated. The presence of metastasis, unknown cause of death, HIV, or widespread infection precludes donation. Donors with hepatitis C are sometimes accepted for hepatitis C–positive recipients. A combination of factors such as hypertension, advanced age, elevated serum creatinine, oliguria, or dependence on pressor support may exclude a donor. Preimplantation biopsies can be performed on an individual basis when there is concern about the function of a donor kidney. **Expanded criteria donors (ECDs)** are defined by any donor older than 60 years, or any donor older than 50 years with two of the following: terminal serum creatinine greater than 1.5, cerebrovascular accident as a cause of death, or preexisting hypertension. ECD kidneys have a higher risk of graft failure but still provide survival benefit compared to dialysis in selected populations, and are commonly used in older recipients or those who may not be expected to have extended survival on dialysis. In **donation after cardiac death (DCD)**, organs are recovered from a donor who has undergone cardiac death after a period of circulatory arrest, usually in the setting of a withdrawal of care in the hospital. Although longer warm ischemia times lead to an increase in delayed graft function (DGF), DCD kidneys have similar long-term survival and function when compared to kidneys from donors with brain death.

C. Predictors of outcome

Recipient factors, donor factors, and donor/recipient compatibility all influence long-term graft survival. Recipients who are younger, have low levels of PRA, have spent less time on dialysis, and who are employed or college educated have superior graft survival. Recipients who have been transplanted preemptively, that is, before dialysis started, also have superior long-term graft survival. Race and ethnicity may affect graft survival for both donors and recipients, with nonblack donor kidneys and nonblack, non-Hispanic recipients of grafts having the longest graft survival. Kidneys from living related or unrelated donors survive longer on average than deceased donor kidneys. Other donor qualities that positively affect outcomes include younger age and shorter cold ischemia time. Finally, factors of donor and recipient compatibility also affect outcomes: better HLA matching, CMV serologic status matching, and equivalent donor/recipient body mass index all have positive affects on long-term graft survival.

III. IMMUNOLOGY AND PHARMACOTHERAPY

A. Immunology

A basic review of the mechanisms of immune recognition and response to an allograft is helpful to better understand the patient who has undergone kidney transplantation as well as the pharmacologic agents used to prevent allograft rejection.

1. **Major histocompatibility complex (MHC)**

Cells in the tissues of mammals, birds, and bony fish express MHC surface molecules, which are crucial for the immune system to be able to recognize and respond to a foreign antigen. In humans, these MHC molecules are located on the short arm of chromosome 6 and encode for proteins termed the *HLAs*. MHC molecules serve two basic functions: they identify self from nonself and coordinate the T-cell receptor (TCR) recognition of the antigen-MHC complex. The MHC molecules are divided into two groups: class I and class II. MHC class I molecules appear on the surface of all cells and are known as *HLA-A, B,* and *C*. MHC class II molecules appear on antigen presenting cells (APCs) and are termed *HLA-DR, DP,* and *DQ*. One MHC *haplotype* is inherited from each parent as a locus containing each of the six genetically linked HLA molecules. In kidney transplantation, only the HLA-A, B, and DR are determined due to their immunogenicity. A "zero-antigen mismatched kidney" has no mismatches in either locus for HLA-A, B, and DR, although mismatches may be present at HLA-C, DP, DQ, or at other minor antigens. Although advances in immunosuppression have narrowed advantages for well-matched transplants, a 2-haplotype-identical transplant from a family member or a zero-antigen mismatched deceased donor transplant confers a graft survival benefit compared to transplants with lesser degrees of matching.

2. **Antigen-Presenting Cells**

APCs are distributed in a ubiquitous manner in body tissues and allow T cells to recognize foreign antigens. Monocytes, macrophages, dendritic cells, and activated B cells can all serve as APCs. Either by phagocytosis or through surface immunoglobulin (Ig) (B cells), APCs capture foreign antigens, degrade and process them into peptides, and express these foreign peptides on MHC class II surface molecules. Through TCR interactions and various downstream events, the T cell is then able to coordinate an immune response to this foreign antigen.

3. **T cells**

T cells are processed in the thymus and are central to cellular immunity and allograft recognition and rejection. These properties make them a common target of drugs designed to prevent rejection. Central to the immune response is the ability of the T cell to recognize foreign antigens through a surface TCR. These receptors recognize antigens through either indirect or direct pathways. The *indirect pathway* involves TCR recognition of a foreign antigen that is presented by a self-MHC molecule located on an APC surface. The *direct pathway* refers to the ability of some T-cell populations to recognize foreign MHC that is not presented with self MHC on an APC.

There are two major classes of T cells: T-helper cells which express CD4 surface molecules (CD4$^+$), and cytotoxic T cells which express CD8. (CD8$^+$). CD4$^+$ cells recognize MHC class II molecules on the surface of APCs, whereas CD8$^+$ cells are restricted to recognition of MHC class I. CD4$^+$ cells are activated after recognition of a foreign antigen (e.g., foreign MHC from a kidney transplant). They then initiate an immune response to foreign peptides by secreting cytokines important in B-cell proliferation and activation and cytotoxic T-cell activation. CD8$^+$ T cells kill cells bearing foreign antigen through the use of cytotoxic molecules such as perforins, granzymes, and Fas, which triggers apoptosis in the targeted cell.

4. T cell and APC interactions

T cells and APCs have a number of important interactions central to allograft recognition and rejection. *Signal 1* is the term for initial binding of the T cell to the APC through interactions between the TCR/CD3 complex and foreign peptide expressed in MHC. Signal 1 is a calcium-dependent process and results in calcineurin activation. Although signal 1 alone will cause anergy, the addition of **signal 2**, also known as *costimulation*, will lead to an immune response. The best understood costimulation signal is between CD28 on the T-cell surface and B7 on the APC surface. CD28/B7 activation leads to intracellular signaling, interleukin 2 (IL-2) production, and T-cell activation. While CD28 is expressed on resting T cells, the T-cell surface molecule cytotoxic T lymphocyte antigen-4 (CTLA-4) immunoglobulin is expressed only on activated T cells. CTLA-4 binds preferentially to B7 and eventually inactivates the immune response, thereby providing potent negative feedback. Another costimulatory molecule, CD40, is found on APCs and activated B cells, and binds to CD40 ligand (CD40L) on T cells. The CD40/CD40L pathway is important in Ig production and class switching by B cells.

5. B cells

B cells develop at multiple sites of the body, including the liver, spleen, and lymph nodes. In response to T-cell signals for activation and proliferation, they produce Igs. A naive B cell produces IgM and, after class switching, is able to produce IgG, IgA, or IgA. Depending on their class, antibodies mediate opsonization for phagocytosis or antibody-dependent cellular cytotoxicity, and can fix complement. B cells and antibodies are important in the processes of hyperacute rejection (immediate allograft destruction due to preformed antibodies), and donor-specific antibodies have been implicated in both antibody-mediated (humoral) rejection and chronic allograft nephropathy (CAN).

B. Pharmacotherapy

In the last two decades, the number of immunosuppressive agents available has increased greatly. Commonly used agents, their mechanism of action, and common toxicities appear in Table 13-1. Agents can be used for *induction* therapy at the time of transplant, as *maintenance* therapy to prevent rejection of the allograft, or for the treatment of *acute rejection*.

1. **The calcineurin inhibitors,** cyclosporine A (CsA) and tacrolimus (FK506), are a mainstay of maintenance immunosuppression. Cyclosporine and tacrolimus have similar side effects, but hyperlipidemia, hypertension, hirsutism, and gingival hyperplasia are more common with cyclosporine, and posttransplant diabetes mellitus (PTDM) and neurotoxicity may be more common with tacrolimus. They both cause significant nephrotoxicity. Tacrolimus has also been advocated as the maintenance agent of choice for steroid-resistant acute rejection.

2. One **target of rapamycin (TOR) inhibitor,** sirolimus, is currently used in kidney transplantation for maintenance therapy and for calcineurin inhibitor withdrawal. Important toxicities include hypertriglyceridemia, hypercholesterolemia, cytopenias, pneumonitis, delayed wound healing, lymphoceles, and diarrhea. Sirolimus may also potentiate the toxicity of calcineurin inhibitors.

3. **The antiproliferatives.** Mycophenolate mofetil (MMF), mycophenolic acid (MPA), or azathioprine can be used in combination with calcineurin inhibitors and corticosteroids for maintenance immunosuppression. MMF and MPA often cause diarrhea and gastrointestinal discomfort, can be associated with cytopenias, and may be associated with an increased risk of tissue-invasive CMV. It is still not clear if MPA, an enteric-coated version, leads to decreased gastrointestinal side effects. Azathioprine, a purine analog, provides less selective lymphocyte inhibition and can be associated with cytopenias and neoplasias.

4. **Corticosteroids** are used during induction, as maintenance therapy, and for the treatment of acute rejection. Their effectiveness is complicated by a variety of well-known side effects, including hypertension, glucose intolerance, weight gain, cataracts, poor wound healing, osteoporosis, and osteonecrosis. Although

TABLE 13-1 Commonly Used Drugs in Renal Transplantation

Class and drugs	Mechanism	Toxicity	Indication
Calcineurin inhibitors			
Cyclosporin	Binds cyclophilin and blocks action of calcineurin	Hypertension, hyperlipidemia nephrotoxicity, neurotoxicity hirsuitism, gingival hyperplasia	M
Tacrolimus	Binds to FKBP, inhibiting action of calcineurin	PTDM, neurotoxicity side effects similar to cyclosporine	M
TOR inhibitors			
Sirolimus	Binds to FKBP and inhibits mTOR effects, cytokine signaling, cell cycling, and CD28-mediated costimulation	Elevated cholesterol and triglycerides, cytopenias, acne, wound healing, pneumonitis	M, CIW
Antiproliferatives			
Azathioprine	6-MP release *in vivo*, interferes with DNA synthesis, cell cycling	Cytopenias, diarrhea, hepatotoxic, neoplasias	M
Mycophenolate mofetil (MMF)	Inosine monophosphate dehydrogenase inhibitors, blocks *de novo* purine synthesis	Diarrhea, GI discomfort, cytopenias, invasive CMV	M
Mycophenolic acid (MPA)	Multiple sites of action; cytokine production, T-cell proliferation, leukocyte traffic, others	HTN, PTDM, hyperlipidemia, obesity, infection, osteoporosis, AVN	I, M, AR
Corticosteroids			
Antibody therapies			
Antithymocyte globulin	Rabbit polyclonal Ab against thymocytes	Allergic reaction, leukopenia	I, AR
Muromonab/CD3	Mouse monoclonal Ab against CD3 on TCR	Cytokine release syndrome	I, AR
Daclizumab	Humanized (90%) monoclonal Ab against CD25, the α subunit of IL-2 receptor	Low incidence of side effects: fever, chills, allergy	I
Basiliximab	Partially humanized (75%) monoclonal Ab, same target as daclizumab		I
Alemtuzumab	Humanized monoclonal Ab against CD52 on lymphocytes and monocytes	Lymphopenia, autoimmune syndromes, infection, delayed rejection	I

Ab, antibody; AR, acute rejection; AVN, avascular necrosis; CIW, calcineurin inhibitor withdrawal; FKBP, FK binding protein; GI, gastrointestinal; HTN, hypertension; I, induction; IL-2, interleukin 2; M, maintenance; 6-MP: 6-mercaptopurine; PTDM, posttransplant diabetes mellitus; TCR, T-cell receptor; TOR, target of rapamycin.

corticosteroid withdrawal and avoidance have been explored (see section V.C.2), they remain a mainstay of current immunosuppression.

5. **Antibody therapies** are available for many indications in kidney transplantation, including acute humoral rejection, steroid-resistant acute rejection, and induction in patients with elevated PRA, repeat transplant, positive B-cell cross match, ABO incompatibility, or other situations involving high immunologic risk. *Polyclonal antibody preparations (antithymocyte globulin and antilymphocyte globulin)* are used for induction and acute rejection. These compounds are developed by injecting human thymic extracts into rabbits or, less commonly, horses, and purifying the antibodies produced. These preparations neutralize lymphocytes by multiple antibody-mediated mechanisms, with a sustained effect on proliferation. Toxicities are related to immunosuppression, heterogeneity of preparations, allergic or anaphylactoid responses to nonhuman preparations, and cytopenias. *Muromonab/CD3 (OKT3)* is a murine monoclonal Ab against the CD3 complex of the TCR. Given intravenously for 7 to 14 days, it is available for induction therapy and for the treatment of acute rejection. Toxicities include a cytokine release syndrome, which can sometimes be complicated by capillary leak and pulmonary edema. Aseptic meningitis, serum sickness, profound immunosuppression, and lymphoproliferative disorders are less common side effects. *Daclizumab and basiliximab* are 90% and 75% humanized monoclonal antibodies to the CD25 portion of the IL-2 receptor. These agents are used for induction therapy and prevention of acute rejection. Administration has decreased the incidence of acute rejection with minimal side effects. Despite lacking a U.S. Food and Drug Administration (FDA) indication for transplantation, *alemtuzumab* is used for induction of immunosuppression in many centers, often with steroid avoidance and immunosuppression-reduction protocols. Alemtuzumab is associated with profound lymphopenia, susceptibility to infection, and autoimmune syndromes. Furthermore, a change in type and timing of rejection may be seen, including monocyte-induced and humoral rejections, with a delaying of rejections past the early posttransplant months.

6. **Drug interactions**

Although it is not possible to list all possible drug interactions, it is important for the clinician to be aware of general types of interactions when initiating new therapies or witnessing unexpected toxicities. In general, interactions can result from changes in absorption, metabolism, excretion, or through additive or synergistic toxicity with agents that have similar side effects. Agents that can decrease the absorption of immunosuppressive agents include antacids, cholestyramine, and food, whereas promotility agents can increase absorption. Metabolism of tacrolimus and cyclosporine occurs through cytochrome P-450-3A4; therefore, agents that affect this system can alter calcineurin inhibitor levels or altered metabolism of the interacting agent, leading to toxicity or inadequate levels. Examples of these agents include azole antifungals, calcium channel blockers, anticonvulsants, protease inhibitors, some antimicrobials, and grapefruit juice. Statin clearance may be decreased due to cytochrome P-450 interactions, resulting in myopathy and rhabdomyolysis. Antimicrobials and other agents should be dosed according to kidney function as in any patient, with added attention to agents which affect cyclosporine or tacrolimus metabolism. Drugs that cause synergistic or additive toxicities include allopurinol, trimethoprim/sulfamethoxazole, angiotensin-converting enzyme (ACE) inhibitors, or ganciclovir with azathioprine, all potentially causing myelosuppression. Also, nonsteroidal anti-inflammatory drugs (NSAIDs) and ACE inhibitors may have additive effects on glomerular hemodynamics with calcineurin inhibitors. Anticoagulation or antiplatelet therapies require more cautious monitoring due to frequent thrombocytopenia and multidrug therapy in many transplant recipients. Although this summary is not exhaustive, cautious attention to these possibilities can prevent morbidity from drug interactions.

IV. TRANSPLANTATION

A. Induction

With few exceptions, kidney transplant recipients will receive a brief course of high-dose steroids at the time of transplantation, followed by a taper to the initial maintenance dose. Either for perceived increased risk of rejection or by local protocol, antibody therapy may be given during induction. Increased risks of rejection may be seen in those with high PRA, previous transplants, and African-Americans. Available antibody-based therapies include antithymocyte globulin, IL-2 receptor antagonists, alemtuzumab, and muromonab/CD3 (OKT3) (see section IV.B.5).

B. Donor nephrectomy

Living donor kidneys can be recovered in either an open or laparoscopic approach, each with its own advantages and disadvantages. The left kidney is most often selected due to its longer renal vein and accessibility. Laparoscopic donation rates have increased due to technical advancement and donor preferences. In general, laparoscopic donation has advantages of a shorter hospital stay, quicker return to work, and less pain, but can come with higher costs, longer operative time, and a learning curve to decrease rates of morbidity to equal that of open nephrectomy. Deceased donor kidneys are removed together with a patch of aorta and inferior vena cava as part of a multiorgan recovery. The organs are then separated and stored in hypothermic preservation solution until implantation. Pulsatile perfusion may be used, especially in ECD or DCD kidneys.

C. Transplant surgery

The transplanted kidney is placed in either the right or left iliac fossa. The renal vein and artery are both connected through an end-to-side anastomosis, the donor vein usually being connected to the external iliac vein and the donor artery to the external iliac artery. The ureter is implanted into the bladder, and the bladder mucosa is pulled over the ureter to create a tunnel which prevents reflux and urine leak. A ureteral stent is often placed at the time of surgery to ensure patency and prevent urine leak. Lymphatics are ligated to prevent postoperative lymphocele formation. A Foley catheter is placed at the time of surgery and maintained for up to 5 days postoperatively. Kidney transplantation in the absence of donor ischemia or technical complications is usually accompanied by prompt urine formation.

V. POSTOPERATIVE MANAGEMENT

A. Immediate postoperative care

of the transplant recipient involves close monitoring of urine output, fluid administration, and vital signs. Many centers use algorithms, which replace the urine output with half normal saline or similar solution. Hourly central venous pressure (CVP) measurements are often done as part of routine monitoring, with target CVP of 7 to 10 mm per Hg. The brisk diuresis that can ensue in a transplant recipient can cause disturbances in potassium, magnesium, calcium, and phosphorus. The effect of elevated parathyroid hormone along with a suddenly functioning kidney also contributes to these abnormalities. Insulin requirements may increase in diabetic patients or those without prior diabetes due to the presence of steroids, calcineurin inhibitors, and improved clearance of insulin by the transplanted kidney. An uncomplicated patient with a functioning kidney can usually ambulate by postoperative day 1 or 2, and the diet can be advanced as tolerated. By postoperative day 5, the Foley catheter can be removed and the patient can be discharged if he or she is free of other complications.

B. Complications

can occur as a result of technical problems related to surgery, infections, disorders of kidney function, or other routine postoperative complications. Surgical complications include problems with each of the aspects of the transplant: the vascular anastomoses, urologic complications, lymphocele, and wound complications.

1. Urologic complications include urine leak, obstruction, and reflux. Routine stenting at many centers may be responsible for a decrease in the incidence of urologic complications. *Urine leak* can occur in approximately 2% of transplants. It is usually due to ureteral necrosis caused by interruption of blood supply but can be at the site of bladder implantation or the calyces. The clinical presentation is one of decreased urine output, pain, fever, abdominal tenderness,

swelling, and a perinephric fluid collection by ultrasonography. Fluid aspiration reveals a high creatinine that far exceeds the plasma creatinine. The diagnosis can be confirmed by nuclear scan or computed tomographic (CT) urography demonstrating extravasation into local tissues. Temporary Foley catheterization and ureteral stenting followed by surgical repair are the usual management. *Ureteric obstruction* is usually secondary to ureteral ischemia but can be due to multiple other factors. Imaging by ultrasonography, cystogram, or other studies usually leads to a diagnosis; the obstruction can be relieved by ureteral repair, stenting, or nephrostomy. *Vesicoureteral reflux* into the transplanted ureter is less common since the introduction of submucosal tunneling of the ureter through the bladder.

2. **Arterial or venous thrombosis** are uncommon but may occur as a result of pre-existing hypercoagulability or technical difficulty, and should be suspected when sudden deterioration develops in a previously functioning transplant. While venous thromboses can occasionally be reversed by surgery or thrombolysis, vascular thromboses most often lead to graft loss.

3. **Lymphocele** presents as an asymptomatic cystic fluid collection. It may, however, cause graft obstruction and reduced kidney function, pain, or lower extremity edema and deep vein thrombosis (DVT) due to compression of the ileofemoral vessels. Lymphoceles are distinguished from urine leaks as fluid aspiration yields a fluid creatinine equal to serum creatinine. The aspirated fluid should also be sent for cell count and Gram stain to rule out hematoma or abscess. Lymphoceles can be aspirated but may require surgical repair (marsupialization) if they are recurrent.

4. **Wound complications** may stem from the problems detailed earlier, or due to infection. Clinical suspicion is necessary, as immunosuppression masks both the symptoms and increases the risk of wound infections. Prompt drainage and antibiotic administration are central to treatment.

5. **Infections** in the first postoperative month are similar to those in other post-operative patients but occur more frequently in immunosuppressed patients. Lung, urine, and wound infections, and infections related to dialysis catheters are common culprits. Infections of fluid collections (lymphocele, urinoma, and hematoma) may also occur. Opportunistic and other infections are discussed in section VI.

C. Maintenance immunosuppression

1. Conventional therapy

Since 1995, the available options for maintenance immunosuppression have been expanded with the introduction of MMF, tacrolimus, cyclosporine microemulsion, and sirolimus. Standard therapy in the United States consists of a calcineurin inhibitor, an antiproliferative or TOR inhibitor, and corticosteroids. The calcineurin inhibitors, tacrolimus and cyclosporine, have similar efficacy in patient and graft survival, but with slightly different toxicity profiles. Tacrolimus has also lowered both the incidence and severity of acute rejection in head-to-head comparisons. One approach is to maintain target trough levels of cyclosporine that are highest (300 ng per mL) in the first month, with gradual tapering to 150 to 250 ng per mL by 6 months and 100 to 200 ng per mL after 12 months. Similarly, target tacrolimus levels are 10 to 12 ng per mL in the first month, 7 to 9 ng per mL for months 1 to 5, and 5 to 7 ng per mL after 6 months. Target levels may need to be lower in patients receiving sirolimus, and are often individualized based on age, PRA, matching, rejection history, and the presence of infection. MMF and sirolimus have largely supplanted azathioprine in clinical use, as both result in less acute rejection. The third agent used in combination regimens is corticosteroids; they are usually tapered rapidly to 20 mg daily by 1 to 2 weeks post transplant. They are then gradually tapered to 5 to 10 mg daily by month 6. The availability of multiple agents has allowed clinicians to choose a regimen that best fits a patient's profile of immunologic risk and perceived susceptibility to side effects. For example, patients with second transplants or poor matching who are at greater risk for rejection may be placed on tacrolimus. However, an obese patient with a family history of diabetes but with low immunologic risk may be placed on cyclosporine or chosen for a steroid withdrawal protocol in an attempt to reduce the risk of PTDM.

2. Alternative regimens

The toxicities of corticosteroids and calcineurin inhibitors have led to corticosteroid withdrawal or avoidance and calcineurin inhibitor withdrawal. Meta-analysis of late steroid withdrawal, however, has been associated with acute rejection and graft loss, particularly in African-Americans. In contrast, trials of early withdrawal or avoidance of steroids in low-risk patients have shown promise but lack long-term results. Although recent randomized trials utilizing induction and rapid discontinuation of steroids have demonstrated similar graft survival at 4 years, trends toward increased acute rejection and CAN mean that steroid withdrawal remains controversial. Calcineurin inhibitor withdrawal is another goal due to nephrotoxicity and other side effects. A meta-analysis of studies revealed that calcineurin inhibitor withdrawal was again associated with an increased risk of acute rejection, especially in African-Americans. However, more recent trials with sirolimus-based regimens have allowed for calcineurin inhibitor withdrawal in low- to moderate-risk patients and led to FDA approval for this indication. However, calcineurin inhibitor avoidance has largely been disappointing, with increased acute rejection and decreased tolerability.

VI. RENAL COMPLICATIONS

In addition to DGF, acute rejection, recurrent disease, and CAN, patients who have undergone kidney transplantation are susceptible to kidney failure from all the causes that affect the general population. In the initial 48 hours after transplantation, technical causes related to surgery or DGF are most common. After 48 hours, the approach to a patient with kidney dysfunction should rule out hypovolemia, medication toxicity, and urinary tract obstruction, and should attempt to uncover causes of acute tubular necrosis (ATN) such as hypotension, sepsis, or radiocontrast. Evaluation for acute rejection should take place if clear causes are not found.

A. Delayed Graft Function

DGF is commonly defined as the requirement for dialysis in the first 7 days after transplantation. It occurs in 20% to 25% of deceased donor transplants but is uncommon in living donor transplants. Although technical factors or other events that affect kidney function can cause DGF, it is most commonly a result of postischemic ATN, caused by donor hypovolemia or hypotension, or prolonged cold or warm ischemia during recovery and preservation. DGF adds to the cost and length of hospitalization and is associated with decreased short- and long-term graft survival. To determine the cause of graft dysfunction in the early postoperative period, a kidney ultrasonography should be performed to rule out technical causes, and the timing of kidney biopsy to rule out acute rejection should be guided by the patient's immunologic risk.

B. Acute rejection

Rejection refers to an immunologic response by the recipient to the transplanted organ. There are several types of acute rejection. *Hyperacute rejection* is rare and is caused by preformed antibodies against donor antigen, leading to immediate graft destruction after perfusion. *Accelerated acute rejection* usually occurs 2 to 3 days after transplant, and often is an antibody-mediated process that takes place in presensitized patients with prior transplants, transfusions, or pregnancies. *Acute cellular rejection* is a T-cell–mediated response that may occur at any time, but is most common from 5 to 7 days post transplant until 4 weeks after transplant, with a gradual lessening of risk in the first 6 months. Clinically, the spectrum of low-grade fever; a swollen, tender allograft; and oliguria are not seen commonly with modern immunosuppression. Therefore, frequent laboratory monitoring and a high incidence of suspicion are necessary to diagnose acute rejection. Acute rejection typically presents as a decrease in kidney function, as measured by the serum creatinine. However, rejection can occur without discernable changes in kidney function, a process referred to as *subclinical rejection.* Some centers perform routine "protocol biopsies" to evaluate for subclinical rejection and other graft abnormalities. Current regimens incorporating newer agents have lowered the incidence of acute rejection in the first year to 20% or lower, have improved 1-year deceased donor allograft survival to approximately 90%, and may be responsible for some of the improvement in long-term outcomes. The diagnosis of acute rejection requires an ultrasound-guided kidney biopsy, with application of the Banff criteria to grade the severity of rejection or disclose other pathology. Pathologic features are interstitial infiltration with lymphocytes, tubulitis, and endarteritis. Treatment of acute rejection is usually a 3- to 5-day course of high-dose intravenous steroids or a 5- to 10-day course of antithymocyte globulin in steroid-refractory or more severe rejection. Although most acute rejection can be reversed, its occurrence remains a powerful predictor of long-term graft survival. Patients who do not experience acute rejection may experience graft survival that is two to three times longer than those who experience rejection episodes. The term *acute humoral rejection* reflects increased understanding of the importance of anti-HLA antibodies in early rejections, and is also called *antibody-mediated rejection*. It is distinguished by peritubular capillary staining with the complement-split product C4d, detection of donor-specific antibodies, demonstration of tissue injury by biopsy, and kidney dysfunction. This process is often resistant to steroids and antibody therapies, and portends a worse prognosis than cellular rejection. It has been managed with plasmapheresis, intravenous immunoglobulin (IVIG), immunoadsorption, rituximab, and tacrolimus/MMF rescue, but optimal therapy is not established.

C. Recurrent disease

The diagnosis of recurrent disease is guided by the clinical scenario and knowledge of which diseases tend to recur in kidney transplants. In patients with glomerulonephritis, for example, recurrent disease is the third most common cause of graft loss, after CAN and death with a functioning allograft. Recurrent nephritis may present as proteinuria, nephrotic syndrome, microscopic hematuria, and loss of function. It can be differentiated from other causes (chronic allograft dysfunction, *de novo* glomerular disease) by kidney biopsy. In the patient who has undergone transplantation, the important variables are the frequency of recurrence and frequency of graft loss due to recurrence. For example, focal and segmental glomerulosclerosis (FSGS) and type I membranoproliferative glomerulonephritis (MPGN) recur in 20% to 60% of patients, and commonly may lead to graft loss. Alternatively, IgA nephropathy, type II MPGN, and type 1 diabetes recur in 50%, 50% to 100%, and up to 100% of recipients, but are uncommon causes of graft loss. Systemic lupus erythematosus (SLE) may also recur microscopically in kidney allografts but rarely is clinically important. Autosomal dominant polycystic kidney disease (ADPKD) does not recur in an allograft from a donor lacking the PKD mutation. Although recurrent disease caused only 3% of first graft losses in a recent European report, 48% of patients who lost one graft due to recurrence also lost a second graft.

D. Interstitial fibrosis and tubular atrophy (IFTA)/CAN

IFTA is a pathologic description of the most common findings in CAN, a non-specific syndrome that appears clinically as progressive kidney failure, proteinuria, and hypertension. The etiology for this disorder is unknown, but a combination of immunologic and nonimmunologic factors have been implicated, thereby explaining replacement of the term *chronic rejection*. Pathologically, glomerular and vascular changes occur in addition to IFTA. Despite advances in treatment of acute rejection and other areas of transplantation, up to 40% of grafts experience CAN, and it is the most common cause of graft loss after 1 year. The importance of immune mechanisms in the development of CAN is underscored by the reality that acute rejection episodes, anti-donor HLA antibodies, poor matching, and C4d staining all correlate with the incidence of CAN. However, there are important nonimmune risks that also correlate with the development of CAN. These include donor age, prolonged ischemia time, size mismatching, hypertension, hyperlipidemia, proteinuria, and smoking. Some of these risks implicate low nephron dose and hyperfiltration injury as a contributing factor. The allograft response to injury may cause the release of proinflammatory and profibrotic growth factors and cytokines, such as transforming growth factor β (TGF-β), platelet-derived growth factor (PDGF), and others, worsening the cascade of CAN. Premature senescence (aging) has also been implicated. Although calcineurin-inhibitor induced nephrotoxicity has similar effects on kidney function, there are conflicting results on their use and the risk of CAN. Treatment of CAN is not currently well defined; control of blood pressure and lipids are advocated, and ACE inhibition appears safe and helpful by retrospective analysis. Immunosuppressive strategies are not generally effective, but trials of novel regimens aimed at prevention of CAN are ongoing.

VII. MEDICAL CARE OF THE TRANSPLANTED PATIENT

The success of kidney transplantation and the growing population of transplant recipients are unfortunately accompanied by the complications from comorbid diseases and side effects of long-term immunosuppression. Patients often die with functioning grafts due to cardiovascular disease, infections, and malignancy, and these and other conditions contribute to a spectrum of common disorders in transplantation.

A. Infectious diseases

In the patient who has undergone transplantation, typical signs and symptoms of infection may be absent, and coinfections are common, necessitating increased scrutiny. Infections after kidney transplantation occur in patterns that are important to recognize. Immediately after transplant, patients are at risk for common postoperative infections: wound infections, pneumonia, line, and urinary infections. The first 6 months after transplant is marked by a risk of opportunistic infections due to more intense immunosuppression, especially after antibody induction. For this reason, patients usually receive prophylaxis against *pneumocystis carinii pneumonia* (PCP) for at least 6 months, and for CMV for 3 to 6 months if they are at risk (see next section). Some centers provide prophylaxis for fungal infections. After 6 months, the risk of opportunistic infections is lower but remains present, and patients remain at risk for more frequent and severe infections with community-acquired pathogens. Some common pathogens and principles specific to kidney transplantation will be reviewed.

1. Immunosuppression during infection

There are no clear guidelines for decreasing immunosuppression during infection. Furthermore, many infections carry an increased risk of acute rejection due to upregulation of immune surveillance and activity. In general, mild infections treated with appropriate antimicrobials can be managed without a change in immunosuppression. However, more severe infections may require decreasing or stopping antiproliferative medications (sirolimus, MMF, azathioprine) and reductions in calcineurin-inhibitor dosing. Severe or life-threatening infections should include attention to the requirement for stress doses of corticosteroids, which are often adequate to decrease the risk of rejection during an illness. Reduction of immunosuppression is best done with careful monitoring of graft function along with the consultation of transplant physicians.

2. Cytomegalovirus

CMV is a human herpes virus that is common in the general population but usually does not lead to serious morbidity without immunosuppression. A potential organ recipient who has not been exposed to CMV is at risk for a primary infection if transplanted with a CMV-positive organ, and a recipient who has been exposed before transplant is at risk for reactivation or superinfection, especially if receiving antibody induction. Therefore, the risk of CMV infection is tied to serologic status of the donor and recipient, with rates as high as 50% to 70% in donor-positive/recipient-negative patients not receiving prophylaxis, and 20% to 30% in patients who were exposed before transplant. CMV infection is uncommon in donor-negative/recipient-negative transplants. Therefore, donor-positive/recipient-negative patients and recipient-positive patients generally receive prophylaxis for CMV for 3 to 6 months, usually with valganciclovir. CMV infection leads to morbidity related directly to infection, but also increases the risk of acute rejection, graft loss, and death. Clinically, the disease often presents as low-grade fever, leukopenia and/or thrombocytopenia, and malaise. Tissue invasion can occur in 5% to 15% of infections, with syndromes of pneumonitis, hepatitis, esophagitis, and diarrhea being most common. Polymerase chain reaction (PCR)-based testing is the most sensitive diagnostic technique, but other options exist, including biopsy of affected tissues. Standard therapy is intravenous ganciclovir, a nucleoside analog, although ganciclovir resistance can develop.

3. **BK virus (BKV) nephropathy (polyomavirus)**
    Human BK virus (BKV) is a polyoma virus that is present as a latent infection in most of the population and has tropism for the genitourinary tract. During immunosuppression, the virus can reactivate. In patients who have undergone kidney transplantation, BKV most commonly causes a syndrome of decreased kidney function and interstitial nephritis, which appears clinically and pathologically similar to acute rejection. Because discovery at the time of nephropathy may be too late to prevent graft loss, current practices emphasize screening for BK viruria and viremia using PCR-based testing. "Decoy cells" may also be found in the urine. Immunohistochemical techniques and the presence of viral inclusions can be used to confirm the diagnosis through kidney biopsy. It is important to suspect BKV nephropathy when presumed acute rejection does not respond to steroids or occurs after 6 months, as increasing the intensity of immunosuppression may lead to graft loss. The mainstay of management is decreasing the intensity of immunosuppression, which may stabilize BKV-related kidney dysfunction but increase the risk of acute rejection. IVIG, cidofovir, and leflunomide have been used anecdotally with varying success in subjects with ongoing viremia or declining kidney function despite immunosuppression reduction.

4. **Hepatitis B and C**
    Although the incidence of hepatitis B in patients with ESRD has been declining due to immunization, isolation techniques, and screening of transfused blood, hepatitis C infections are relatively common, affecting up to 7% of recent U.S. deceased donor transplant recipients. There is no consensus on management or outcome of either disease in respect to kidney transplantation. For hepatitis B, patients with antigenemia usually receive evaluation and liver biopsy before transplant, as antiviral therapies may be more effective before transplantation. For hepatitis C, the effects on outcomes and management are somewhat controversial. Data suggest that hepatitis C infection increases the risk of graft loss, death, and PTDM. Although many patients have mild, indolent disease, there are reports of rapid progression to cirrhosis and liver failure after kidney transplantation. A complicating factor is that interferon therapy increases the risk of acute rejection. Most patients with hepatitis C should receive liver biopsy to exclude cirrhosis and should have consideration of interferon therapy before transplantation.

5. **Other infections**
    Urinary infections are common after kidney transplantation, and pyelonephritis of the transplanted kidney can lead to decreased kidney function. Pulmonary infections from both common and uncommon pathogens are the most common cause of tissue-invasive infection. Although the list of pathogens affecting patients is too long to mention, differential diagnosis should include fungal diseases such as *Cryptococcus, Candida,* and endemic fungi, mycobacterial disease, nocardia, *pneumocystis carinii,* viral pathogens, and others.

6. **Immunization**
    Potential transplant recipients should receive immunization against influenza, pneumococcus, hepatitis B, and varicella if they are seronegative. After transplant, many centers wait 6 months before any immunizations because of theoretic risks of stimulating the immune system and increasing the risk of rejection. Also, the vaccines may be less effective in this time period. The oral polio, typhoid, varicella, yellow fever, and Bacillus Calmette-Guérin (BCG) vaccines are live vaccines that are contraindicated after kidney transplant due to their ability to cause disease in immunocompromised hosts. However, the

live measles-mumps-rubella (MMR) vaccine can be given after 6 months if indicated. Vaccination for influenza, pneumococcus, hepatitis A and B, and tetanus/diphtheria should be given as indicated. The role of human papilloma virus (HPV) vaccine in transplant candidates requires elucidation.

B. Cardiovascular disease

Cardiovascular disease is the most common cause of death in patients with a functioning allograft. Ischemic coronary artery disease, congestive heart failure, and left ventricular hypertrophy are all more common in patients with kidney disease, and cerebrovascular disease is another important cause of morbidity and mortality. Therefore, efforts at improving outcomes after kidney transplantation have been appropriately shifted to focus on cardiovascular risks. Efforts at preventing cardiovascular events begin with pretransplant evaluation, risk stratification, and intervention when necessary. After transplantation, attention is given to modification of existing risk factors and careful evaluation and treatment of new symptoms or disease.

1. Hypertension

Since the introduction of calcineurin inhibitors, hypertension has been present in 70% to 90% of patients after kidney transplant. Hypertension not only represents a modifiable cardiovascular risk factor but also is correlated with graft loss. Clinicians should aim for a target blood pressure below 130/80 mm Hg as indicated by current recommendations for patients with chronic kidney disease. The choice of agents after kidney transplantation is controversial and complicated by interpretation of fluctuations in kidney function that occur with diuretics, ACE inhibitors, and angiotensin receptor blockers (ARBs). In general, β-blockers and dihydropyridine calcium channel blockers are used in the early posttransplant period due to their lack of drug interactions and effects on kidney function. Many patients require diuretics because of salt retention due to corticosteroids, calcineurin inhibitors, and other blood pressure medication. ACE inhibitors and ARBs are often avoided early after transplantation due to effects on renal hemodynamics and serum creatinine. However, these agents may be an important addition to attenuate hypertension and cardiovascular risk and are often given in patients with CAN.

2. Hyperlipidemia

Lipid abnormalities occur in at least 50% of transplant recipients and represent an important modifiable cardiovascular risk factor. Hypertriglyceridemia, high low-density lipoprotein (LDL), and low high-density lipoprotein (HDL) often occur as part of a metabolic syndrome which is common after transplantation. Corticosteroids, calcineurin inhibitors, and sirolimus may all play important roles in worsening lipid profiles. Despite concerns about rhabdomyolysis due to drug interactions, there is now prospective data from randomized controlled trials indicating that statins (specifically, fluvastatin) prevent cardiac death and nonfatal myocardial infarction after kidney transplantation without effects on graft survival. Other therapies such as niacin, fibrates, and binding resins have been used as well. As always, attention to drug interactions must be given, especially regarding the risk of rhabdomyolysis (statins, fibrates, and calcineurin inhibitors) and decreased or enhanced absorption (binding resins and ezetimibe).

3. Diabetes mellitus

a. Background

Diabetes is a major independent risk factor for cardiovascular disease, is present in 30% to 40% of patients before transplant, and develops after transplant in 2.5% to 35% of nondiabetic patients depending on pretransplant risk factors and the immunosuppressive regimen. Complications from diabetes have important effects on patient outcomes, leading to cardiovascular and infectious morbidity, renal allograft loss and decreased function, as well as decreased patient survival. In patients with diabetes preceding transplant, control may be worsened by corticosteroids, calcineurin inhibitors, and the decreased half-life of endogenous and exogenous insulin due to improved kidney function. Rigorous control of diabetes is likely to decrease diabetic complications, based on accumulated evidence in other populations. A target glycosylated hemoglobin target of 6.5 to 7.0 is likely to be associated with improved outcomes.

b. PostTransplant Diabetes Mellitus

PTDM, also called *new onset diabetes after transplantation*, complicates a substantial percentage of kidney transplants, and is associated with poorer patient outcomes. Risks for PTDM include increasing age, obesity, family history of diabetes, African-American or Hispanic race/ethnicity, hepatitis C infection, and abnormal glucose tolerance. Corticosteroids have well-known adverse effects on insulin resistance, and calcineurin inhibitors are diabetogenic, likely due to a combination of β-cell toxicity and promotion of insulin resistance. The definition of PTDM has varied in the past, but consensus has established that it should be defined similarly as the general population: a fasting glucose greater than 126 mg per dL, symptoms of diabetes with any glucose above 200 mg per dL, or a 2-hour oral glucose tolerance test value above 200 mg per dL. Fasting plasma glucose should be routinely monitored after transplant because the incidence of PTDM is high. Prevention of diabetes through weight loss and exercise in patients at risk should be attempted, and treatment of new-onset diabetes should follow established guidelines.

4. Other cardiovascular risk factors

Smoking is obviously an important modifiable cardiovascular risk factor, and evidence is accumulating that smoking also influences deterioration of kidney function and is a risk for graft loss. At any stage in the transplant process, counseling, formal smoking cessation programs, and pharmacologic agents should be offered to encourage smoking cessation. Anemia is present in many patients both before and after transplant, and may be under-recognized and undertreated. Anemia is correlated with left ventricular hypertrophy and cardiovascular disease; therefore, diagnosis and treatment based on cause is probably appropriate.

C. Malignancy

Malignancy is an important complication of immunosuppression, probably due to effects on immune surveillance of abnormal tumor cell populations and viral-mediated cancers. The intensity of immunosuppression, including exposure to antilymphocyte antibodies, are important factors determining risk for malignancy. Nonmelanoma skin cancers, especially squamous cell carcinomas, have a particularly high incidence and aggressiveness in transplant patients compared to the general population. HPV has been partially implicated in these cancers. Therefore, patients with transplants are counseled to avoid the sun, use protective sunscreens and clothing, and to see a dermatologist at least once yearly. After skin cancers, posttransplant lymphoproliferative disorders (PTLDs) are the next most common malignancy. These lymphomas are associated with Epstein-Barr virus (EBV) infection and usually contain EBV DNA. Risks are increased after T-cell depleting antibody therapies. These malignancies are often managed with reduction in immunosuppression, but aggressive tumors, particularly when monoclonal, may require systemic chemotherapy. Similarly, women are at increased risk of cervical squamous cell carcinomas related to HPV infection and require yearly Pap smears with increased frequency of surveillance and attention if there are any abnormalities. Vulvar, perineal, and anogenital cancers are also more frequent after transplantation. Hepatitis B and C may lead to hepatocellular carcinoma, and Kaposi's sarcoma, caused by human herpes virus 8, is another viral-mediated cancer that affects transplant recipients. Renal cell carcinoma occurs in 4% of transplant candidates, perhaps due to acquired cystic kidney disease. Screening native kidneys for disease has been advocated. Other solid tumors, such as breast, lung, and colon cancer show modest elevation in risk compared to the general population. Given the risks of malignancy in transplantation, age-appropriate screening should occur before placement on the waiting list, and should continue for the patient's lifetime.

D. Bone disease

1. Preexisting bone disease

The clinical picture after kidney transplantation is often complicated by the presence of preexisting bone disease. Most commonly, secondary hyperparathyroidism leads to osteitis fibrosa, imparting a risk of bone loss and fracture. Other causes of preexisting bone disease include adynamic (low turnover) bone disease, aluminum-related osteomalacia, and β_2-microglobulin–associated arthropathy. Furthermore, diabetic patients have decreased bone mineral density compared to other populations. Although aluminum and β_2-microglobulin–related bone disease are no longer common, many patients will undergo transplant with established bone loss and increased fracture risk.

2. Posttransplant bone disease

It is well established that up to 9% of bone density is lost in the first 6 to 12 months after transplantation. Furthermore, osteopenia and osteoporosis are present in a substantial number of patients who have undergone transplantation after long-term follow-up. Kidney transplant recipients carry an increased risk of fracture of 3% to 4% per year for the first 3 years after transplant, declining somewhat after that time. Fracture risk is increased in both males and females and is particularly increased in older females. There are many contributing factors to the milieu that supports bone loss. Steroids are known to induce osteopenia and osteoporosis through effects on calcium absorption and excretion, aggravation of secondary hyperparathyroidism, hypogonadism, and effects on bone turnover. Cyclosporine, secondary hyperparathyroidism, renal phosphate wasting, uremia, and gonadal hormones are other contributing factors to bone loss. Another syndrome affecting transplant recipients is avascular osteonecrosis, especially of the femoral head, which is associated with steroid use. Patients present with bone pain but may be asymptomatic. Often patients require operative intervention including replacement of the affected joint.

3. Management

The timing and frequency of measuring bone mineral density is not well defined, but should be performed at some established interval due to the risk of fractures. Control of secondary hyperparathyroidism before transplant is important. After transplant, calcium and vitamin D supplements are recommended unless hypercalcemia is present. Parathyroidectomy is usually reserved for patients with symptomatic or persistent hypercalcemia or with persistent (greater than 1 to 2 years) hyperparathyroidism. Cinacalcet has been used with some success in posttransplant hyperparathyroidism. Trials of biphosphonates have been shown to reduce bone loss especially when given immediately after transplant, but indications are not defined and concerns remain regarding promotion of adynamic bone disease. Weight-bearing exercise is a low-cost intervention that should be recommended for all patients.

E. Hematologic disease

Hematologic disorders are common after transplantation and have multifactorial origins. Anemia and posttransplant erythrocytosis are common and are covered in subsequent text. Leukopenia and thrombocytopenia are often seen as complications of antiproliferative medication, CMV or other viral infections, or any of a number of primary diseases.

1. Anemia

Anemia is common after kidney transplantation, occurring in 30% to 40% of patients in some series. Furthermore, it has been correlated with an increased risk of cardiovascular events and death and therefore may be an important prognostic factor. It is more common in the early posttransplant period but is also present in high frequency in patients with decreased kidney function. An obvious factor involved in the presence of anemia is decreased production of erythropoietin, especially when graft function is impaired. Iron deficiency, ACE inhibitors, ARBs, MMF, and azathioprine have also been associated with anemia after transplantation. Recurrent or *de novo* hemolytic uremic syndrome can be a dramatic cause of anemia and graft loss and may be associated with calcineurin inhibitors and other medications. Although prospective data are needed, it seems prudent to correct anemia depending on the underlying etiology, including administration of erythropoietin to those with chronic kidney disease stages III–V.

2. Posttransplant erythrocytosis (PTE)

PTE, a hematocrit above 51%, occurs in 5% to 15% of kidney transplant recipients. The etiology of the disorder is not clear, but erythropoietin- and nonerythropoietin-dependent mechanisms have been implicated. It is more common in smokers, those without acute rejection episodes, and patients with diabetes. This condition can usually be managed by treatment with ACE inhibitors s or ARBs. Occasionally, phlebotomy may be necessary if the hematocrit cannot be lowered below 56%.

F. Pregnancy

Years of experience in kidney transplantation have allowed some understanding of pregnancy after transplantation. Most women are counseled to avoid pregnancy for some time after the transplant, usually 6 months to 2 years. Fertility is improved after transplantation, and attention should be given to contraception. In mothers at high risk for primary CMV infection, pregnancy should probably be delayed until an antibody response has occurred and viremia has cleared. Kidney function, if normal at the time of conception, is probably not adversely affected during pregnancy. However, the risk of a pregnancy-related deterioration in kidney function is increased when renal insufficiency is present. Glucose intolerance may also complicate pregnancy, leading to gestational diabetes or increased insulin requirements in those with diabetes. Immunosuppression should be maintained at levels similar to nonpregnant women, but levels should be checked frequently as changes in pharmacokinetics are unpredictable. Prednisone is unlikely to be teratogenic, and calcineurin inhibitors and azathioprine have minimal to small risks. Animals and human studies indicate that MMF may be teratogenic, and sirolimus has limited experience in pregnancy. Fetal outcomes after kidney transplantation include a significant risk of preterm delivery (50%) and growth restriction (40%), but these outcomes may be more closely related to decreased kidney function than the transplant *per se*. After delivery, breast-feeding may not be recommended in patients taking calcineurin inhibitors, but discussion of the risks and benefits should occur on an individual basis.

Suggested Readings

Chan L, Gaston R, Hariharan S. Evolution of immunosuppression and continued importance of acute rejection in renal transplantation. *Am J Kidney Dis* 2001; 38(6 Suppl 6):S2–S9.

Hariharan S, Johnson CP, Bresnahan BA, et al. Improved graft survival after renal transplantation in the United States, 1988 to 1996. *N Engl J Med* 2000;342(9):605–612.

Kasiske BL, Chakkera HA, Louis TA, et al. A meta-analysis of immunosuppression withdrawal trials in renal transplantation. *J Am Soc Nephrol* 2000;11(10):1910–1917.

Meier-Kriesche HU, Schold JD, Srinivas TR, et al. Lack of improvement in renal allograft survival despite a marked decrease in acute rejection rates over the most recent era. *Am J Transplant* 2004;4(3):378–383.

Oberbauer R, Segoloni G, Campistol JM, et al. Early cyclosporine withdrawal from a sirolimus-based regimen results in better renal allograft survival and renal function at 48 months after transplantation. *Transpl Int* 2005;18(1):22–28.

Chan L, Wiseman A, Wang W, et al. Outcomes and complications of renal transplantation, Chapter 98. In: Schrier RW, ed. *Diseases of the kidney and urinary tract*, 8th ed, Vol. III. Lippincott Williams & Wilkins, 2006:2553–2611.

USRDS 2007 Annual Data Report. http://www.usrds.org/adr.htm. 2007.

Wolfe RA, Ashby VB, Milford EL, et al. Comparison of mortality in all patients on dialysis, patients on dialysis awaiting transplantation, and recipients of a first cadaveric transplant. *N Engl J Med* 1999;341(23):1725–1730.

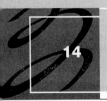

14

THE PATIENT WITH KIDNEY DISEASE AND HYPERTENSION IN PREGNANCY

Phyllis August

$\mathcal{I}$n most instances, pregnancy in women with renal disorders is successful, provided kidney function is well preserved and hypertension absent.

I. **THE KIDNEY FUNCTION AND BLOOD PRESSURE (BP) IN NORMAL PREGNANCY.** The anatomy and function of the kidneys and lower urinary tract are altered during gestation. Physiologic alterations in volume homeostasis and BP control also occur, and recognizing this is a prerequisite for the appropriate interpretation of data from pregnant patients with renal disease or hypertension (Table 14-1).

A. **Anatomic and functional changes in urinary tract.** Kidney length increases approximately 1 cm during normal gestation. The major anatomic alterations of the urinary tract during pregnancy, however, are seen in the collecting system, where calyces, renal pelves, and ureters dilatate often giving the erroneous impression of obstructive uropathy. The dilation is accompanied by hypertrophy of ureteral smooth muscle and hyperplasia of its connective tissue, but whether bladder reflux is more common in gravidas is unclear. The cause of the ureteral dilation is disputed. Some researchers favor hormonal mechanisms, whereas other researchers believe that it is obstructive in origin. Clearly, as pregnancy progresses, assumption of a supine or upright posture may cause ureteral obstruction when the enlarged uterus entraps the ureters at the pelvic brim (Fig. 14-1). These morphologic changes result in stasis in the urinary tract and a propensity of pregnant women with asymptomatic bacteriuria to develop pyelonephritis, especially in women with a history of prior urinary tract infection (UTI).

Acceptable norms of kidney size should be increased by 1 cm if estimated during pregnancy or the immediate puerperium, and reductions of renal length noted several months postpartum need not be attributed to renal disease. Rarely, ureteral dilation is of sufficient magnitude to cause a "distension" syndrome (characterized by abdominal pain, and on occasion small increments in serum creatinine levels presenting in late gestation; these resolve with the placement of ureteral stents). Also, because dilation of the ureters may persist until the 12th postpartum week, elective ultrasonographic or radiologic examination of the urinary tract should be deferred, if possible, until after this time.

B. **Renal hemodynamics.** The changes in renal hemodynamics in gestation are the most striking and clinically significant of all the urinary tract alterations of pregnancy.

1. **Glomerular filtration rate (GFR) and renal plasma flow (RPF)** increase to levels 30% and 50% above nongravid values during pregnancy. Increments in GFR that are already present during the early days after conception reach a maximum during the first trimester. The basis for the increase in GFR and RPF is unknown. Animal studies suggest that renal vasodilation [mediated by nitric oxide (NO)] leading to increased glomerular plasma flow is a contributing, but not the sole, factor. RPF is greatest at midgestation, declining somewhat in the third trimester. Although increments in GFR measured by the infusion of inulin appear to be sustained until term, 24-hour creatinine clearance declines during the last 4 weeks of pregnancy, accompanied by increases in serum creatinine levels of 15% to 20%.

The increase in GFR has important clinical implications. Because creatinine production is unchanged during pregnancy, increments in its clearance result

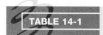

TABLE 14-1	Renal Changes in Normal Pregnancy	

Alteration	Manifestation	Clinical relevance
Increased renal size	Renal length approximately 1 cm greater on radiographs	Postpartum decreases in size should not be mistaken for parenchymal loss
Dilation of pelves, calyces, and ureters	Resembles hydronephrosis on renal ultrasonography or intravenous pyelography (more marked on right)	Not to be mistaken for obstructive uropathy; elective evaluation should be deferred to the 12th postpartum wk; upper urinary tract infections are more virulent; retained urine leads to collection errors
Increased renal vasodilation	Glomerular filtration rate and renal plasma flow increase 35%–50%	Serum creatinine and urea nitrogen values decrease during normal gestations; >0.8 mg/dL creatinine already suspect; protein, amino acid, and glucose urinary excretion all increase
Changes in acid–base metabolism	Renal bicarbonate threshold decreases	Serum bicarbonate is 4 to 5 μmol/L lower in normal gestation
Renal water handling	Osmoregulation altered	Serum osmolality decreases 10 mOsm/L (serum sodium decreases 5 mEq/L) during normal gestation
—	Osmotic thresholds for thirst and AVP decrease; the metabolic clearance of AVP increases markedly; high levels of vasopressinase circulating	Increased metabolism of AVP may cause transient diabetes insipidus in pregnancy

AVP, arginine vasopressin.

in decreased serum levels. Using the Hare method, one group of investigators observed that true serum creatinine, which averaged 0.67 mg per dL in nongravid women, decreased to 0.46 mg per dL during gestation [to convert to SI units (μmol per L), multiply serum creatinine (mg per dL) by 88.4]. In studies that also measured creatinine chromogen (which yielded results resembling those reported in most clinical laboratories), values were 0.83 mg per dL in nonpregnant women and decreased to 0.74, 0.58, and 0.53 mg per dL in the first, second, and third trimester of pregnancy, respectively. Therefore, values considered normal in nongravid women may reflect decreased renal function during pregnancy. For example, in gravid women, concentrations of serum creatinine exceeding 0.8 mg per dL or of serum urea nitrogen that are greater than 13 mg per dL suggest the need for additional evaluation of renal function.

2. **Other consequences of the increased renal hemodynamics.** Increased GFR and RPF also alter urinary solute content. For example, excretion of glucose, most amino acids, and several water-soluble vitamins increases, and these increments in the nutrient content of urine may be a factor in the enhanced

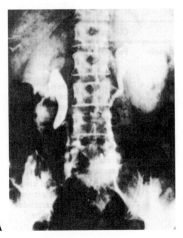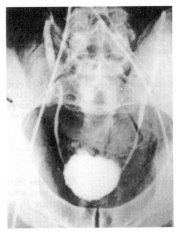

A   B

Figure 14-1. Intravenous pyelogram. **A:** Ureteral dilation of pregnancy. The right ureter is sharply cut off at the pelvic brim where it crosses the iliac artery (the iliac sign). **B:** Relationship between the ureters and iliac arteries can be demonstrated in postmortem studies. Note the iliac sign at the pelvic brim on the right. (From Dure-Smith P. Pregnancy dilation of the urinary tract. *Radiology* 1970;96:545. Reprinted with permission.)

susceptibility of gravidas to UTIs. Urinary protein excretion also increases during gestation, but the fate of albumin excretion is more complex and disputed.

C. Acid–base regulation in pregnancy. Renal acid–base regulation is altered during gestation. The bicarbonate threshold decreases, and early morning urines are often more alkaline than those in the nongravid state. In addition, plasma bicarbonate concentrations decrease approximately 4 μmol per L, averaging 22 μmol per L. This change most likely represents a compensatory renal response to hypocapnia, because pregnant women hyperventilate and their P_{CO_2} averages only 30 mm Hg. The mild alkalosis (arterial pH averages 7.44) found in pregnancy is in accord with this view. Because steady-state P_{CO_2} and HCO_3 levels are already diminished, pregnant women are, in theory, at a disadvantage when threatened by sudden metabolic acidosis [e.g., lactic acidosis in preeclampsia, diabetic ketoacidosis, or acute renal failure (ARF)]; however, they respond with appropriate increments in urinary titratable acid and ammonia after an acid load, and proton regeneration is already evident at blood pH levels higher than those in similarly tested nonpregnant women. Finally, when managing gravidas with pulmonary disorders, it should be noted that a P_{CO_2} of 40 mm Hg, normal in nonpregnant women, signifies considerable carbon dioxide retention in pregnancy.

D. Water excretion. After conception, a rapid decrease in plasma osmolality levels of 5 to 10 mOsm per kg below that of nongravid subjects occurs. If this decrease occurred in a nonpregnant woman, she would cease secreting antidiuretic hormone and enter a state of water diuresis; however, gravidas maintain this new osmolality, diluting and concentrating urine appropriately when the woman is subjected to water loading or dehydration. This suggests a resetting of the osmoreceptor system, and, indeed, clinical studies demonstrate that the osmotic thresholds for both thirst and arginine vasopressin (AVP) release are decreased in pregnant women. Furthermore, the plasma of pregnant women contains large quantities of a placental enzyme (vasopressinase) capable of destroying substantial quantities of AVP *in vitro*; moreover, the *in vivo* production and metabolic clearance of AVP hormone are increased fourfold after midgestation.

The changes in osmoregulation and AVP metabolism may be responsible for two unusual syndromes of transient diabetes insipidus that complicate pregnancy.

One, in which polyuria is responsive to both AVP and deamino-8-D-arginine vasopressin (dDAVP), probably occurs in women with unapparent partial central diabetes insipidus whose disease is brought to the fore by the increment in hormonal disposal rates during late gestation. The other disorder, in which the marked polyuria continues despite large doses of AVP, is responsive to dDAVP, an analog resistant to inactivation by vasopressinase. These gravidas may have excessively high circulating levels of this aminopeptidase enzyme due to increased activation.

E. **Volume regulation.** Most healthy women gain approximately 12.5 kg during the first pregnancy and 1 kg less during subsequent pregnancies. Most of the increment is fluid, with total body water increasing 6 to 8 L, 4 to 6 L of which is extracellular. Plasma volume increases 50% during gestation, the largest rate of increment occurring during midpregnancy, whereas increments in the interstitial space are greatest in the third trimester. A gradual cumulative retention of approximately 900 mEq of sodium occurs in pregnancy; this is distributed between the products of conception and the maternal extracellular space. These alterations in maternal intravascular and interstitial compartments produce apparent hypervolemia, yet the gravida's volume receptors sense these changes as normal. Therefore, when salt restriction or diuretic therapy limits this physiologic expansion, maternal responses resemble those in salt-depleted nonpregnant women. This is one compelling reason for the reluctance to recommend sodium restriction or diuretics during pregnancy. Pregnant women are now advised to salt their food to taste, and some researchers believe that a liberal sodium intake is beneficial during gestation. Another physiologic adaptation that appears to influence sodium balance during pregnancy is the marked stimulation of the renin-angiotensin-aldosterone system. Aldosterone levels are markedly increased during pregnancy, despite normal BP and normal potassium balance. It is likely that the increased aldosterone secretion is a compensatory mechanism to counteract the increase in sodium excretion that would be expected as a result of the large increase in GFR and RPF. Arterial vasodilation that causes relative arterial underfilling, as occurs in pregnancy, is known to stimulate the renin-angiotensin-aldosterone system. Moreover, increases in aldosterone balance the natriuretic effects of the large increases in progesterone during pregnancy.

F. **BP regulation.** Mean BP starts to decrease early in gestation, with diastolic levels in midpregnancy averaging 10 mm Hg less than measurements postpartum. In later pregnancy, BP increases, gradually approaching nonpregnancy values near term. Because cardiac output rises quickly in the first trimester and remains relatively constant thereafter, the decrease in pressure is due to a marked decrement in systemic vascular resistance. The slow rise toward nonpregnant levels after a midtrimester nadir is interesting, because it demonstrates that increasing vasoconstrictor tone is a feature of late gestation in healthy women as well as in women in whom preeclampsia is developing. The cause of the decrease in systemic vascular resistance during pregnancy is obscure. Studies of arterial compliance in pregnancy demonstrate early rises, perhaps due to alterations in vessel ground substance. Elevations of plasma estrogen and progesterone to concentrations that may relax smooth muscle occur, and increments in vasodilating prostaglandins and relaxin are also present during gestation. Hormonally mediated increases in endothelial NO production may also contribute to the vasodilation in pregnancy. Despite lower BP, the levels of all components of the renin-angiotensin system are increased during pregnancy. Exaggerated hypotensive responses to converting enzyme inhibition in normal gravidas suggest that the increased renin-angiotensin system in pregnancy is a normal physiologic response to decreased BP and increased sodium excretion.

Lack of awareness of the fluctuation in BP during normal gestation may lead to diagnostic errors. For example, women with mild essential hypertension often experience a decrease in BP during early pregnancy, and BP may even approach normal levels. They may be then erroneously labeled preeclamptic in the last trimester, when frankly elevated pressures occur.

G. **Mineral metabolism.** Serum calcium levels decrease in pregnancy, in conjunction with a decrement in circulating albumin concentrations. Ionized calcium levels, however, remain in the normal nonpregnant range. Striking changes relating to calcium regulatory hormones also occur during normal pregnancy. Production of 1,25, dihydroxyvitamin D_3 increases as early as the first trimester, reaching circulating levels that are approximately two times nonpregnant values. Gastrointestinal absorption of calcium increases, resulting in an "absorptive hypercalciuria," with 24-hour urine excretion often exceeding 300 mg per day (in appropriately nourished individuals). Intact parathyroid hormone levels are lower during normal pregnancy.

II. CLINICAL EVALUATION OF RENAL FUNCTION IN PREGNANCY

A. Examination of the urine. The association of proteinuria with eclampsia was first noted in the 1840s, and the science of prenatal care advanced dramatically when physicians began to systematically examine the urine of gravidas, primarily for albuminuria. In certain instances, latent renal disease is first uncovered by the detection of excessive protein excretion or microscopic hematuria during a routine prenatal evaluation.

Healthy nonpregnant women excrete considerably less than 100 mg of protein in the urine daily, but due to the relative imprecision and variability of testing methods used in hospital laboratories, proteinuria is not considered abnormal until it exceeds 150 mg per day. During pregnancy, protein excretion increases, and excretion up to 300 mg per day may still be normal. On occasion, a healthy gravida can excrete more than that amount. In pregnancy, the gold standard for evaluation of abnormal proteinuria is the 24-hour urine protein measurement. A 24-hour protein excretion of greater than 300 mg is abnormal in pregnancy and correlates with a urine dipstick 1+ protein measurement. Although commonly used to detect proteinuria, urine dipstick testing is susceptible to error due to variations in urine concentration; therefore, if the level of suspicion is high, 24-hour urine testing should be performed. Total protein/creatinine ratio has been shown to accurately estimate 24-hour urine protein excretion in nonpregnant patients. In pregnancy, however, the urine protein/creatinine ratio does not adequately exclude the equivalent of 0.3 g per 24-hour proteinuria and underestimates severe proteinuria.

Few attempts have been made to quantitate the urine sediment in pregnancy. The excretion of both red and white blood cells may increase during normal gestation, and one to two red blood cells per high-powered field is acceptable in a urinalysis.

B. Renal function tests. The clearance of endogenous creatinine, the most satisfactory approximation of GFR in nongravid subjects, is equally useful for assessing renal function in gravidas. Gravidas, as well as nonpregnant women, show little variation (approximately 10% per day) in urinary creatinine excretion and, presumably, in creatinine production, which in a given woman is similar both during and after gestation. The lower limit of normal creatinine clearance during gestation should be 30% greater than the average of 110 to 115 mL per minute for nongravid women. Calculation of GFR by serum creatinine–based formulae are confounded by increasing maternal weight which is not muscle weight, and neither Modification of Diet in Renal Disease (MDRD) nor Cockroft-Gault GFR estimates have been validated in pregnancy.

Acid excretion and urinary concentration and dilution are similar in gravid and nonpregnant women. Therefore, tests such as ammonium loading (rarely indicated in gestation) give values similar to those in nongravid women. When examining urinary diluting ability, the clinician should be aware that supine posture can interfere with this test. Therefore, studies to detect minimal urinary osmolal concentrations should be performed with the patient lying on her side. However, although lateral recumbency is the required position for prenatal measurement of most renal function parameters, this posture interferes with tests of concentration. For example, a urine osmolality that was 800 mOsm per kg after overnight dehydration may decrease to 400 mOsm per kg within 1 hour through fluid mobilization from the extremities during bed rest, thereby resulting in volume-induced inhibition of AVP secretion, a mild osmotic diuresis, or both. These observations demonstrate the importance of upright posture, such as quiet sitting, when maximum urinary concentration is measured in pregnancy.

C. **Role of renal biopsy in pregnancy.** Percutaneous renal biopsy is performed infrequently during gestation. In fact, pregnancy was once considered a relative contraindication to the procedure because of early reports of excessive bleeding and other complications in gravid women. It is now evident that if the renal biopsy is performed in women with well-controlled BP and normal coagulation indices, morbidity is similar to that of nonpregnant patients. Renal biopsy should be considered only when renal function suddenly deteriorates remote from term and no obvious cause is present. This is because certain forms of rapidly progressive glomerulonephritis, when diagnosed early, may respond to aggressive treatment such as steroid pulses and, perhaps, plasma exchange. Another situation in which biopsy may be recommended is symptomatic nephrotic syndrome. Although some might consider a therapeutic trial of steroids in such cases, it may be prudent to determine beforehand whether the lesion is likely to respond to steroids, because pregnancy is itself a hypercoagulable state prone to worsening by such treatment. Biopsy can usually be deferred when proteinuria alone develops in a normotensive woman with well-preserved renal function who has neither marked hypoalbuminemia nor intolerable edema. These women can usually be evaluated at more frequent intervals, and monitored for signs of either deterioration in renal function or development of superimposed preeclampsia, and renal biopsy deferred to the postpartum period. Similarly, there is rarely a need for renal biopsy during pregnancy in women with normal renal function and asymptomatic microscopic hematuria, when neither stone nor tumor is suggested by ultrasonography. Later in pregnancy (after 30 weeks) biopsy is rarely indicated and almost always should be deferred until after delivery.

III. RENAL DISEASE IN PREGNANCY

A. **Asymptomatic bacteriuria.** UTI is the most common renal problem occurring in pregnancy. The urine of gravidas supports bacterial growth better than that of nonpregnant women because of its increased nutrient content. This, as well as ureteral dilation, stasis, and occasional obstruction, would be expected to increase the susceptibility of pregnant women to UTI. Surprisingly, this is not the case, and, with the exception of certain high-risk groups (diabetic patients and gravidas with sickle cell trait), the prevalence of asymptomatic bacteriuria during gestation varies between 4% and 7%, a value similar to that in sexually active nonpregnant women. The natural history of asymptomatic UTIs is, however, quite different in pregnancy.

Although in the nonpregnant state asymptomatic bacteriuria is quite benign, progression to overt cystitis or pyelonephritis occurs in up to 40% of affected gravidas. Therefore, screening all pregnant women for the presence of asymptomatic bacteriuria and treating those with positive urine cultures are important.

1. **Method of urine collection.** Pregnant women contaminate midstream urine specimens more frequently. The incidence can be reduced by the use of multiple vulval washings combined with carefully supervised collection procedures. In some women, suprapubic aspiration is required to differentiate contamination from true infection. Pregnancy is not a contraindication to this procedure.

If the urine is sterile at the beginning of pregnancy, it usually remains so until term. Still, a small number (1% to 2%) of gravidas whose original urine cultures are negative subsequently have bacteriuria. Abnormal urinalysis and the presence of dysuria do not differentiate between contamination and true infection. For example, dysuria occurs in 30% of gravidas whose urines are sterile, and the urine may be infected and still contain fewer than two leukocytes per high-power field.

2. **Method of treatment.** The optimum way to manage asymptomatic UTI in pregnancy has not been precisely defined. In the earlier literature, some authors recommended continuous antibiotic treatment from the time the bacteriuria was detected until delivery. This was based on the belief that the relapse rate was high, and that most bacteriuric women have renal parenchymal involvement as opposed to bladder infection. However, it is now apparent that one-half of these infections involve only the bladder, and most of these patients are cured by standard short-course (or even single-dose) therapy. More than 90% of the uropathogens involved are aerobic gram-negative rods, usually *Escherichia coli*,

and the physicians recommend a 4- to 7-day course of the antibiotic to which the cultured organism is sensitive, preferably a short-acting sulfa drug, nitrofurantoin, amoxicillin, a cephalosporin, or a single dose of fosfomycin. This approach, when combined with surveillance for recurrent bacteriuria, has been shown to be quite effective.

3. **Importance of postpartum evaluation.** Asymptomatic UTI has been linked to premature labor, hypertension, and anemia during gestation, but these assertions have not been proved. On the other hand, an increased incidence of occult urinary tract pathology is present in these gravidas. Therefore, women with bacteriuria during pregnancy may benefit from evaluation of their urinary tract postpartum, especially those in whom the infection is resistant to therapy.

B. **Symptomatic bacteriuria.** The clinical approach to symptomatic UTI during gestation differs from that for asymptomatic bacteriuria.

1. **Acute pyelonephritis.** Pyelonephritis was a cause of maternal death in the preantibiotic era, and 3% of pregnant patients in a more recently reported series developed septic shock. At one time, symptomatic UTIs complicated almost 2% of all gestations, but prenatal screening combined with rapid treatment of asymptomatic bacteriuria has reduced this incidence to approximately 0.5%. The bacteriology of these infections resembles that in asymptomatic patients (predominantly *E. coli*), and most cases present after midpregnancy. The clinical presentation of pyelonephritis in pregnancy can be dramatic. As noted in the preceding text, the disease caused maternal deaths in the preantibiotic era, and upper UTIs in gravidas are associated with exaggerated effects of endotoxemia, including shock, respiratory distress syndrome, marked renal dysfunction, and hematologic and liver abnormalities. Symptomatic UTIs have also been implicated in the etiology of intrauterine growth restriction, prematurity, congenital anomalies, and fetal demise; however, most studies reporting these associations were not adequately controlled for potential confounders. The treatment of pyelonephritis should be aggressive and is best performed in the hospital.

Most patients with pyelonephritis respond quickly, with defervescence within 48 to 72 hours. Once afebrile for 48 hours, oral therapy may be started and continued to complete 10 to 14 days of treatment. Continuous low-dose suppressive therapy during the remainder of pregnancy is recommended because of the high rate of recurrence. An alternative approach, frequent surveillance for recurrent infection with prompt treatment when significant bacteriuria is identified, has been claimed to be as effective as suppressive therapy.

2. **Perirenal abscess and renal abscess formation or carbuncle,** although infrequent complications of gestation, should be considered in the differential diagnosis of postpartum fever. It is important to recognize that a high incidence of positive urine cultures occurs in the postpartum period—perhaps 17% to 20% in the first few days after delivery, decreasing to 4% after the third postpartum day. These cases, which resolve spontaneously, may reflect a temporary breakdown in the normal host antibacterial mechanisms in the immediate postpartum period rather than true infection.

3. **Antibiotic use in pregnancy.** The first-choice antibiotic for symptomatic infections changes from decade to decade because of the rapid emergence of resistant strains, thereby resulting in the use of drugs that have not yet withstood the test of time for safety in pregnancy. The physicians continue to recommend starting treatment with cephalosporins, because a significant percentage of community-acquired *E. coli* infections are resistant to ampicillin. For routine cystitis, nitrofurantoin is often effective and is acceptable during pregnancy.

The physician should also be aware of problems specific to the use of antibiotics in obstetrics and anticipate the potential fetal toxicity of agents that cross the placental barrier. (Information concerning drug safety during pregnancy is listed in the *Physicians' Desk Reference*, which is updated annually.) In brief, sulfa drugs should not be used near term, because they may precipitate kernicterus in the newborn. The anti–folic acid activity of trimethoprim has been associated with anomalies such as cleft palate in animals, and this combination drug should also be avoided, at least before midpregnancy.

Aminoglycosides such as gentamicin may be used in pregnancy. Fluoro-quinolones cross the placenta and should be avoided if possible. Tetracyclines are contraindicated because they deposit in fetal bones and teeth and may cause severe reactions in the mother, including hepatic failure. Nitrofurantoin is contraindicated at term because of risk of hemolytic disease in the newborn.

C. Acute renal failure

1. **Incidence.** Before 1970, the incidence of ARF in pregnancy severe enough to require dialytic therapy was estimated at between 1 in 2,000 and 1 in 5,000 gestations, and it represented a considerable proportion of cases reported in large series. Since then, the number of patients with ARF from obstetric causes has declined markedly, and the incidence is now estimated to be less than 1 in 20,000 pregnancies. This trend, attributed to the liberalization of abortion laws and improvement of prenatal care, has not been shared by the poorer and less industrialized nations, in which such patients comprise up to 25% of referrals to dialysis centers and in which renal failure in pregnancy continues to be an important cause of maternal and fetal mortality.

   The frequency distribution of ARF during gestation was bimodal, with one peak early in pregnancy (12 to 18 weeks) comprising most of the cases associated with septic abortion, and a second peak between gestational week 35 and the puerperium, primarily due to preeclampsia and bleeding complications, especially placental abruption.

2. **Causes.** ARF in pregnancy can be induced by any of the disorders leading to renal failure in the general population, such as acute tubular necrosis (ATN). Early in pregnancy, the most common problems are prerenal disease due to hyperemesis gravidarum, and ATN resulting from a septic abortion. Several different uncommon disorders can lead to ARF later in pregnancy. Mild to moderately severe preeclampsia is not usually associated with renal failure, because renal function is generally maintained in the normal or near-normal range for a nonpregnant woman. A variant of preeclampsia, the *H*emolysis, *E*levated *L*iver Enzymes, and *L*ow *P*latelet count (HELLP) syndrome (see section VI.B.) may be associated with significant renal dysfunction, especially if not treated promptly.

   a. **Thrombotic microangiopathy.** An important and difficult differential diagnosis is that of ARF in late pregnancy in association with microangiopathic hemolytic anemia and thrombocytopenia. Pregnancy is considered to be a risk factor for thrombotic thrombocytopenia purpura/hemolytic uremic syndrome (TTP/HUS). However, whether the pathogenesis of these disorders in pregnancy is similar to that in nonpregnant individuals is unclear. TTP/HUS is rare in pregnancy, and must be distinguished from the HELLP variant of preeclampsia, a much more common condition. The distinction of these syndromes is important for therapeutic and prognostic reasons, but considerable overlap exists in their clinical and laboratory features. Features that may be helpful in making the diagnosis include timing of onset and the pattern of laboratory abnormalities, which in TTP may include decreased levels of a von Willebrand cleaving protease. Preeclampsia typically develops in the third trimester, with only a few cases developing in the postpartum period, usually within a few days of delivery. TTP usually occurs antepartum, with many cases developing in the second trimester, as well as the third. HUS is usually a postpartum disease. Symptoms may begin antepartum, but most cases are diagnosed postpartum.

   Preeclampsia is much more common than TTP/HUS, and it is usually preceded by hypertension and proteinuria. Renal failure is unusual even with severe cases, unless significant bleeding or hemodynamic instability, or marked disseminated intravascular coagulation (DIC) occurs. In some cases, preeclampsia develops in the immediate postpartum period, and when thrombocytopenia is severe, it may be indistinguishable from

HUS. However, preeclampsia spontaneously recovers, whereas HUS only infrequently improves.

In contrast to TTP/HUS, preeclampsia may be associated with mild DIC and prolongation of prothrombin and partial thromboplastin time. Another laboratory feature of preeclampsia/HELLP syndrome that is not usually associated with TTP/HUS is marked elevations in liver enzymes. The presence of fever is more consistent with a diagnosis of TTP than preeclampsia or HUS. The main distinctive features of HUS are its tendency to occur in the postpartum period and the severity of the associated renal failure. Treatment of preeclampsia/HELLP syndrome is delivery and supportive care. More aggressive treatment is rarely indicated. Treatment of TTP/HUS includes plasma infusion or exchange and other modalities used in nonpregnant patients with these disorders, although clinical trials of these modalities in pregnancy have not been performed.

b. Bilateral **renal cortical necrosis is extremely rare and** may be induced by abruptio placenta or other clinical events complicated by severe obstetric hemorrhage (e.g., uterine rupture). Both primary DIC and severe renal ischemia have been proposed as the initiating events. Affected patients typically present with oliguria or anuria, hematuria, and flank pain. Ultrasonography or computed tomographic (CT) scanning may demonstrate hypoechoic or hypodense areas in the renal cortex. Most patients require dialysis, but 20% to 40% have partial recovery of renal function.

c. Acute pyelonephritis. Some pregnant women may develop ARF in association with pyelonephritis.

d. Acute fatty liver of pregnancy (fatty infiltration of hepatocytes without inflammation or necrosis) is a rare complication of pregnancy that is associated with significant azotemia. Women with this disorder often complain of anorexia and occasionally of abdominal pain in the third trimester. Clinical features suggesting preeclampsia, including hypertension and proteinuria, are not uncommon. Laboratory test results reveal elevations in liver enzymes, hypoglycemia, hypofibrinogenemia, and prolonged partial thromboplastin time. Delivery is indicated, and most patients improve shortly afterwards.

e. Urinary tract obstruction. Pregnancy is associated with dilation of the collecting system, which is not usually associated with renal dysfunction. Rarely, complications such as large uterine fibroids, which may enlarge in the setting of pregnancy, can lead to obstructive uropathy. Uncommonly, acute urinary tract obstruction in pregnancy is induced by a kidney stone. Diagnosis can usually be made by ultrasonography. Often the stones pass spontaneously, but occasionally cystoscopy is necessary for insertion of a stent to remove a fragment of stone and relieve obstruction, particularly if there is sepsis or a solitary kidney.

3. The **management** of ARF occurring in gestation or immediately postpartum is similar to that in nongravid subjects (see Chapter 11), but several points peculiar to pregnancy deserve emphasis. Because uterine hemorrhage near term may be concealed and blood loss underestimated, any overt blood loss should be replaced early. Gravidas should be slightly overtransfused to forestall the development of acute tubular or cortical necrosis. Both peritoneal dialysis and hemodialysis have been successfully used in patients with obstetric-related ARF. Neither pelvic peritonitis nor the enlarged uterus is a contraindication to the former method. In fact, this form of treatment is more gradual than hemodialysis and therefore less likely to precipitate labor. Because urea, creatinine, and other metabolites that accumulate in uremia traverse the placenta, dialysis should be undertaken early, with the aim of maintaining the blood urea nitrogen at approximately 50 mg per dL. In essence, the advantages of early dialysis in nongravid patients are even more important for the pregnant patient, making arguments for prophylactic dialysis quite compelling. Excessive fluid removal should be avoided, because it may contribute to hemodynamic compromise, reduction of uteroplacental perfusion, and premature labor. Some obstetricians and perinatologists recommend continuous fetal monitoring during hemodialysis treatments, starting at midpregnancy. Finally, the physician should be aware of potential dehydration in the neonate, because the newborn usually undergoes a brisk urea-induced diuresis.

D. Pregnancy in women with preexisting renal disease. The current approach to management of pregnancy in women with chronic kidney disease (CKD) is primarily based on retrospective studies. Nevertheless, several generalizations can be made and some guidelines presented regarding gestation in women with chronic kidney dysfunction (Table 14-2).

1. Prognosis. Counseling and managing women with CKD is based on the following general approach: Fertility and ability to sustain an uncomplicated pregnancy relate to the degree of functional impairment, and whether hypertension is present, and not to the underlying disorder.

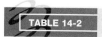

TABLE 14-2	**Summary of Pregnancy in Women with Preexisting Renal Disease[a]**

Disease	Comments
Chronic glomerulonephritis and focal and segmental glomerular sclerosis (FSGS)	Increased incidence of high blood pressure, usually later in gestation, but usually no adverse effect results if renal function is preserved and hypertension is absent before gestation; some cases of exacerbation in pregnancy have been reported in women with immunoglobulin A nephropathy, membranoproliferative glomerulonephritis, and FSGS
Systemic lupus erythematosus (SLE)	Controversial: prognosis is most favorable if disease is in remission 6 mo or more before conception
Vasculitis	Case reports of Wegener's GN suggest acceptable outcomes if disease is in remission and renal function is normal; scleroderma and polyarteritis may be associated with severe and accelerated hypertension during pregnancy
Diabetic nephropathy	No adverse effect on the renal lesion. Increased frequency of infections; high incidence of heavy proteinuria and hypertension near term; optimal time for pregnancy is when renal function is normal, hypertension absent, and albuminuria is <300 mg/d
Vesicoureteral reflux	Bacteriuria in pregnancy may lead to exacerbation; urinary infection is common
Polycystic kidney disease	Few problems when function is preserved and hypertension is absent; however, the incidence of preeclampsia is increased
Urolithiasis	Ureteral dilation and stasis do not seem to affect natural history, but infections can be more frequent; stents have been successfully placed during gestation
Previous urologic surgery	Urinary tract infection is common with urinary diversion, and renal function may undergo reversible decrease; cesarean section might be necessary to avoid disruption of the continence mechanism if artificial sphincters or neourethras have been constructed
After nephrectomy, solitary pelvic kidneys	Pregnancy is well tolerated; might be associated with other malformations of the urogenital tract; dystocia occurs rarely with a pelvic kidney

GN, glomerulonephritis.
[a]Generalizations are for women with only mild renal dysfunction (serum creatinine level less than 1.5 mg per dL) and without hypertension at conception.

| TABLE 14-3 | **Pregnancy and Renal Disease: Functional Renal Status and Prospects**[a] | | |

| | Category | | |
	Mild	**Moderate**	**Severe**
Prospects	Cr <1.5 mg/dL	Cr 1.5–3.0 mg/dL	Cr >3.0 mg/dL
Pregnancy complications	25%	47%	86%
Successful obstetric outcome	96% (85%)	90% (59%)	47% (8%)
Long-term sequelae	<3% (9%)	25% (71%)	53% (92%)

Cr, creatinine.
[a]Estimates are based on 1,862 women with 2,799 pregnancies (1973 to 1992) and do not include collagen diseases. Numbers in parentheses refer to prospects when complication(s) develop before 28 weeks' gestation.
(From Davison JM, Lindheimer MD. Renal disorders. In: Creasy RK, Resnick RK, eds. *Maternal–fetal medicine,* 3rd ed. Philadelphia: WB Saunders, 1994. Reprinted with permission.)

a. **Degree of impairment.** Patients are arbitrarily considered in three categories: preserved or mildly impaired renal function (serum creatinine less than or at 1.5 mg per dL), moderate renal insufficiency (creatinine 1.5 to 3.0 mg per dL), and severe renal insufficiency (creatinine higher than or equal to 3 mg per dL).

   In Table 14-3 the maternal and fetal prognosis in each category are summarized. Pregnancy is hazardous in the presence of moderate or severe renal dysfunction, because up to 40% of pregnancies in the former category are complicated by either difficult to control hypertension or sudden declines in GFR, which may not reverse after delivery. An even higher incidence of serious maternal problems occurs when renal insufficiency is severe. This is especially true for women receiving dialytic therapy, in whom fewer than 50% of the gestations succeed, and problems of extreme prematurity plague many of those that do. Notably, although prognosis is based primarily on the degree of functional impairment, the underlying disease may also play a role. Therefore, all authorities recommend against pregnancy in women with scleroderma and periarteritis nodosa.

b. **Level of BP.** The BP level at the time of gestation is an important prognostic index. In the absence of hypertension, the natural history of most established renal parenchymal disease is unaffected by gestation (although preeclampsia may occur more readily). In contrast, when renal disease and hypertension coexist, the gestation is more likely to be complicated, either by severe increments in BP or by additional reductions in renal function. Women with well-controlled BP and only mild renal dysfunction may have relatively uncomplicated pregnancies; however, they must be seen frequently and should understand that their gestation may be terminated early if renal function deteriorates or if their BP becomes difficult to control.

E. **Proteinuria.** Urinary protein excretion, which increases in normal pregnancy, may increase markedly in pregnant women with underlying parenchymal renal disease. In one large series, one-third of the patients with preexisting renal disease developed nephrotic-range proteinuria during gestation. These increments do not necessarily reflect worsening of the underlying kidney disease.

   1. **Renal hemodynamics.** Gravidas with kidney disorders who have only minimal renal dysfunction usually experience increments in GFR during gestation, although levels do not reach those seen in healthy pregnant women. Therefore, a decrement in serum creatinine level early in pregnancy is a good prognostic sign. If serum creatinine levels before conception exceed 1.5 mg per dL, decrements during gestation are less common, and, as noted, the prognosis of such pregnancies is more guarded.

F. Glomerulonephritis. Glomerulonephritides in women of childbearing age include immunoglobulin (Ig) A nephropathy, focal and segmental glomerulosclerosis, membranoproliferative glomerulonephritis, minimal change nephritis, and membranous nephropathy. Data that support the notion that histologic subtype confers a specific prognosis for pregnancy are absent. Rather, when kidney function is normal and hypertension absent, prognosis is good. Absence of gravidas in large epidemiologic surveys of poststreptococcal glomerulonephritis is remarkable and has led to speculations that pregnancy protects women from this disease. However, this form of immune complex nephritis does occur rarely in gestation, in which it may mimic preeclampsia. Its prognosis is favorable, because in those instances in which the occurrence of acute poststreptococcal glomerulonephritis during gestation was properly documented, renal function recovered rapidly and the pregnancy usually had a successful outcome.

G. Collagen vascular disease

    1. Lupus nephritis. The effect of gestation in women with lupus erythematosus who have renal involvement is difficult to evaluate, in part because of the unpredictable course of the disease regardless of pregnancy. Activity of the disease in the 6 months before conception is often a useful prognostic guide (the longer the remission the better the outlook). Although most pregnancies, in the presence of preserved function, proceed uneventfully or are accompanied by only transient functional declines, in approximately 10%, gestation appears to cause permanent renal damage and to accelerate the renal disease. Also, placental transmission of maternal autoantibodies is associated with an increased frequency of spontaneous abortion in these women, and certain anticytoplasmic antibodies [especially anti-Sjögren's syndrome antigen (ASS-A/Ro)] cause a neonatal lupus syndrome characterized by congenital heart block, transient cutaneous lesions, or both. Women with systemic lupus erythematosus (SLE) have a high incidence of detectable levels of antiphospholipid antibodies (anticardiolipin antibodies and lupus anticoagulant). High titers of these antibodies are associated with several complications of pregnancy, including spontaneous fetal loss, hypertensive syndromes indistinguishable from preeclampsia, and thrombotic events including deep vein thrombosis, pulmonary embolus, myocardial infarction, and strokes. Also, pregnant women with circulating antiphospholipid antibodies can manifest a rare form of rapid renal failure postpartum, associated with glomerular thrombi. Therefore, women with SLE should be screened for antiphospholipid antibodies early in gestation. The therapeutic approach when gravidas manifest antiphospholipid antibodies is disputed, and many would not treat asymptomatic patients who manifest low titers. However, when titers are elevated (more than 40 GPL IgG antiphospholipid level), most authorities prescribe aspirin (80 to 325 mg per day). Heparin in combination with aspirin is recommended for patients with a history of thrombotic events and may also be advisable when titers are higher than 80 GPL.

        A flare of lupus nephritis may be difficult to distinguish from preeclampsia when a woman with a history of lupus develops worsening renal function, proteinuria, and hypertension. Elevation in liver enzymes and new-onset severe hypertension is more consistent with preeclampsia. Hypocomplementemia, and severe nephritic syndrome without hypertension, is more consistent with lupus nephritis. Often, a flare of nephritis in the third trimester appears to trigger "superimposed preeclampsia," and improvement in BP and proteinuria occurs only after delivery. However, in the presence of abnormal serologic testing, it is often reasonable to treat worsening proteinuria and azotemia with increased prednisone in the hope that it will improve, particularly if the fetus is immature. However, close maternal and fetal surveillance is of utmost importance, and delivery should be considered in the setting of obvious signs of HELLP syndrome, accelerating hypertension and/or azotemia, and other signs of worsening maternal condition.

        Previously, patients with lupus nephropathy were believed to be prone to relapse in the immediate puerperium, and some physicians still start or increase steroid treatment during and after delivery. Such views of "stormy puerperium" are now disputed, and most authorities institute or change therapy only if signs of increased or *de novo* disease activity appear.

2. Pregnancy in patients with other **vasculitides** has only rarely been reported. Several successful pregnancies in women with Wegener's granulomatosis have been reported. Women may be treated with corticosteroids, azathiaprine, cyclosporine, and intravenous immunoglobin (IVIg) with safety. Cyclophosphamide is contraindicated in pregnancy. Such pregnancies are high risk and should be managed by a multidisciplinary team, and when possible women should be advised to wait until their disease is in remission before contemplating pregnancy. Polyarteritis nodosa **and scleroderma with renal involvement** are rare and potentially dangerous conditions in pregnancy because of the associated hypertension, which may become malignant.

H. **Diabetic nephropathy.** Diabetes is one of the most common medical disorders encountered during pregnancy, and most cases are due to gestational diabetes. Preexisting diabetes poses significant risks to pregnancy. Many younger women with pregestational diabetes have type 1 diabetes, and if their disease has been present for 10 to 15 years, they may show early signs of diabetic nephropathy. Women with microalbuminuria rather than macroalbuminuria, well-preserved kidney function, and normal BP have a good prognosis for pregnancy, although they are at increased risk for transient, pregnancy-associated increases in proteinuria, preeclampsia, and urinary infection. Women with type 1 diabetes with microalbuminuria and normal kidney function and normotension should be encouraged *not* to postpone pregnancy because of the worse prognosis once overt nephropathy develops. Published studies of pregnancy and nephropathy associated with type 2 diabetes are lacking. However, given the increasing prevalence of this condition, it is an important area for future study.

The effects of gestation in diabetic patients with overt nephropathy are similar to those in women with other forms of renal parenchymal disease. Prognosis is determined by the degree of hypertension and renal functional impairment.

I. **Nephrotic-range proteinuria during pregnancy.** The most common cause of nephrotic-range proteinuria (more than 3.5 g per day) in late pregnancy is preeclampsia, a diagnosis that may be missed when diastolic pressures are between 85 and 95 mm Hg. The fetal prognosis in preeclampsia with heavy proteinuria is poorer than in other preeclamptic states, but maternal prognosis is similar. Most of the usual causes of nephrotic syndrome, including membranous nephropathy, proliferative or membranoproliferative glomerulonephritis, minimal change disease, diabetic nephropathy, amyloidosis, and focal segmental glomerulosclerosis have been described in gravidas. The pros and cons of renal biopsy during pregnancy have already been mentioned.

One should not confuse physiologic changes during gestation with the exacerbation of a disease causing the nephrotic syndrome; many women with a variety of non-nephrotic renal disorders develop heavy proteinuria when pregnant. Such increments in urinary protein may relate to the increased renal hemodynamics, alterations in the glomerular barrier, and possibly a rise in renal vein pressure. Other alterations in pregnancy that simulate symptoms accompanying nephrotic syndrome include decrements in serum albumin (approximately 0.5 to 1.0 g per dL), increments in the levels of cholesterol and other circulating lipids, and edema, which can occur at one time or another in up to 80% of normal gestations.

Diuretic therapy for treatment of edema should be used with caution during pregnancy, particularly when BP is not elevated. The concern is that intravascular volume depletion might impair uteroplacental perfusion. Exceptions to this, however, are women with hypertension, in whom diuretics may be necessary to control BP.

Prognosis in most nephrotic gravidas with preserved function is good; however, there is some evidence to suggest that fetal outcome may be worse in the setting of significant and sustained maternal proteinuria. Focal segmental glomerulosclerosis, a frequent cause of nephrotic syndrome in women of childbearing age, is a disease the natural history of which during gestation remains disputed. Some claim pregnancy leads to irreversible functional loss and hypertension-sustained postpartum; others find the natural history of this entity in pregnancy similar to that of most other disorders.

J. Tubulointerstitial disease

1. **Vesicoureteral reflux (VUR).** Reflux nephropathy due to VUR may cause CKD in young women. A prospective study of 54 pregnancies in 46 women with reflux nephropathy found that preeclampsia occurred in 24% and was more common in women with hypertension. Nine (18%) experienced deterioration in kidney function during pregnancy, and those with preexisting reduced kidney function were at greater risk. One-third of the infants were delivered preterm, and 43% had VUR. These high-risk women should be screened with urine cultures, and should be treated promptly when infections are present with consideration to suppressive antibiotic therapy for the duration of pregnancy in some cases.

2. **Adult dominant polycystic kidney disease** may remain undetected in gestation. Careful questioning of gravidas for a family history of renal problems and ultrasonography may lead to its earlier detection. Patients with minimal functional impairment have few complications, but are at increased risk for preeclampsia. They are also prone to UTIs, and it may therefore be prudent to culture their urines more frequently. Hypertension usually accompanies or antedates the onset of functional deterioration, and pregnancy in such gravidas is more hazardous.

Some women with autosomal dominant polycystic kidney disease have cysts in their livers that may enlarge with repeated pregnancy as well as with oral contraceptive use. A high incidence of cerebral aneurysms also occurs in certain affected families. When aware of such family clustering, usually identified by a history of subarachnoid hemorrhages among relatives, the patient should undergo screening using magnetic resonance angiography (MRA). If an aneurysm is detected, neurosurgical consultation should be obtained, and the obstetrician may wish to avoid natural labor. All these patients should undergo genetic counseling before pregnancy to ensure they are aware that 50% of their offspring are at risk. Finally, predicting the fetal outcome using molecular probes on cells cultured from the amniotic fluid is possible.

3. **Solitary kidneys.** Women with solitary kidneys appear to tolerate gestation well. However, if the nephrectomy was performed for nephrolithiasis or chronic pyelonephritis, the remaining kidney may be infected. Patients with these conditions must be carefully scrutinized by frequent examination and culture of the urine throughout pregnancy and in the puerperium.

K. Pelvic kidneys may be associated with other malformations of the urogenital tract of the mother. In addition, dystocia may occur when the kidney is in the true pelvis.

L. Urolithiasis and hematuria. The prevalence of urolithiasis in gestation varies between 0.03% and 0.35% in the Western hemisphere. Many of the stones contain calcium, and some are infective in origin. A survey of 148 gestations in 78 nonselected stone formers suggest that pregnancy has little influence on the course of stone disease (although women with renal calculi may have an increased incidence of spontaneous abortions). It should be noted that most of the reported series focus on women whose calculi are mainly of the noninfective variety, and little is known of the natural history of the more serious infected struvite stones during gestation. In any event, UTI in the presence of nephrolithiasis requires prompt and prolonged treatment (3 to 5 weeks), followed by suppressive therapy through the immediate puerperium, because the calculus may represent a nidus of infection resistant to sterilization.

Experience with cystinuria in pregnancy is limited, but most women with this disease also do well in gestation. D-Penicillamine as used in these patients appears to have no apparent adverse effects on mother or fetus.

Renal calculi are among the most common causes of abdominal pain (of nonobstetric origin) requiring hospitalization during gestation, and, when complications suggest the need for surgical intervention, pregnancy should not be a deterrent to x-ray examination. If the stone obstructs the ureter, intervention with ureteral stenting, percutaneous nephrostomy, or rarely, surgery, is indicated. Spontaneous gross or microscopic hematuria occasionally complicates an otherwise uneventful gestation. The differential diagnosis includes all causes of hematuria in nongravid patients (see Chapter 8), but frequently no etiology is demonstrable, and the bleeding subsides postpartum. It has been suggested that these events are due to the rupture of small veins around the dilated renal pelvis. Hematuria may or may not occur in subsequent gestations. In any event, investigation of the hematuria can often be deferred until after delivery, and noninvasive techniques such as ultrasonography and magnetic resonance imaging are helpful in arriving at such decisions.

IV. RENAL TRANSPLANTATION

A. Menstruation and fertility resumes in most women from 1 to 12 months after kidney transplant. Pregnancy is not uncommon following kidney transplantation and the risk to mother and baby is much lower in this population than in pregnant patients on dialysis. Although pregnancy has become common after transplantation, there is little other than case reports, series, and voluntary databases to guide practice; a Consensus Conference generated a report in 2005 summarizing the literature and generated practice guidelines as well as identified gaps in knowledge. Most pregnancies (greater than 90%) that proceed beyond the first trimester succeed. However, there are maternal and fetal complications due to immunosuppressant effects, preexisting hypertension, and kidney dysfunction. These include maternal complications of glucocorticsteroid therapy such as impaired glucose tolerance, hypertension (47% to 73%), preeclampsia (30%), and increased infection. Fetal complications include a higher incidence of preterm delivery and intrauterine growth restriction with lower birth weight. Best practice guidelines have outlined criteria for considering pregnancy in kidney transplant recipients and it is suggested that those contemplating pregnancy should meet the following:

- Good health and stable kidney function for 1 to 2 years after transplantation with no recent acute or ongoing rejection or infections
- Absent or minimal proteinuria (less than 0.5 g per day)
- Normal BP or easily managed hypertension
- No evidence of pelvicalyceal distention on ultrasonography before conception
- Serum creatinine less than 1.5 mg per dL
- Drug therapy: prednisone 15 mg daily or less, azathioprine 2 mg per kg or less, cyclosporine less than 5 mg per kg per day.

Although cyclosporine levels tend to decrease during pregnancy, there is no information regarding whether or not drug dosage should be increased. Tacrolimus has not been used as widely in pregnancy as cyclosporine, although growing experience suggests that it is safe, with a similar side effect profile to cyclosporine. Considerations regarding hypertension and growth restriction are important; there is no established BP target, although 140/90 mm Hg is suggested and antihypertensives should be switched to those safe in pregnancy. Mycophenolate mofetil has been reported to be embryotoxic in animals and is associated with ear and other deformities in humans. This drug should be discontinued before conception, and women should be switched to azathioprine if indicated. Sirolimus causes delayed ossification in animal studies, and although successful liveborn human outcomes have been reported, its use is contraindicated in humans until more data are available. Finally, data from the National Transplantation Pregnancy Registry and the European Dialysis and Transplant Association suggest that in women with stable, near-normal kidney function, pregnancy rarely negatively affects the graft, although there may be minor increases in serum creatinine postpartum compared with prepregnancy creatinine. On the other hand, women with significantly reduced transplant function antepartum are at risk for irreversible deterioration after delivery, as observed with CKD in native kidneys. Rejection is difficult to diagnose in pregnancy and kidney biopsy may be required; the consensus opinion is that corticosteroids and IVIg are safe treatments for acute rejection, but the safety of antilymphocyte globulins and rituximab in pregnancy is unknown.

V. DIALYSIS. Fertility is reduced in patients undergoing dialysis, due to abnormalities of pituitary luteinizing hormone (LH) release leading to anovulation. Pregnancy that does occur in patients undergoing maintenance dialysis is extremely high risk, and conception should be strongly discouraged due to very high fetal mortality; in large surveys only 42% to 60% of such pregnancies result in a live-born infant. Prematurity, very low birthweight, and intrauterine growth restriction are common, and approximately 85% of infants born to women who conceive after starting dialysis are born before 36 weeks' gestation. The single most important factor influencing fetal outcome in patients on dialysis is the maternal plasma urea level. In patients undergoing hemodialysis, both the number of dialysis sessions per week as well as the time per session must be increased to a minimum of 20 hours per week, aiming for a predialysis urea of 30 to 50 mg per dL (5 to 8 mmol per L). Heparinization should be minimized to prevent obstetric bleeding. Dialysate bicarbonate should be decreased to 25 mEq/L, in keeping with the expected lower bicarbonate levels of pregnancy. If peritoneal dialysis is being used, decreasing exchange volumes by increasing exchange frequency or cycler use are recommended. Adequate calorie and protein intake is required; 1 g per kg per day protein intake plus an additional 20 g per day has been suggested. After the first trimester, maternal "dry" weight should be increased by approximately 1 lb (400 g) per week to adjust for the expected progressive weight increase in pregnancy. Antihypertensive therapy should be adjusted for pregnancy by discontinuing angiotensin-converting enzyme (ACE) inhibitors and angiotensin receptor blockers (ARBs), and aiming for maintenance of maternal diastolic pressure of 80 to 90 mm Hg, using methyldopa, labetalol, and sustained release nifedipine in standard doses to achieve target. Anemia should be treated with supplemental iron, folic acid, and erythropoietin. Erythropoietin is safe in pregnancy, and pregnancy-related erythropoietin resistance requires a dose increase of approximately 50% to maintain hemoglobin target levels of 10 to 11 g per dL. Owing to placental 25-hydroxyvitamin D_3 conversion, decreased supplemental vitamin D may be required and should be guided by levels of vitamin D, parathyroid hormone, calcium, and phosphorus. Magnesium supplementation may be needed to maintain serum magnesium level at 5 to 7 mg per dL (2 to 3 mmol per L). Low-dose aspirin has been suggested to prevent preeclampsia. Babies born to mothers on dialysis may require monitoring for osmotic diuresis in the immediate postpartum period if maternal urea was high at the time of delivery.

VI. HYPERTENSIVE DISORDERS OF PREGNANCY. Hypertension during gestation remains a major cause of morbidity and death in both mother and child.

A. Of the many **classifications** proposed for hypertension complicating pregnancy, that of the Committee on Terminology of the American College of Obstetricians and Gynecologists (1972) has been the most useful. The National High Blood Pressure Education Program in the United States endorsed this system in 1990 and again in 2000. The four categories of hypertensive disorders in pregnancy are:

1. Preeclampsia.   Preeclampsia, characterized by hypertension, proteinuria, edema, and, at times, coagulation and liver function abnormalities, occurs in late pregnancy (after 20 weeks), primarily in nulliparas. Third-trimester hypertension is defined as a BP of 140/90 mm Hg or greater (Korotkoff V) sustained for 4 to 6 hours.

Attempts have been made to categorize this disease as severe (e.g., diastolic and systolic pressures of 110 and 160 mm Hg or greater, heavy proteinuria, oliguria, and neurologic symptoms) or mild. Because a patient with seemingly mild preeclampsia (e.g., a teenage gravida with a systolic BP of 140/85 mm Hg and trace proteinuria) may suddenly convulse (in which case the disease is called *eclampsia*, a complication associated with maternal mortality), terms such as *mild* and *severe* may be misleading. Hypertension during late pregnancy in a nullipara, whether or not other signs are present, is sufficient reason to consider hospitalization and treatment as if the patient were potentially preeclamptic.

2. Chronic hypertension.   Most women in this category have essential hypertension, but in some the elevated BP is secondary to such conditions as renal artery stenosis, coarctation of the aorta, renal disease, primary aldosteronism, and pheochromocytoma. Evidence of arteriolar disease and knowledge that hypertension was present before conception or early in gestation are helpful in establishing a diagnosis. Cocaine abuse may masquerade as chronic hypertension in pregnancy. Pheochromocytoma has a catastrophic outcome during pregnancy; therefore, measurement of plasma metanephrines should be considered in selected hypertensive gravidas not previously evaluated.

3. **Chronic hypertension with superimposed preeclampsia.** Hypertensive women are at increased risk for the development of superimposed preeclampsia, and, when this occurs, maternal and fetal morbidity and mortality are greater than when preeclampsia develops in a previously normotensive woman. Many of the maternal deaths attributable to hypertensive disease occur in previously hypertensive women with superimposed preeclampsia.

4. **Gestational hypertension**, which is high BP appearing first after midpregnancy, is distinguished from preeclampsia by the absence of proteinuria. This category is broad, and includes women who later develop diagnostic criteria for preeclampsia, as well as women with chronic hypertension in whom BP decreased in early pregnancy, masking the true diagnosis. Gestational hypertension that resolves postpartum, and which was not in retrospect preeclampsia, is more likely to occur in women who develop essential hypertension later in life.

5. The physician should be aware that on rare occasions convulsions and hypertension may develop after delivery. So-called late postpartum eclampsia (hypertension and convulsions 48 hours to weeks after delivery) is poorly understood, and is treated by hospitalization, magnesium sulfate, and supportive care.

B. **Pathophysiology of preeclampsia.** Preeclampsia is a syndrome the manifestations of which affect many organ systems, including brain, liver, kidney, blood vessels, and placenta. Therefore, while the focus may be on hypertension and proteinuria, we must always be aware that such signs and symptoms may be minimal whereas other, life-threatening syndromes develop, including convulsions and liver failure, both often associated with thrombocytopenia, as well as signs of DIC.

The placenta may be critically involved in the genesis of preeclampsia, and failure of cytotrophoblastic invasion of the uterine spiral arteries is one of the earliest changes in this disorder. Therefore, these vessels do not undergo the expected transformation into the dilated blood vessels characteristic of normal placentation. This aberration may underlie the poor placental perfusion and growth restriction characteristic of preeclampsia. The reason for the failure of the trophoblast to invade the uterine spiral arteries is obscure. Research has focused on the abnormal modulation of cytotrophoblast adhesion molecules, integrins, and abnormal vascular endothelial growth factor (VEGF) receptor–ligand interactions. The abnormal placentation leading to the maternal syndrome of preeclampsia is believed to occur early in pregnancy (10 to 20 weeks' gestation). Finally, a growing body of evidence has implicated the production of antiangiogenic factors in the genesis of preeclampsia. Women with preeclampsia have been found to have increased circulating levels of a soluble, splice variant of a receptor for VEGF called *sFlt-1*. SFlt-1 is believed to be released from the placenta into the maternal blood, and by binding to VEGF causes decreased bioavailability of VEGF, maternal vascular endothelial cell dysfunction, and the characteristic clinical features such as hypertension and proteinuria. Experimental administration of sFlt-1 to pregnant rats recapitulates the classic renal histologic findings of glomerular endotheliosis. Current studies are in progress to determine whether measurement of sFlt-1 is a useful test for either screening or early diagnosis of preeclampsia.

The mediators of hypertension in preeclampsia are not clearly understood. Evidence suggests that vasoconstriction results from a complex interplay of hormonal and vascular alterations. The renin–angiotensin system is stimulated in normal pregnancy and relatively suppressed in women with preeclampsia. However, patients with preeclampsia are more sensitive to the pressor effects of angiotensin II, and therefore this pressor peptide may play a role in their elevated BP. Aldosterone levels are also lower in preeclamptic women than in women with normal pregnancies, although still higher than nonpregnant levels.

Alterations in vascular endothelial cell function are important features of the pathophysiology of preeclampsia. Endothelial cells produce a variety of substances important in modulating vascular tone and coagulation (e.g., NO, prostacyclin, and endothelin). Animal studies of gestational hypertension as well as clinical studies in women suggest that decreased NO and prostacyclin, and increased endothelin, in addition to antiangiogenic factors mentioned earlier are both sequelae as well as contributory factors leading to vasoconstriction, platelet aggregation, and increased intravascular coagulation and finally, the maternal clinical manifestations of preeclampsia.

The ability to excrete sodium may be impaired in preeclampsia, but the degree to which this occurs varies, as severe disease can occur in the absence of edema (the "dry preeclamptic" patient). Even when edema is marked, plasma volume is below that for normal pregnancy, and hemoconcentration is often present. This latter phenomenon may relate to the development of a "leaky" vasculature (therefore, hypoalbuminemia in this disease may have three components: renal protein loss, liver dysfunction, and extravasation from the intravascular to the interstitial space). A decrement or suboptimal increase in intravascular volume also appears to precede the onset of overt hypertension.

Cardiac output is often decreased, and central venous and pulmonary capillary wedge pressures are normal or low. Therefore, high BP is maintained by a marked increase in peripheral resistance. The alterations in cardiac output, combined with the decrements in intravascular volume, and the fact that placental perfusion is decreased in preeclampsia are major reasons why diuretic use is discouraged in this disease.

In one variant of preeclampsia, HELLP, coagulation abnormalities, and liver dysfunction predominate, whereas hypertension and proteinuria may be minimal. This syndrome is life threatening because platelet counts may plunge far below 100 mm^3, whereas transaminase and lactic acid dehydrogenase levels rise above 1,000 units per L and evidence of a marked microangiopathic hemolytic anemia appears on the peripheral blood smear, all in less than 24 hours. Early recognition of this HELLP variant and prompt termination of gestation are important; such action avoids substantial maternal morbidity.

The pathogenesis of the eclamptic convulsion is also poorly understood. Vasospasm, ischemia, and local hemorrhage may all play a role. The importance of hypertension *per se* in the genesis of the seizures is debated, because convulsions may be observed in women whose BP is only mildly elevated. Descriptions of the syndrome of reversible posterior leucoencephalopathy syndrome, which is characterized by altered cerebrovascular autoregulation, endothelial dysfunction, and dramatic clinical sequelae in the setting of elevated BP, may be relevant to eclampsia.

C. **Kidney function and morphology in preeclampsia**
1. **GFR and RPF.** Both GFR and RPF decrease in preeclampsia. The decrements approximate 25% in most instances, so that the GFR of preeclamptic women often remains above pregravid values. However, in rare instances, large decreases in function may occur and, on occasion, lead to acute tubular or cortical necrosis.
2. **Uric acid.** Changes occur in the renal handling of urate in preeclampsia. A decrease in the clearance of uric acid, accompanied by increments in blood levels of this solute, may occur weeks before any clinical signs of the disease appear. In pregnancy, serum urate levels above 4.5 mg per dL are suspect [to convert to SI units (μmol per L), multiply mg per dL by 59.48]. The level of hyperuricemia also correlates with the severity of the preeclamptic renal lesion, as well as with fetal outcome.
3. Increased **proteinuria**, which may be moderate or heavy, is a feature of preeclampsia, and the diagnosis is suspect in its absence. The magnitude of proteinuria does not appear to affect maternal prognosis, but protein excretion in the nephrotic range is associated with greater fetal loss.
4. **Calcium.** Studies have demonstrated that renal calcium handling is altered in preeclampsia, and that in contrast to normotensive gravidas, or those with chronic or transient hypertension, patients with preeclampsia demonstrate marked hypocalciuria. The basis for this abnormality is unknown. Levels of 1,25 vitamin D are lower, and parathormone higher when compared with normal pregnancy.

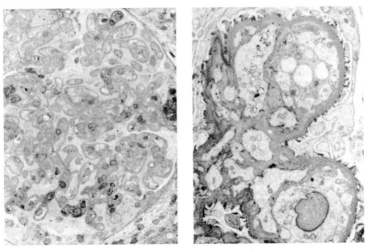

A   B

Figure 14-2. A: Electron micrograph demonstrating complete capillary obliteration by a swollen endothelial cell. Note, however, that the basement membrane is normal and the epithelial foot processes are intact. **B:** Micrograph showing glomerulus from a preeclamptic kidney. Swollen endothelial and mesangial cells that display prominent vacuolization encroach on the capillary lumina. (Courtesy of B. H. Spargo, M.D.)

    5. Preeclampsia is accompanied by a characteristic histologic lesion: **glomerular capillary endotheliosis** (Fig. 14-2). In women diagnosed clinically as preeclamptic, this lesion is present in only approximately 85% of biopsies obtained from primiparas and in considerably fewer biopsies from multiparas. The remaining patients have evidence of nephrosclerosis or another parenchymal disease. Glomerular endotheliosis is characterized by swollen glomerular capillary endothelial cells with the appearance of a "bloodless glomerulus." Some claim that preeclampsia is a cause of focal glomerular sclerosis, but others believe preeclampsia lesions to be completely reversible, with the presence of focal glomerular sclerosis reflecting preexisting nephrosclerosis or primary renal disease. Women with glomerular endotheliosis alone tend to have uneventful subsequent gestations, but when focal glomerular sclerosis or alterations in the renal vessels are present, hypertension is more likely to recur in later pregnancies.

D. Management of preeclampsia

    1. Hospitalization. Ambulatory treatment is risky in the management of preeclampsia. Therefore, suspicion of the disease is sufficient to consider hospitalization. Such an approach diminishes the frequency of convulsions and other consequences of diagnostic error. In general, fetal maturity is evaluated; if the gestation is near term, induction is the therapy of choice, whereas attempts to temporize are made if the pregnancy is at an earlier stage. Rest is an extremely important part of the therapeutic regimen, which must be prescribed rather than suggested. Termination of pregnancy should be considered when signs of impending eclampsia (e.g., hyperreflexia, headaches, and epigastric pain) develop or persist; BP cannot be controlled; serum creatinine, urea nitrogen, and uric acid rise; laboratory evidence suggests DIC or abnormal liver function (increased transaminases); or specific obstetric test results suggest fetal jeopardy. When signs of impending convulsions (eclampsia) are present, parenteral magnesium sulfate is the drug of choice.

    2. Treatment of hypertension. The approach to treatment of high BP in gravidas is disputed. As noted, morphologic examination of preeclamptic placentae demonstrates decreased trophoblastic invasion of the uterine spiral arteries, causing these vessels to be more constricted than normal. Thus, perfusion of the placenta is compromised. Therefore, aggressive reduction in maternal BP may decrease uteroplacental perfusion even further (i.e., poor autoregulation of uterine blood flow). Thus, large decrements in the mother's mean pressure should be avoided, especially in acute emergencies. Data on human pregnancy are limited, but they suggest that decrements in maternal pressure may indeed reduce placental perfusion. Others have argued that, based on evidence obtained from animal studies, uterine blood flow is autoregulated, and therefore hypertension should be aggressively treated. Assuming that autoregulation of uterine blood flow exists, a critical but unanswered question is how quickly it takes place, because fetuses may be damaged by short periods of ischemia. Therefore, the author prescribes the careful use of parenteral hydralazine or labetalol, in addition to close maternal scrutiny and fetal monitoring, when acute hypertension exceeds diastolic levels of 100 mm Hg or systolic levels of 150 mm Hg (Table 14-5). This approach is successful in most gravidas. Long-acting oral calcium channel blockers have also been used to treat acute hypertension associated with preeclampsia.

Diazoxide can be used in rare resistant cases and should be administered only in small doses (30 mg at a time). Sodium nitroprusside should be avoided, because cyanide poisoning and fetal death have been observed in laboratory animals. ACE inhibitors and ARBs should not be used in pregnancy.

3. Treatment of the eclamptic convulsion. Several large clinical trials have demonstrated that magnesium sulfate is superior to other anticonvulsants for prevention of recurrent eclamptic convulsions, and also for primary prevention of eclampsia in women with preeclampsia. The usual protocol is to administer a loading dose of 4 g magnesium sulfate, infused over 15 minutes, followed by a sustaining infusion of 1 to 2 g per hour, aiming to achieve plasma levels of 2 to 4 μmol per L. Because the incidence of convulsion is highest in the immediate puerperium, it is common practice to begin magnesium sulfate immediately after delivery and continue it for 24 hours.

E. Prevention of preeclampsia. Many strategies have been investigated in well-conducted clinical trials (including thousands of women) of antiplatelet therapy, nutritional supplementation, and antioxidant vitamins for the prevention of preeclampsia. These trials, and subsequent meta-analyses, demonstrate a small (10% to 15% reduction in relative risk) benefit for low-dose aspirin for prevention of preeclampsia and meaningful adverse maternal and fetal outcomes. With respect to nutritional strategies, calcium supplementation appears to have a small benefit in women ingesting a baseline low calcium diet, and not much benefit in women ingesting a normal calcium diet. To date, antioxidant supplementation with vitamins C and E have not shown benefit in three large randomized controlled trials

Although prevention of preeclampsia is usually not possible, avoidance of severe complications may be accomplished by early recognition of the disease before such complications develop. If early signs are detected, hospitalization should be strongly considered to permit close monitoring of the patient. If preeclampsia is detected early, bedrest and close monitoring of maternal and fetal condition may enable prolongation of pregnancy in some cases.

F. The hypertensive patient without preeclampsia. Pregnancies in women with chronic hypertension are associated with increased maternal as well as fetal risks. Complications include superimposed preeclampsia, placental abruption, acute tubular and cortical necrosis, retardation of intrauterine growth, and midtrimester fetal death. Such events seem to correlate with the age of the gravida and the duration of her high BP. Therefore, most of these complications occur in women older than 30 years or with evidence of end-organ damage. Conversely, most women (approximately 85%) with essential hypertension have uncomplicated and successful gestations.

Women with chronic hypertension often have reductions in BP by midpregnancy, so that their BP may not exceed that observed in normotensive pregnant women. The failure of this decrement to occur, or increases in BP in early or midtrimester pregnancy, indicates a guarded prognosis for the gestation. Fetal outcome is poorer in hypertensive women with superimposed preeclampsia than in previously normotensive women with this complication, and the combination of chronic hypertension and preeclampsia increased the risk for cerebral hemorrhage. Patients with chronic hypertension and superimposed preeclampsia should be hospitalized and their hypertension controlled. Delivery should be considered if either maternal or fetal condition is unstable.

1. **Antihypertensive therapy.** Guidelines for antihypertensive therapy during gestation are less clear than those for nonpregnant hypertensive women. For the latter, compelling data exist from large population studies to document the benefits of lowering BP with medication, even in women with only mild hypertension. During pregnancy, however, although maternal safety remains the primary concern, there is also a desire to minimize exposure of the fetus to drugs, given their unknown long-term effects on growth and development. A systematic review of clinical trials of hypertension found only 13 randomized clinical trials comparing antihypertensive therapy to either no treatment or placebo in women with chronic hypertension. The most commonly used drug, methyldopa, was given to just more than 200 subjects. Six trials showed no reduction in perinatal mortality with antihypertensive treatment, whereas three reported a trend toward lower perinatal mortality with treatment. A debatable issue is whether lowering BP will prevent superimposed preeclampsia, but little or no convincing evidence supports this contention. Therefore, it is permissible to tolerate higher BP levels during gestation that do no harm in the short term, while limiting use of antihypertensive drugs. In this respect, most pregnant women with chronic hypertension have only mild or very moderate elevations in BP and require little or no medication at all. However, "appropriate" or "tolerable" levels of BP for these patients during gestation seem to have been set empirically, and multicenter clinical trials are needed to support or reject such practices.

Whether mild degrees of hypertension during gestation should be treated is not generally agreed on. Although one group claimed that such therapy decreases the incidence of superimposed preeclampsia, most would withhold treatment

TABLE 14-4	**Guidelines for Treating Severe Hypertension Near Term or during Labor**

Regulation of blood pressure
The degree to which blood pressure should be decreased is disputed; maintaining diastolic levels between 90 and 100 mm Hg is recommended

Drug therapy
Labetalol, administered intravenously, is an effective and safe agent for preeclamptic hypertension; start with 20 mg and repeat the dose every 20 min, up to 200 mg, until desired blood pressure is achieved. Side effects include headache

Hydralazine administered intravenously may also be used; start with low doses (5 mg as an intravenous bolus), then administer 5 to 10 mg every 20–30 min to avoid precipitous decreases in pressure; side effects include tachycardia and headache

Calcium channel blockers (*long acting*) have been used, p.o.

Diazoxide should be used only in the rare instance that hydralazine, labetalol, or calcium channel blockers have been unsuccessful; small doses (30 mg at a time) have been reported to be effective; side effects include arrest of labor and neonatal hypoglycemia

Refrain from using *sodium nitroprusside*, because fetal cyanide poisoning has been reported in animals; however, maternal well-being should dictate the choice of therapy

Prevention of convulsions
Parenteral *magnesium sulfate* is the drug of choice for preventing eclamptic convulsions; therapy should be continued for 12–24 hr postpartum, because one-third of women with eclampsia have convulsions during this period

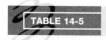

TABLE 14-5	Antihypertensive Drugs used to Treat Chronic Hypertension in Pregnancy

α_2-Adrenergic receptor agonists

Methyldopa is the most extensively used drug in this group. Its safety and efficacy are supported by evidence from randomized trials and a 7.5-year follow-up study of children born to mothers treated with methyldopa

β-Adrenergic receptor antagonists

These drugs, especially *atenolol* and *metoprolol*, appear to be safe and efficacious in late pregnancy, but fetal growth retardation has been reported when treatment was started in early or midgestation. Fetal bradycardia can occur, and animal studies suggest that the fetus's ability to tolerate hypoxic stress may be compromised

α-Adrenergic receptor and β-adrenergic receptor antagonists

Labetalol appears to be as effective as methyldopa, but no follow-up studies of children born to mothers given labetalol have been carried out, and concern about maternal hepatotoxicity still exists

Calcium channel blockers

Several small studies and reviews suggest that both dihydropyridines (long acting) as well as verapamil and diltiazem are safe and effective in pregnancy

Direct acting vasodilators

Hydralazine is frequently used as adjunctive therapy with methyldopa and β-adrenergic receptor antagonists. Rarely, neonatal thrombocytopenia has been reported; The experience with *minoxidil* is limited, and this drug is not recommended

Angiotensin-converting enzyme (ACE) inhibitors

Captopril causes fetal death in diverse animal species, and several ACE inhibitors have been associated with oligohydramnios and neonatal renal failure when administered to humans; do not use at any time in pregnancy

Angiotensin II receptor blockers

These drugs have not been used in pregnancy; in view of the deleterious effects of blocking angiotensin II generation with ACE inhibitors, angiotensin II receptor antagonists are also considered to be contraindicated in pregnancy

Diuretics

Diuretics may be used in women with salt sensitive hypertension and/or renal disease; attempts should be made to use the lowest possible dose and avoid volume depletion

until diastolic levels are at least 15 mm Hg above borderline hypertension (defined in the author's clinics as 75 mm Hg in the second trimester and 85 mm Hg in late gestation). Very young gravidas, however, may require treatment at lower levels. Tables 14-4 and 14-5 summarize current knowledge on the use of antihypertensive drugs in pregnancy. The available information regarding the safety and efficacy of these medications in pregnant women is limited.

A reasonable strategy, based on available data, is to treat maternal hypertension when BP exceeds 145 to 150 mm Hg systolic, 95 to 100 mm Hg diastolic. Exceptions, however, include parenchymal renal disease and evidence of target organ damage (e.g., retinopathy and cardiac hypertrophy), in which therapy is recommended once levels are 90 mm Hg or more.

The argument of whether to treat is debatable when only fetal well-being is considered. Some evidence suggests fetal benefits when mild to moderate hypertension is treated with antihypertensive drugs during pregnancy.

In summary, the unknown but potential hazards of antihypertensive treatment during pregnancy are sufficient reasons for withholding drug treatment when mild hypertension (systolic 140 to 150 mm Hg, diastolic levels of 90 to 95 mm Hg) is present, particularly during the initial trimester. As noted, many of these patients experience a physiologic decrease in BP that on occasion reaches normotensive levels. Patients with evidence of renal disease or end-organ damage require the initiation of treatment at lower levels (less than 90 mm Hg).

Suggested Readings

Armenti VT, Radomski JS, Moritz MJ, et al. Report from the National Transplantation Pregnancy Registry (NTPR): outcomes of pregnancy after transplantation. *Clin Transpl* 2004;103–114.

August P, Mueller FB, Sealey JE, et al. Role of renin-angiotensin system in blood pressure regulation in pregnancy. *Lancet* 1995;345(8954):896–897.

Cadnapaphornchai MA, Ohara M, Morris KG, et al. Chronic NOS inhibition reverses systemic vasodilation and glomerular hyperfiltration in pregnancy. *Am J Physiol Renal Physiol* 2001;280(4):F592–F598.

Chapman AB, Johnson AM, Gabow PA, et al. Pregnancy outcome and its relationship to progression of renal failure in autosomal dominant polycystic kidney disease. *J Am Soc Nephrol* 1994;5(5):1178–1185.

Chapman AB, Zamudio S, Woodmansee W, et al. Systemic and renal hemodynamic changes in the luteal phase of the menstrual cycle mimic early pregnancy. *Am J Physiol* 1997;273(5 Pt 2):F777–F782.

Chen HH, Lin HC, Yeh JC, et al. Renal biopsy in pregnancies complicated by undetermined renal disease. *Acta Obstet Gynecol Scand* 2001;80(10):888–893.

Clowse ME, Magder L, Witter F, et al. Hydroxychloroquine in lupus pregnancy. *Arthritis Rheum* 2006;54(11):3640–3647.

Conde-Agudelo A, Villar J, Lindheimer M, et al. World Health Organization systematic review of screening tests for preeclampsia. *Obstet Gynecol* 2004;104(6):1367–1391.

Conrad KP, Debrah DO, Novak J, et al. Relaxin modifies systemic arterial resistance and compliance in conscious, nonpregnant rats. *Endocrinology* 2004;145(7):3289–3296.

Davison JM, Shiells EA, Philips PR, et al. Serial evaluation of vasopressin release and thirst in human pregnancy. Role of human chorionic gonadotrophin in the osmoregulatory changes of gestation. *J Clin Invest* 1988;81(3):798–806.

Davison JM, Sheills EA, Philips PR, et al. Metabolic clearance of vasopressin and an analogue resistant to vasopressinase in human pregnancy. *Am J Physiol* 1993;264 (2 Pt 2):F348–F353.

Derksen RH, Bruinse HW, de Groot PG, et al. Pregnancy in systemic lupus erythematosus: a prospective study. *Lupus* 1994;3(3):149–155.

Duley L. Evidence and practice: the magnesium sulphate story. *Best Pract Res Clin Obstet Gynaecol* 2005;19(1):57–74.

Duley L, Henderson-Smart DJ, Knight M, et al. Antiplatelet agents for preventing preeclampsia and its complications. *Cochrane Database Syst Rev* 2004;(1):CD004659.

Erkan D. The relation between antiphospholipid syndrome-related pregnancy morbidity and non-gravid vascular thrombosis: a review of the literature and management strategies. *Curr Rheumatol Rep* 2002;4(5):379–386.

Fesenmeier MF, Coppage KH, Lambers DS, et al. Acute fatty liver of pregnancy in 3 tertiary care centers. *Am J Obstet Gynecol* 2005;192(5):1416–1419.

Gammill HS, Jeyabalan A. Acute renal failure in pregnancy. *Crit Care Med* 2005;33 (Suppl 10):S372–S384.

Haase M, Morgera S, Budde K, et al. A systematic approach to managing pregnant dialysis patients—the importance of an intensified haemodiafiltration protocol *Nephrol Dial Transplant* 2006;20(11):2537–2542.

Hofmeyr GJ, Atallah AN, Duley L, et al. Calcium supplementation during pregnancy for preventing hypertensive disorders and related problems. *Cochrane Database Syst Rev* 2006;3:CD001059.

Holley JL, Reddy SS. Pregnancy in dialysis patients: a review of outcomes, complications, and management. *Semin Dial* 2003;16(5):384–388.

Khan KS, Wojdyla D, Say L, et al. WHO analysis of causes of maternal death: a systematic review. *Lancet* 2006;367(9516):1066–1074.

Le Ray C, Coulomb A, Elefant E, et al. Mycophenolate mofetil in pregnancy after renal transplantation: a case of major fetal malformations. *Obstet Gynecol* 2004;103 (5 Pt 2):1091–1094.

Maynard S, Min JY, Merchan J, et al. Excess placental soluble fms-like tyrosine kinase 1 (sFlt1) may contribute to endothelial dysfunction, hypertension, and proteinuria in preeclampsia. *J Clin Invest* 2003;111:649–658.

McKay DB, Josephson MA. Pregnancy in recipients of solid organs—effects on mother and child. *N Engl J Med* 2006;354(12):1281–1293.

National High Blood Pressure Education Program Working Group. National High Blood Pressure Education Program Working Group report on high blood pressure in pregnancy. *Am J Obstet Gynecol* 2000;183:S1–S22.

Prakash J, Kumar H, Sinha DK, et al. Acute renal failure in pregnancy in a developing country: twenty years of experience. *Ren Fail* 2006;28(4):309–313.

Rossing K, Jacobsen P, Hommel E, et al. Pregnancy and progression of diabetic nephropathy. *Diabetologia* 2002;45(1):36–41.

Ruiz-Irastorza G, Lima F, Alves J, et al. Increased rate of lupus flare during pregnancy and the puerperium: a prospective study of 78 pregnancies. *Br J Rheumatol* 1996;35(2):133–138.

Rumbold AR, Crowther CA, Haslam RR, et al. Vitamins C and E and the risks of preeclampsia and perinatal complications. *N Engl J Med* 2006;354(17):1796–1806.

Smith WT, Darbari S, Kwan M, et al. Pregnancy in peritoneal dialysis: a case report and review of adequacy and outcomes. *Int Urol Nephrol* 2005;37(1):145–151.

Sturgiss SN, Wilkinson R, Davison JM, et al. Renal reserve during human pregnancy. *Am J Physiol* 1996;271(1 Pt 2):F16–F20.

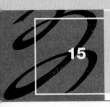

15 THE PATIENT WITH HYPERTENSION

Charles R. Nolan

I. **DEFINITION AND CLASSIFICATION OF HYPERTENSION.** The definition of hypertension is somewhat arbitrary, because blood pressure (BP) is not distributed bimodally in the population. Instead, the distribution of BP readings in the population is unimodal, and an arbitrary level of BP must be defined as the threshold above which hypertension can be diagnosed. The correlation between the levels of systolic BP and diastolic blood pressure (DBP) and cardiovascular risk has long been recognized. It has become clear that in patients older than 50, systolic BP of more than 140 mm Hg is a much more important cardiovascular disease risk factor than is DBP. Increasing BP clearly has an adverse effect on mortality over the entire range of recorded pressures, even those generally considered to be in the normal range. Lifespan and health are progressively reduced as BP rises. The goal of identifying and treating high BP is to reduce the risk of cardiovascular disease and associated morbidity and mortality. In this regard, classifying hypertension in adults is useful in identifying high-risk individuals and providing guidelines for follow-up and treatment of hypertension. The seventh report of the Joint National Committee (JNC) on Prevention, Detection, Evaluation, and Treatment of High Blood Pressure (JNC 7) has established criteria for the diagnosis and classification of BP in adult patients (Table 15-1). The optimal BP in an individual who is not acutely ill is lower than 120/80 mm Hg. Individuals with a systolic BP of 120 to 139 mm Hg or a DBP of 80 to 89 mm Hg should be considered as prehypertensive; these patients require health-promoting lifestyle modifications to prevent cardiovascular disease. Patients with prehypertension are at twice the risk of developing hypertension as those with lower values. Although normotensive by definition, these prehypertensive patients should be rechecked annually to exclude the development of hypertension. Hypertension is arbitrarily defined as a systolic BP of 140 mm Hg or greater or a DBP of 90 mm Hg or greater, or by virtue of the patient taking antihypertensive medications. The stage of hypertension (stage 1 or 2) is determined by the levels of both systolic BP and DBP (Table 15-1). This classification should be based on the average of two or more BP readings at each of two or more visits after the initial BP screening. When systolic BP and DBP fall into different categories, the higher category should be selected to classify the individual's BP.

II. **EPIDEMIOLOGY OF HYPERTENSION.** Data from the National Health and Nutrition Examination Survey (NHANES 1999 to 2000) indicate that approximately 31.3% of the adult population in the United States has hypertension. The prevalence of hypertension increases sharply with age (18 to 34, 6%; 35 to 44, 16%; 45 to 54, 31%; 55 to 64, 48%; 65 to 74, 65%; and older than 75 years, 78%). Worldwide more than 1 billion individuals have hypertension. At least 65 million (31.3%) adults in the United States had hypertension in the 1999 to 2000 NHANES survey compared to 50 million (28.9%) for 1988 to 1994. The 30% increase in the total number of adults with hypertension was almost fourfold greater that the 8.3% increase in total prevalence rate. The increasing burden of hypertension is not only the result of the increased size of the population but also reflects the increased prevalence of obesity and the overall aging of the population. Data from the Framingham Heart Study indicate that even individuals who are normotensive at 55 years have a 90% lifetime risk for developing hypertension. As the mean age in the general population increases, the prevalence of hypertension will no doubt increase further unless effective preventative measures are implemented. Many hypertensive patients have a positive family history of parental hypertension. The mode of inheritance is complex and probably polygenic in most instances. Black men and women have a twofold higher prevalence of hypertension

TABLE 15-1	Classification of Blood Pressure (BP) for Adults[a]

BP classification[b]	Systolic BP (mm Hg)[c]		Diastolic BP (mm Hg)[c]
Normal	<120	and	<80
Prehypertension	120–139	or	80–89
Stage 1 hypertension	140–159	or	90–99
Stage 2 hypertension	≥160	or	≥100

[a]Adults aged 18 years and older.
[b]Classification should be based on the mean of two or more properly measured seated blood pressure readings obtained on each of two or more office visits.
[c]When systolic and diastolic BP fall into different categories, classify based on the higher category. (Adapted with permission from Chobanian AV, Bakris GL, Black HR, et al. The seventh report of the Joint National Committee on prevention, detection, evaluation and treatment of high blood pressure. The JNC 7 Report. *JAMA* 2003;289:2560–2572.)

(30%) than white men and women (15%) in a sampling of almost 18,000 American adults aged 48 to 75 years in the NHANES data. Prevalence appears to be equal in men and women in most surveys. Obese individuals have significantly more hypertension than nonobese individuals. In childhood, obesity is a major cause of hypertension. More than one-half of the adult population is overweight [body mass index (BMI) of 25 to 29.9] or obese (BMI greater than or equal to 30). Data from NHANES III show that the among men and women, whites, blacks, and Mexican Americans, the prevalence of hypertension and the mean levels of systolic BP and DBP increase as BMI increases at ages younger than 60 years. Overall, the prevalence of hypertension in adults with BMI greater than or equal to 30 is 41.4% for men and 37.8% for women, respectively; compared with 14.9% for men and 15.2% for women with BMI less than or equal to 25. Further proof of the significant relationship between body weight and BP is found in the observation that BP falls with even modest weight reduction. The intake of dietary salt (sodium chloride) has significant effects on BP, especially in patients with other factors predisposing to the development of hypertension, such as advancing age, obesity, adult-onset diabetes, positive family history of hypertension, black race, or underlying renal disease. Numerous epidemiologic studies have shown that the dietary intake of salt correlates with the average BP in a population. Northern Japanese fishermen who ingest 450 mEq of sodium daily have a 40% prevalence of hypertension. In contrast, indigenous Alaskan populations and the Yanomamo Indians in Brazil and Venezuela, who have dietary intake of 1 mEq of sodium daily, do not develop hypertension at any age. Intersalt, an international epidemiologic study, examined the relation between dietary sodium intake (based on 24-hour urinary sodium excretion) and BP in more than 10,000 individuals aged 20 to 59 years from 52 countries around the world. The results demonstrate a significant correlation between median systolic BP and DBP and dietary sodium intake. These observations can be explained based on the role of abnormal renal sodium handling in the pathogenesis of hypertension, which is discussed in section IV. The therapeutic implications of these observations include dietary sodium restriction as part of nonpharmacologic therapy and the recommendation of thiazide diuretics as first-line drug therapy for the treatment of hypertension in most patients. Despite the known cardiovascular risks of untreated hypertension and the widespread availability of effective pharmacologic treatment, the identification and effective control of hypertension remains a significant public health problem in the United States. From the 1976 to 1980 NHANES survey (NHANES II) to the 1991 to 1994 survey (NHANES III, phase 2), the percentage of hypertensive Americans who are aware that they have high BP increased from 51% to 68%. Among persons with hypertension, the prevalence of treatment increased from 31% to 54% during the same period. The number of persons with high BP controlled to below 140/90 mm Hg increased from 10% in NHANES II to 27% in

NHANES III. Alarmingly, data computed for 1999 to 2000 reveal that more than 65% of patients with hypertension still have inadequate control of their BP. The continued high prevalence of hypertension and hypertension-related complications such as stroke, cardiovascular complications, heart failure, and end-stage renal disease (ESRD) represent a major public health challenge.

III. **CARDIOVASCULAR DISEASE RISK.** The relationship of BP to cardiovascular risk is continuous and independent of other cardiovascular risk factors. Beginning at 115/75 mm Hg and across the entire BP range, each increment of 20/10 mm Hg doubles the risk of cardiovascular disease. The overall risk of cardiovascular morbidity and mortality in patients with hypertension is determined not only by the stage of hypertension but also by the presence of other risk factors, such as smoking, hyperlipidemia, and diabetes, and by the existence of target organ damage (Table 15-2). The major target organs affected by hypertension are the heart, peripheral vasculature, central nervous system, kidney, and the eye. Most of the consequences of hypertension are the result of progressive vascular injury. Hypertension accelerates atherosclerotic vascular disease and aggravates the deleterious effects of diabetes, smoking, and hyperlipidemia on the aorta and its major branches. Atherosclerotic disease results in significant morbidity from myocardial infarction (MI), atherothrombotic cerebral infarction, peripheral vascular disease with claudication, and renal disease due to ischemia or cholesterol embolization. Hypertensive renal disease may result from hypertension-induced vasculitis in the setting of malignant hypertension or more insidious renal injury from long-standing essential hypertension with benign hypertensive

 TABLE 15-2   **Cardiovascular Risk Factors and Target Organ Damage**

Major risk factors
  Hypertension[a]
  Cigarette smoking
  Obesity (BMI)[b] >30[a]
  Physical inactivity
  Dyslipidemia[a]
  Diabetes mellitus[a]
  Microalbuminuria or estimated GFR[c] <60 mL/min
  Age (older than 55 yr for men, older than 65 yr for women)
  Family history of premature cardiovascular disease (men younger than 55 yr or women younger than 65 yr)
Target organ damage
  Heart
    Left ventricular hypertrophy
    Angina or prior myocardial infarction
    Prior coronary revascularization
    Heart failure
  Brain
    Prior stroke or transient ischemic attack
  Chronic kidney disease
  Peripheral arterial disease
  Retinopathy (Table 15-8)

BMI, body mass index; GFR, glomerular filtration rate.
[a]Components of the metabolic syndrome associated with insulin resistance and hyperinsulinemia.
[b]BMI indicates body mass index calculated as weight in kilograms divided by the square of height in meters.
[c]GFR indicates glomerular filtration rate.
(Adapted with permission from Chobanian AV, Bakris GL, Black HR, et al. The seventh report of the Joint National Committee on prevention, detection, evaluation and treatment of high blood pressure. The JNC 7 Report. *JAMA* 2003;289:2560–2572.)

nephrosclerosis. Hypertension is also an important cofactor in the progression of other renal diseases, especially diabetic nephropathy. Hypertension may also cause cerebrovascular disease in the form of lacunar infarction or intracerebral hemorrhage. Left ventricular hypertrophy (LVH) and congestive heart failure (CHF), often due to isolated diastolic dysfunction, are the result of the heightened peripheral vascular resistance (afterload) imposed by systemic hypertension. In clinical trials, antihypertensive therapy has been associated with significant reductions in the incidence of stroke (35% to 40%), MI (20% to 25%), and heart failure (50%). It has been estimated that in patients with stage 1 hypertension (systolic BP 140 to 159 mm Hg and/or DBP 90 to 99 mm Hg) and additional cardiovascular risk factors, achieving a sustained 12 mm Hg reduction in systolic BP for 10 years will prevent one death for every 11 patients treated. In the setting of preexisting cardiovascular disease or target organ damage, treatment of nine patients would prevent one death.

IV. PATHOGENESIS OF HYPERTENSION. Experiments with isolated, perfused kidneys demonstrate that the magnitude of urinary sodium excretion is a direct function of the renal arterial perfusion pressure. The level of perfusion pressure may alter sodium excretion by changing the peritubular hydrostatic pressure. Therefore, an increase in perfusion pressure should increase peritubular hydrostatic pressure with a resultant decrease in sodium reabsorption. Micropuncture studies in the rat have shown an inverse relationship between renal perfusion pressure and proximal sodium reabsorption. It has been argued that if this pressure natriuresis mechanism operates in a normal manner, in the presence of hypertension, profound volume depletion would result. The fact that this does not occur suggests that in every hypertensive state, a shift in the pressure natriuresis curve must occur so that a higher perfusion pressure is required to achieve any given level of natriuresis. In this regard, Guyton et al. have postulated that this shift in the pressure natriuresis curve is the fundamental underlying pathophysiologic abnormality that leads to essential hypertension and virtually all secondary forms of hypertension (Fig. 15-1). If a primary renal defect in natriuresis does exist in hypertension, then, to avert disaster due to persistent positive sodium balance with inexorable fluid accumulation, compensatory mechanisms must be invoked that restore sodium balance. These compensatory processes restore sodium balance and normal extracellular fluid (ECF) volume but, in the process, cause systemic hypertension.

Guyton's hypothesis states that the most important and fundamental mechanism in determining the long-term control of BP is the renal fluid–volume feedback mechanism. In simple terms, through this basic mechanism, the kidneys regulate arterial pressure by altering renal excretion of sodium and water, thereby controlling circulatory volume and cardiac output. Changes in BP, in turn, directly influence the renal excretion of sodium and water, thereby providing a negative feedback mechanism for the control of ECF volume, cardiac output, and BP. The hypothesis is that derangements in this renal fluid–volume pressure control mechanism are the fundamental cause of virtually all hypertensive states (Fig. 15-1). In every hypertensive state, an underlying abnormality exists in the intrinsic natriuretic capacity of the kidney, so that the daily salt intake cannot be excreted at a normal BP, and the development of hypertension is necessary to induce a pressure natriuresis that allows the kidney to excrete the daily salt intake. Normal sodium balance and ECF volume are maintained, but at the expense of systemic hypertension. The underlying cause for the abnormality in the natriuretic capacity depends on the etiology of hypertension. In essential hypertension, some underlying abnormality increases renal avidity for sodium. In patients with obesity and insulin resistance (metabolic syndrome), hyperinsulinemia increases proximal tubular sodium reabsorption. Increased angiotensin II levels and sympathetic nervous system activity also enhance sodium reabsorption. Mineralocorticoids enhance distal tubular sodium reabsorption. Renal parenchymal disease causes nephron loss, resulting in a natriuretic defect. Abnormalities in renal endothelin or nitric oxide (NO) levels may also impair natriuresis. To date, each of the genetic causes of hypertension that have been elucidated has been shown to relate to an abnormality of renal sodium handling. For example, Liddle's syndrome results from enhanced distal tubular sodium reabsorption due to an abnormality in sodium channels in the distal

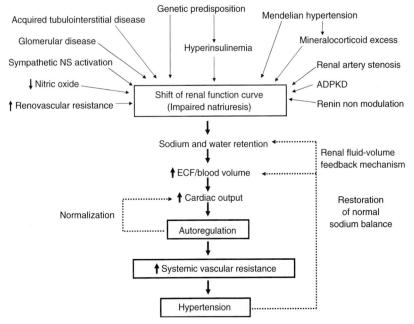

Figure 15-1. Abnormal renal sodium handling in the pathogenesis of hypertension (Guyton's hypothesis). In the setting of essential hypertension, primary renal disease, mineralocorticoid excess, or insulin resistance with hyperinsulinemia, a defect in the intrinsic natriuretic capacity of the kidney is present that prevents sodium balance from being maintained at a normal level of BP. Initially, this impairment in natriuresis leads to increases in extracellular fluid (ECF) volume and cardiac output. However, this hemodynamic state is short lived. Circulatory autoregulation occurs to maintain normal perfusion of the tissues, resulting in an increase in the systemic vascular resistance (SVR). The increase in SVR leads to systemic hypertension. With pressure-induced natriuresis, the renal fluid–volume feedback mechanism returns sodium balance, ECF volume, and cardiac output to normal. Systemic hypertension can be conceptualized as an essentially protective mechanism that prevents life-threatening fluid overload in the setting of reduced renal natriuretic capacity. Normal salt balance and fluid volume are maintained, but at the expense of systemic hypertension. (ADPKD, autosomal dominant polycystic kidney disease; NS, nephrotic syndrome; AII, angiotensin II.) (Adapted with permission from Nolan CR, Schrier RW. The kidney in hypertension. In: Schrier RW, ed. *Renal and electrolyte disorders*, 6th ed. Philadelphia: Lippincott Williams & Wilkins, 2003.)

nephron. Cross-transplant experiments in hypertensive and normotensive rat strains validate the importance of the kidney in the pathogenesis of hypertension, because the presence or absence of hypertension depends on the donor source of the kidney. Guyton's hypothesis states that this decreased natriuretic capacity of the kidney initially leads to renal salt and water retention, ECF volume expansion, and increased cardiac output with hypertension. This phase of volume expansion and high cardiac output is short lived. In the setting of high cardiac output, autoregulatory vasoconstriction of each vascular bed matches the blood flow to the metabolic requirements of the tissues. This phenomenon of circulatory autoregulation leads to an increase in systemic vascular resistance (SVR). Therefore, hypertension that was initially caused by high cardiac output becomes high-SVR hypertension.

The development of hypertension represents a protective mechanism, because it induces the kidney to undergo a pressure natriuresis and diuresis, thereby restoring normal salt balance and returning ECF volume to normal. This mechanism explains why an underlying problem with sodium excretion, as in salt-sensitive hypertension, is manifest as high-SVR hypertension without evidence of overt fluid overload. Support for this hypothesis is found in animal models of mineralocorticoid-induced hypertension. To substantiate the role of direct pressure-induced natriuresis in the regulation of sodium balance in mineralocorticoid hypertension, Hall et al. compared the systemic BP and natriuretic effect of aldosterone infusion in a dog model in which the renal perfusion pressure was either allowed to increase or mechanically servocontrolled to maintain renal artery pressure at normal levels. In the intact animal, continuous aldosterone infusion caused a transient period of sodium and water retention with a mild increase in BP. This sodium retention lasted only a few days, however, and was followed by an escape from the sodium-retaining effects of aldosterone and a restoration of normal sodium balance. In contrast, when the renal perfusion pressure was servocontrolled to maintain normal renal perfusion pressure during aldosterone infusion, no aldosterone escape occurred, and a relentless increase in sodium and water retention occurred, accompanied by severe hypertension, edema, ascites, and pulmonary edema. When the servocontrol device was removed and the renal perfusion pressure was allowed to rise to the systemic level, a prompt natriuresis and diuresis ensued, with the restoration of sodium balance and a fall in BP. These observations highlight the pivotal role of BP in the regulation of renal sodium and water excretion. Moreover, the observation that abnormal renal sodium handling is central in the pathogenesis of all forms of hypertension provides a sound pathophysiologic rationale for the JNC 7 recommendation regarding thiazide-type diuretics as first-line antihypertensive therapy in most patients.

V. DIAGNOSTIC EVALUATION OF HYPERTENSION. Detection of hypertension begins with proper measurement of BP at each health care encounter. Repeated BP measurements are used to determine whether initial elevations persist and require prompt attention or have returned to normal values and require only periodic surveillance. BP measurement should be standardized as follows: After at least 5 minutes of rest, the patient should be seated in a chair with the back supported and one arm bared and supported at heart level. The patient should refrain from smoking or ingesting caffeine for 30 minutes before the examination. For an appropriately sized cuff, the bladder should encircle at least 80% of the arm. Many patients require a large adult cuff. Measurements should ideally be taken with a mercury sphygmomanometer. Alternatively, a recently calibrated aneroid manometer or a validated electronic device can be used. The first appearance of sound (phase 1) is used to define systolic BP. The disappearance of sound (phase 5) is used to define DBP. The BP should be confirmed in the contralateral arm. Measurement of BP outside of the physician's office may provide some valuable information with regard to the diagnosis and treatment of hypertension. Self-measurement is useful in distinguishing sustained hypertension from "white coat hypertension," a condition in which the patient's pressure is consistently elevated in the clinician's office but normal at other times. Self-measurement may also be used to assess the response to antihypertensive medications and as a tool to improve patient adherence to treatment. Ambulatory monitoring is useful for the evaluation of suspected white coat hypertension, patients with apparent drug resistance, hypotensive symptoms with antihypertensive medications, and episodic hypertension. However, ambulatory BP measurement is not appropriate for the routine evaluation of patients with suspected hypertension. In elderly patients, the possibility of **pseudohypertension** should always be considered in the diagnostic evaluation of possible hypertension. Pseudohypertension is a condition in which the indirect measurement of arterial pressure using a cuff sphygmomanometer is artificially high in comparison to direct intra-arterial pressure measurement. Failure to recognize pseudohypertension can result in unwarranted and sometimes frankly dangerous treatment. Pseudohypertension can result from Monckeberg's medial calcification (a clinically benign form of arterial calcification) or advanced atherosclerosis with widespread calcification of intimal plaques. In these entities, stiffening of the arterial wall may prevent its collapse by externally applied pressure, resulting in artificially high indirect BP readings affecting both systolic and diastolic measurements. The presence of a positive Osler's maneuver, in which the radial or brachial artery remains palpable despite being made pulseless by proximal inflation of a cuff above systolic pressure, is an important physical examination finding that should suggest the diagnosis. Roentgenograms of the extremities frequently reveal calcified vessels. The diagnosis can only be made definitely by a direct measurement of intra-arterial pressure. Patients with pseudohypertension are often elderly and therefore may have a critical limitation of blood flow to the brain or heart, such that inappropriate BP treatment may precipitate life-threatening ischemic events.

The initial history and physical examination of patients with documented hypertension should be designed to assess lifestyle, identify other cardiovascular risk factors, and identify the presence of target organ damage that may affect prognosis and impact treatment decisions (Table 15-2). Although the vast majority of hypertensive patients have essential (primary) hypertension without a clearly definable etiology, the initial evaluation is also designed to screen for identifiable causes of secondary hypertension (Table 15-3). A medical history should include information about prior BP measurements, to assess the duration of hypertension, and details about adverse effects from any prior antihypertensive therapy. History or symptoms of coronary heart disease, CHF, cerebrovascular disease, peripheral vascular disease, or renal disease should be carefully evaluated. Symptoms suggesting unusual secondary causes of hypertension should be queried, such as weakness (hyperaldosteronism) or episodic anxiety, headache, diaphoresis, and palpitations (pheochromocytoma). Information regarding other risk factors, such as diabetes, tobacco use, hyperlipidemia, physical activity, and any recent weight gain, should be obtained. Dietary assessment regarding the intake of salt, alcohol, and saturated fat is also important. Detailed information should be sought regarding all prescription and over-the-counter medication use, including herbal remedies and illicit drugs, some of which may raise BP or interfere with the effectiveness of antihypertensive therapy. For example, nonsteroidal anti-inflammatory drugs (NSAIDs) impair the response to virtually all antihypertensive agents and increase the risk of hyperkalemia or renal insufficiency with angiotensin-converting enzyme (ACE) inhibitor therapy. Stimulants such as cocaine, ephedra, amphetamines, and anabolic steroids can raise BP. A family history of hypertension, diabetes, premature cardiovascular disease, or renal disease should be sought. A psychosocial history is important to identify family situation, working conditions, employment status, educational level, and sexual dysfunction that may influence adherence to antihypertensive treatment.

Physical examination should include the measurement of height, weight, and calculation of BMI (weight in kilogram divided by the square of height in meters). Funduscopic examination is important to identify striate hemorrhages, cotton wool spots, and papilledema, the characteristic findings of hypertensive neuroretinopathy (HNR), which are indicative of the presence of malignant hypertension. Documentation of

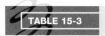

TABLE 15-3	Identifiable Causes of Hypertension

Metabolic syndrome (obesity, insulin resistance, impaired glucose tolerance, dyslipidemia, hypertension)
Obstructive sleep apnea
Drug-induced hypertension (Table 15-7)
Chronic kidney disease
Primary hyperaldosteronism
Renovascular disease
Chronic steroid use or Cushing's syndrome
Pheochromocytoma
Coarctation of the aorta
Thyroid or parathyroid disease

(Adapted with permission from Chobanian AV, Bakris GL, Black HR, et al. The seventh report of the Joint National Committee on Prevention, Detection, Evaluation and Treatment of High Blood Pressure. The JNC 7 Report. *JAMA* 2003;289:2560–2572.)

the presence of arteriosclerotic retinopathy (e.g., arteriolar narrowing, arteriovenous crossing changes, changes in light reflexes) is less important, given its lack of prognostic significance with regard to the potential long-term cardiovascular complications of hypertension. Examination of the neck for carotid bruits, distended neck veins, and thyromegaly is important. Cardiac examination should include investigation for abnormalities of rate or rhythm, murmurs, and third or fourth heart sounds. The lungs should be examined for rales and evidence of bronchospasm. Abdominal examination should include auscultation for bruits (an epigastric bruit present in both systole and diastole suggests renal artery stenosis), abdominal or flank masses (polycystic kidney disease), or increased aortic pulsation (abdominal aortic aneurysm). Peripheral pulses should be examined for quality and bruits. The lower extremities should be examined for edema. A neurologic screening examination is used to identify prior cerebrovascular events. Routine laboratory tests are recommended before the initiation of antihypertensive therapy to identify other risk factors and screen for the presence of target organ damage. These routine tests include blood chemistry (sodium, potassium, creatinine, fasting glucose), lipid profile [total cholesterol, low-density lipoprotein (LDL) and high-density lipoprotein (HDL) cholesterol], and a complete blood cell count. Creatinine clearance should be estimated using either the Cockcroft-Gault or the Modification of Diet in Renal Disease (MDRD) formulae. A urinalysis is used to identify proteinuria or hematuria that would suggest the presence of underlying primary renal disease. A 12-lead electrocardiogram (ECG) is used to identify left atrial enlargement, LVH, or prior MI. Optional tests, depending on the clinical situation, include 24-hour creatinine clearance, 24-hour urine protein or a spot urine protein to creatinine ratio, serum uric acid, glycosylated hemoglobin, and thyroid function tests. An echocardiogram to identify the presence of LVH may be useful in selected patients to determine the clinical significance of labile hypertension. Most patients with hypertension have primary (essential) hypertension in which no clearly definable underlying etiology is apparent.

A. In contrast, a wide variety of uncommon conditions can lead to so-called **secondary hypertension**, some of which are potentially amenable to surgical correction (Table 15-3). Secondary causes of hypertension include underlying chronic kidney disease (CKD), primary hyperaldosteronism (PHA), pheochromocytoma, renovascular hypertension due to fibromuscular dysplasia or atherosclerotic renal artery stenosis, coarctation of the aorta, and Cushing's syndrome. Secondary causes of hypertension amenable to surgical intervention are so uncommon that extensive diagnostic testing is not warranted. Secondary hypertension should be considered when the patient has onset of hypertension at an early age (younger than 30 years) or late age (older than 55 years); inadequate BP in a compliant patient on a three-drug regimen which includes a diuretic (resistant hypertension), previously well-controlled hypertension becomes uncontrolled in a compliant patient; hematuria or proteinuria (underlying renal disease) or elevated serum creatinine (renal disease or ischemic nephropathy due to bilateral renal artery stenosis). The initial history, physical examination, and routine laboratory tests are usually all that is required to evaluate for the possibility of secondary hypertension. A normal estimated creatinine clearance and urinalysis are sufficient to exclude underlying renal disease as a secondary cause of hypertension. Examination for abdominal or flank masses is used to screen for polycystic kidney disease, which can be confirmed by ultrasonographic examination. Because most patients with PHA have unprovoked hypokalemia while not on diuretic therapy, a measurement of serum potassium is a suitable screening test, and routine measurement of aldosterone levels or plasma aldosterone/renin ratio is not necessary. However, some patients with PHA are normokalemic (when not receiving diuretic therapy). Although routine screening of all patients with hypertension for PHA is not warranted, in a patient with drug-resistant hypertension or significant hypokalemia induced by low-dose diuretic therapy, the possibility of PHA should be considered. In this regard, patients with resistant hypertension due to PHA often have a dramatic BP response following the initiation of a mineralocorticoid antagonist (spironolactone or eplerenone). Assessment for any delay or diminution of pulses in the lower extremities, or a discrepancy between arm and leg BP can be used to screen for coarctation of the aorta. A careful assessment for a history of episodic hypertension, associated with headache, palpitations, diaphoresis, and pallor, is all that is usually required to screen for pheochromocytoma. The routine measurement of serum or urine catecholamines is not warranted. Likewise, evaluation for truncal obesity and abdominal purple striae is all that is usually required to screen for Cushing's syndrome; therefore, routine measurement of serum cortisol or cortisol suppression testing is unnecessary. Several tests are notably absent from the recommended list of routine screening tests for secondary hypertension. Hypertensive intravenous pyelography, renal scanning, captopril renography, and arterial digital subtraction angiography all lack sufficient specificity to be of any value as routine screening tests for renovascular hypertension. In this regard, the prevalence of renovascular hypertension in the general hypertensive population is so low that the predictive value of a positive test from any of these procedures is abysmal when used as a general screening test.

VI. TREATMENT OF HYPERTENSION

A. Goals of treatment. The goal of treating hypertension is the reduction of cardiovascular and renal morbidity and mortality. Because systolic BP correlates best with target organ damage and mortality, the primary focus should be on achieving the systolic BP goal. The goal of treatment is a systolic BP less than 140 mm Hg and a DBP less than 90 mm Hg. In hypertensive patients with diabetes or underlying CKD, a BP goal of less than 130/80 mm Hg is recommended.

B. Nonpharmacologic treatment. Lifestyle modification is recommended in the management of all individuals with hypertension, even in those who require antihypertensive drug treatment. All patients should be encouraged to adopt the lifestyle modifications outlined in Table 15-4, especially if they have additional cardiovascular risk factors such as hyperlipidemia or diabetes. Modest weight

| TABLE 15-4 | Lifestyle Modifications to Manage Hypertension |

Modification	Recommendation	Approximate SBP reduction
Weight loss	Maintain normal weight (BMI[a] 18.5–24.9)	5–20 mm Hg/10 kg
Dietary sodium restriction	Limit dietary sodium intake to <100 mEq/d (2.4 g sodium or 6 g sodium chloride)	2–8 mm Hg
Adopt DASH diet	Consume diet rich in fruits, vegetables, and low-fat dairy products with a reduced content of saturated and total fat	8–14 mm Hg
Increase physical activity	Engage in regular aerobic physical activity such as brisk walking (at least 30 min/d, most days of the week)	4–9 mm Hg
Moderate alcohol consumption	Limit consumption to no more than two drinks per day (1 oz or 30 mL ethanol per d; e.g., 24 oz beer, 10 oz wine, 3 oz 80-proof whiskey) in most men, and no more than one drink per day in women and lighter-weight men	2–4 mm Hg

BMI, body mass index; DASH, Dietary Approaches to Stop Hypertension; SBP, systolic blood pressure.
[a]BMI indicates body mass index calculated as weight in kilograms divided by the square of height in meters.
(Adapted with permission from Chobanian AV, Bakris GL, Black HR, et al. The seventh report of the Joint National Committee on Prevention, Detection, Evaluation and Treatment of High Blood Pressure. The JNC 7 Report. *JAMA* 2003;289:2560–2572.)

reduction of as little as 4 kg (10 lb) significantly reduces BP. Anorectic agents should be avoided because they may contain stimulants that raise BP. Obstructive sleep apnea (OSA) is now recognized as an important treatable cause of hypertension. Clues to the presence of OSA include morbid obesity, daytime hypersomnolence, headache, snoring, or fitful sleep. The diagnosis can be confirmed with a sleep study to document apneic episodes. Appropriate treatment with a continuous positive airway pressure (CPAP) device may result in a significant reduction in BP. Dietary sodium intake in the form of sodium chloride (NaCl; table salt) has a strong epidemiologic link to hypertension. Meta-analysis of clinical trials indicates that the limitation of dietary sodium intake to 75 to 100 mEq per day lowers BP over a period of several weeks to a few years. The restriction of sodium intake has been shown to reduce the need for antihypertensive medication, reduce diuretic-induced renal potassium wasting, lead to regression of LVH, and prevent renal stones through a reduction in renal calcium excretion. Average American dietary sodium intake is in excess of 150 mEq per day, most of which (75%) is derived from processed foods. Moderation of sodium intake to a level of less than 100 mEq per day (2.4 g of sodium or 6 g of sodium chloride) is recommended for the nonpharmacologic treatment of hypertension.

Excessive intake of ethanol is an important risk factor for high BP, and it can lead to resistant hypertension. Ethanol intake should be limited to not more than 30 mL (1 oz) per day in men and 15 mL (0.5 oz) per day in women and lighter-weight men. This type of moderate ethanol intake may be associated with a reduction in risk of coronary heart disease.

Regular aerobic exercise can enhance weight loss and reduce the risk for cardiovascular disease and all-cause mortality.

Inadequate potassium intake may increase BP, whereas high dietary potassium intake may improve BP control in patients with hypertension. An intake of 90 mEq per day in the form of fresh fruits and vegetables should be recommended.

An increase in dietary calcium may lower BP in some patients with hypertension, but the effect is negligible. Nonetheless, adequate calcium intake is recommended for general health and osteoporosis prophylaxis.

Smoking cessation and reductions in dietary fat and cholesterol are also recommended to reduce overall cardiovascular risk. Although caffeine may acutely raise BP, tolerance to this effect develops quickly. Most epidemiologic studies have found no direct relationship between caffeine intake and BP.

C. Pharmacologic treatment of hypertension. The decision to treat hypertension with medications after the failure of lifestyle modifications to adequately control BP or initially, as an adjunct to lifestyle modifications, is based on the severity (stage) of hypertension and an assessment of the risk of cardiovascular morbidity, given the presence of other cardiovascular risk factors and preexisting target organ damage or cardiovascular disease (Table 15-2). Reducing BP with drugs clearly decreases cardiovascular morbidity and mortality regardless of age, gender, race, stage of hypertension, or socioeconomic status. Benefit has been demonstrated for stroke, coronary events, heart failure, progression of primary renal disease, prevention of progression to malignant hypertension, and all-cause mortality. Numerous clinical trials have demonstrated that lowering BP with several classes of drugs, including thiazide-type diuretics, ACE inhibitors, angiotensin receptor blockers (ARBs), β-blockers, and calcium channel blockers (CCBs), reduces all the complications of hypertension. Thiazide-type diuretics have been the treatment regimen employed in most large-scale outcome trials. In these trials, including the pivotal Antihypertensive and Lipid Lowering Treatment to Prevent Heart Attack Trial (ALLHAT), thiazide diuretics are unsurpassed in antihypertensive efficacy and for prevention of the cardiovascular complications of hypertension. In ALLHAT, stage 1 or 2 hypertensive patients older than 55 years, with at least one other cardiovascular risk factor, received first-line treatment with chlorthalidone (thiazide-type diuretic), doxazocin (selective α-blocker), amlodipine (CCB), or lisinopril (ACE inhibitor). In this study, 47% of patients were women, 35% were black, 19% were Hispanic, 36% were diabetic, and the mean BMI was approximately 30. The doxazocin arm was terminated prematurely because of an excess risk of CHF. After a mean follow-up of 4.9 years, neither the primary clinical outcome (fatal coronary heart disease or nonfatal MI) nor the secondary outcomes of all-cause mortality, combined coronary heart disease, peripheral arterial disease, cancer, or ESRD had occurred more often in the clorthalidone group than in the amlodipine or lisinopril groups. Furthermore, event rates were significantly lower in the chlorthalidone group than in one or both of the other groups for some of the secondary outcomes (Table 15-5). As expected, patients in the chlorthalidone group developed higher cholesterol levels, lower serum potassium levels, and higher fasting blood glucose levels than patients in other groups. The mean cholesterol was 216 mg per dL at baseline, falling at 4 years to 197 mg per dL in the chlorthalidone group, to 196 mg per dL in the amlodipine group ($p = 0.009$ versus chlorthalidone), and to 195 mg per dL in the lisinopril group ($p < 0.001$ versus chlorthalidone). At 4 years, 8.5% of the chlorthalidone group had developed hypokalemia (serum potassium less than 3.5 mEq per L) compared with 1.9% in the amlodipine group ($p < 0.001$) and 0.8% in the lisinopril group ($p < 0.001$). The incidence of new-onset diabetes (fasting blood glucose greater than 126 mg per dL) was 11.6% with chlorthalidone compared with 9.8% in the amlodipine group ($p = 0.04$) and 8.1% in the lisinopril group ($p < 0.001$). Nonetheless, the presence of these metabolic abnormalities did not translate into more cardiovascular events or deaths in the chlorthalidone group. The public health implications of ALLHAT are enormous. The *2002 Drug Topics Red Book* indicates that generic chlorthalidone costs $15.95 for 100 tablets compared with $97.96 for lisinopril (Prinavil) 10 mg, $102.76 for lisinopril (Zestril) 10 mg, and $145.13 for amlodipine (Norvasc) 5 mg. Using the less expensive generic diuretic to treat the more than 65 million hypertensive patients in the United States could lead to cost savings of billions of dollars annually. On the basis of the results of the ALLHAT and other trials,

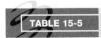

| **TABLE 15-5** | **Results of the Antihypertensive Lipid-Lowering to Prevent Heart Attack Trial** |

Outcome	6-Yr incidence (%)		
	Chlorthalidone	Amlodipine	Lisinopril
Primary outcome			
Coronary heart disease[a]	11.5	11.3	11.4
Secondary outcomes			
All-cause mortality	17.3	16.8	17.2
Stroke	5.6	5.4	6.3[b]
Combined coronary heart disease[c]	19.9	19.9	20.8
Combined cardiovascular disease[d]	30.9	32.0	33.3[b]
Angina	12.1	12.6	13.6[b]
Coronary revascularization	9.2	10.0	10.2[b]
Heart failure	7.7	10.2[b]	8.7[b]
End-stage renal disease	1.8	2.1	2.0
Cancer	9.7	10.0	9.9

[a] Fatal coronary heart disease or nonfatal myocardial infarction.
[b] $p \leq 0.05$.
[c] Combined coronary heart disease death, nonfatal myocardial infarction, coronary revascularization, and hospitalized angina.
[d] Combined coronary heart disease death, nonfatal myocardial infarction, coronary revascularization, angina, heart failure, and peripheral arterial disease.
(Adapted with permission from The ALLHAT Officers and Coordinators for the ALLHAT Collaborative Research Group. Major outcomes in high-risk hypertensive patients randomized to angiotensin-converting enzyme inhibitor or calcium channel blocker vs. diuretic. The Antihypertensive and Lipid-Lowering Treatment to Prevent Heart Attack Trial (ALLHAT). *JAMA* 2002;288:2981–2997.)

the JNC 7 report has recommended that thiazide-type diuretics should be used as initial therapy for most patients with hypertension, either alone or in combination with one of the other classes of drugs (ACE inhibitors, ARBs, β-blockers, or CCBs). An algorithm outlining the approach to treatment of hypertension is shown in Figure 15-2. Diuretic therapy potentiates the antihypertensive effect of most other antihypertensive drugs. For this reason, the drug treatment algorithm outlined in JNC 7 recommends the addition of diuretic as a second-step agent if BP is inadequately controlled with any other drug chosen as a first-line agent. The mechanism of action of thiazide diuretics is to block sodium reabsorption by inhibiting the thiazide-sensitive NaCl cotransporter in the distal tubule. The sustained antihypertensive effect of thiazides, however, is mediated through a reduction in SVR rather than through chronic volume depletion and a reduction of cardiac output, as one might predict. In fact, thiazides do not cause a large, sustained decrease in intravascular volume or negative sodium balance when used for the treatment of hypertension. Within a few days to weeks of the initiation of therapy with thiazide diuretics, salt balance returns toward normal, and total body sodium and intravascular volume returns toward pretreatment levels. This seeming paradox can be understood in the context of Guyton's hypothesis regarding the

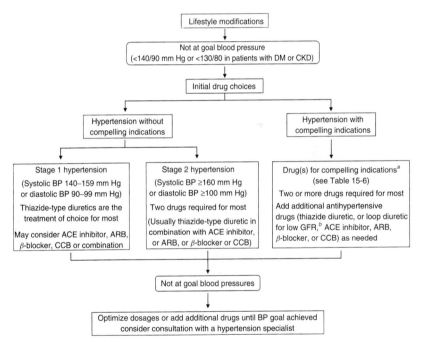

Figure 15-2. Algorithm for treatment of hypertension. [a]Compelling indications are special high-risk conditions for which clinical trials demonstrate benefit of specific classes of antihypertensive drugs: treatment of hypertension in the setting of diabetes, chronic kidney disease, heart failure, high coronary disease risk, post-MI, and for recurrent stroke prevention. [b]In the setting of advanced chronic kidney disease with GFR less than 30 mL per minute or in patients with fluid overload unresponsive to thiazide diuretics, more potent loop diuretic therapy may be required. (ACE, angiotensin-converting enzyme; ARB, angiotensin receptor blocker; BP, blood pressure; CCB, calcium channel blocker; CKD, chronic kidney disease; DM, diabetes mellitus; GFR, glomerular filtration rate.) (Adapted with permission from Chobanian AV, Bakris GL, Black HR, et al. The seventh report of the Joint National Committee on Prevention, Detection, Evaluation and Treatment of High Blood Pressure. The JNC 7 Report. *JAMA* 2003;289:2560–2572.)

pathogenesis of hypertension, whereby the development of systemic hypertension is conceptualized as an essential protective mechanism to maintain normal fluid volume in various disease states in which an underlying renal impairment exists with regard to excreting the daily sodium load at a normal BP (Fig. 15-2). In this context, diuretics lower BP by addressing the primary renal defect in salt excretion, so that systemic hypertension (high SVR) is no longer a prerequisite for maintaining sodium balance. It should be noted that in ALLHAT and most clinical trials, achievement of the desired BP goal often requires treatment with two or more antihypertensive agents. Addition of a second drug from a different class should be implemented when use of a single drug in optimal doses fails to adequately control BP. When the BP is more than 20 mm Hg systolic or 10 mm Hg diastolic above goal, treatment may be initiated with two drugs (usually including a thiazide-type diuretic), either as separate prescriptions or in fixed-dose combinations.

D. Treatment of hypertension in special populations. The presence of certain comorbidities or target organ damage in the individual hypertensive patient may provide a compelling indication for treatment with a certain class of antihypertensive agent, based on favorable outcome data from clinical trials (Table 15-6). In hypertensive patients with diabetes mellitus, thiazide diuretics, β-blockers, ACE inhibitors, ARBs, and CCBs have been shown to reduce cardiovascular disease and the incidence of stroke. In patients with evidence of diabetic nephropathy, ACE inhibitor- or ARB-based treatment regimens have been shown to retard the progression of nephropathy, reduce urine albumin excretion, and slow progression from microalbuminuria to overt proteinuria. CKD is present in patients with estimated glomerular filtration rate (GFR) less than 60 mL per minute or if albuminuria (greater than 300 mg per day or 200 mg albumin per g creatinine on spot urine specimen) is present. ACE inhibitors and ARBs have been shown to slow the progression of both diabetic and nondiabetic CKD. Therefore, these agents should be included as part of the multidrug regimen often required for adequate BP control in CKD. Potent loop diuretics are usually needed in combination with other classes of drugs when the estimated GFR falls below 30 mL per minute. LVH is an independent risk factor for subsequent cardiovascular disease. Regression of LVH occurs with aggressive BP management using all classes of drugs except the direct-acting vasodilators such as hydralazine and minoxidil. Ischemic heart disease is a common form of target organ damage in hypertension. In patients with hypertension and stable angina pectoris, the treatment regimen should include a β-blocker or, alternatively, a long-acting CCB. In patients with acute coronary syndromes (unstable angina or acute MI), hypertension should be treated initially with β-blockers and ACE inhibitors, with the addition of other agents such as thiazide diuretics as needed for BP control. In the chronic BP management of post-MI patients, β-blockers, ACE inhibitors, and aldosterone receptor antagonists have proven to be of highest benefit. In patients with ischemic heart disease, low-dose aspirin therapy and intensive lipid lowering therapy are also indicated. Heart failure represents another special hypertensive patient population; it can occur in the setting of either systolic or diastolic dysfunction. In asymptomatic patients with LV dysfunction, ACE inhibitors and β-blockers are recommended. In patients with symptomatic heart failure or end-stage heart disease, ACE inhibitors, β-blockers, ARBs, and aldosterone receptor blockers (spironolactone or eplerenone) are recommended, along with potent loop diuretics as needed for fluid overload. Treatment of hypertension in patients with cerebrovascular disease requires special consideration. Lowering of BP during the acute phase of an ischemic stroke may worsen ischemia and extend the infarct. However, treatment of chronic hypertension following a cerebrovascular accident with ACE inhibitors and thiazide-type diuretics may reduce the rate of recurrent stroke. The treatment of elderly patients with predominant systolic hypertension should follow the same treatment algorithm. In the Systolic Hypertension in the Elderly Program (SHEP) trial, a double-blind placebo-controlled trial of low-dose chlorthalidone in patients older than 60 years with isolated systolic hypertension (systolic BP greater than 160 mm Hg with DBP less than 90 mm Hg), the relative risks (RRs) of stroke, left ventricular failure,

TABLE 15-6   Clinical Trial and Guideline Basis for Compelling Indications for Treatment with Individual Drug Classes

High-risk condition with compelling indication	Diuretic	β-Blocker	ACE inhibitor	ARB	CCB	Aldosterone antagonist	Clinical trial basis[a]
Diabetes mellitus	■	■	■	■	■	—	ALLHAT, UKPDS, NKF Guideline, ADA Guideline
Chronic kidney disease	—	—	■	■	—	—	Captopril Trial, RENAAL, IDNT, REIN, AASK, NKF Guideline
Heart failure	■	■	■	■	—	■	ACC/AHA Heart Failure Guideline, MERIT-HF, COPERNICUS, CIBIS, SOLVD, AIRE, TRACE, ValHEFT, RALES
High coronary disease risk	■	■	■	—	■	—	ALLHAT, HOPE, ANBP2, LIFE, CONVINCE
Postmyocardial infarction	—	■	■	—	—	■	ACC/AHA Post-MI Guideline, BHAT, SAVE, Capricorn, EPHESUS
Recurrent stroke prevention	■	—	■	—	—	—	PROGRESS

ACC/AHA, American College of Cardiology/American Heart Association; ACE, angiotensin-converting enzyme; ADA, American Diabetes Association; AIRE, Acute Infarction Ramipril Efficacy; ARB, angiotensin receptor blocker; ALLHAT, Antihypertensive and Lipid-Lowering to Prevent Heart Attack Trial; ANBP2, Second Australian National Blood Pressure Study; BHAT, β-Blocker Heart Attack Trial; CCB, calcium channel blocker; CIBIS, Cardiac Insufficiency Bisoprolol Study; CONVINCE, Controlled Onset Verapamil Investigation of Cardiovascular Endpoints; COPERNICUS, Carvedilol Prospective Randomized Cumulative Survival Study; EPHESUS, Eplerenone Post-Acute Myocardial Infarction Heart Failure Efficacy and Survival Study; HOPE, Heart Outcomes Prevention Evaluation Study; INDT, Irbesartan Diabetic Nephropathy Trial; LIFE, Losartan Intervention for Endpoint Reduction in Hypertension Study; MERIT-HT, Metoprolol CR/SL Randomized Intervention Trial in Congestive Heart Failure; MI, myocardial infection; NKF, National Kidney Foundation; PROGRESS, Perindopril Protection against Recurrent Stroke Study; RALES, Randomized Aldactone Evaluation Study; REIN, Ramipril Efficacy in Nephropathy Study; RENAAL, Reduction of Endpoints in Noninsulin Dependent Diabetes Mellitus with the Angiotensin II Antagonist Losartan Study; SAVE, Survival and Ventricular Enlargement Study; SOLVD, Studies of Left Ventricular Dysfunction; TRACE, Trandolapril Cardiac Evaluation Study; UKPDS, United Kingdom Prospective Diabetes Study; ValHEFT, Valsartan Heart Failure Trial.

[a]Compelling indications for certain classes of antihypertensive drugs are based on proven benefit from outcome studies or existing clinical practice guidelines. The compelling indication must be managed in parallel with blood pressure. Patients with these high-risk conditions usually require combination treatment with two to three additional antihypertensive drugs from different classes in order to achieve the recommended blood pressure treatment goal.

(Adapted from Chobanian AV, Bakris GL, Black HR, et al. The seventh report of the Joint National Committee on Prevention, Detection, Evaluation and Treatment of High Blood Pressure. The JNC 7 Report. JAMA 2003;289:2560–2572.)

nonfatal MI or fatal coronary heart disease, and the requirement for coronary artery bypass grafting were all significantly reduced in the active treatment group. Because of the risks of orthostatic hypotension and falls, selective α-blockers should be avoided in the treatment of older individuals with hypertension.

E. **Treatment of hypertension in patients with metabolic syndrome.** In the past, concerns have often been raised that diuretics should not be used as first-line therapy for hypertension because they have unfavorable effects on insulin sensitivity and increase the risk of new-onset diabetes, thereby having the potential to adversely effect cardiovascular and renal outcomes. CCBs, which are metabolically neutral, and ACE inhibitors and ARBs, which improve insulin sensitivity, are therefore considered by many to be superior initial pharmacologic choices for treatment of hypertension. In a recently published subgroup analysis from ALLHAT, metabolic, cardiovascular, and renal outcomes were compared in individuals assigned to initial treatment with thiazide-like diuretic (chlorthalidone), a CCB (CCB, amlodipine), or and ACE inhibitor (lisinopril) in nondiabetic individuals with or without metabolic syndrome. The metabolic syndrome is a clustering of clinical and biochemical characteristics related to insulin resistance and hyperinsulinemia. It is characterized by hypertension, central obesity, dyslipidemia (high triglycerides and low HDL cholesterol levels), and elevated glucose levels. It is estimated that more than 40% of adults older than 60 years in the United States now have this disorder. In this analysis of ALLHAT data, metabolic syndrome was defined by the presence of hypertension plus at least two of the following: BMI greater than or equal to 30 kg per m^2, fasting triglycerides greater than 150 mg per dL, or HDL cholesterol less than 40 mg per dL in men and less than 50 mg per dL in women. Participants with baseline fasting glucose greater than 126 mg per dL or a history of diabetes were excluded. In study participants with metabolic syndrome, at 4 years of follow-up, the incidence of newly diagnosed diabetes (fasting glucose greater than 126 mg per dL) was 17.1% for chlorthalidone, 16.0% for amlodipine ($p = 0.49$ versus chlorthalidone), and 12.6% for lisinopril ($p < 0.05$ versus chlorthalidone). For those without metabolic syndrome, the rate of newly diagnosed diabetes was 7.7% for chlorthalidone, 4.2% for amlodipine, and 4.7% for lisinopril ($p < 0.05$ for both drugs versus chlorthalidone). Among participants with metabolic syndrome, the RRs for the primary outcome (fatal coronary heart disease or nonfatal MI) and the secondary cardiovascular outcomes were not different for amlodipine versus chlorthalidone. However, the risk of heart failure was higher in participants without metabolic syndrome treated with amlodipine [RR for amlodipine versus cholorthalidone, 1.55; 95% confidence interval (CI) 1.25-1.35]. In participants with metabolic syndrome, outcomes were superior with chlorthalidone versus lisinopril for heart failure (RR 1.31; 95% CI, 1.04-1.64) and for the combined cardiovascular disease endpoint (coronary heart disease, stroke, treated angina and heart failure; RR, 1.19; 95% CI, 1.07-1.32). The authors conclude that despite a less favorable metabolic profile, and a higher risk of new-onset diabetes, thiazide-like diuretics are the preferred initial treatment for hypertension in older individuals with the metabolic syndrome, compared with ACE inhibitors and CCBs. Another recent *post hoc* analysis from ALLHAT examined clinical outcomes by race in hypertensive patients with and without metabolic syndrome. Although there were no differences among the four treatment groups (chlorthalidone, amlodipine, lisinopril, and doxazocin) with regard to the primary endpoint (fatal coronary heart disease or nonfatal MI), all three of the newer antihypertensive drugs showed significantly higher rates of heart failure compared with chlorthalidone in metabolic syndrome patients and the results were particularly striking in black participants with metabolic syndrome. The RR for CHF among black subjects with metabolic syndrome was higher for all three newer antihypertensive drugs compared to chlorthalidone (amlodipine, RR 1.5, 95% CI, 1.18-1.90; lisinopril, RR 1.49, 95% CI, 1.17-1.90; doxazocin, RR 1.88, 95% CI, 1.42-2.47). Among black participants, higher rates for combined cardiovascular disease (coronary heart disease, stroke, treated angina, heart failure, or peripheral arterial disease) were observed with lisinopril (RR 1.25, 85% CI, 1.09-1.40) and doxazosin (RR 1.37, 95%

CI, 1.19-1.58) compared with chlorthalidone. Higher rates of stroke were seen with lisinopril (RR 1.37, 95% CI, 1.07-1.76) and doxazosin (RR 1.49, 95% CI, 1.09-2.03) compared with chlorthalidone only in black participants with metabolic syndrome. Remarkably, black patients with metabolic syndrome also had higher rates of ESRD with lisinopril treatment compared with chlorthalidone (RR 1.70, 95% CI, 1.13-2.55). The authors conclude that the magnitude of the excess risk of ESRD (70%), heart failure (49%), and stroke (37%) as well as the increased risk of combined cardiovascular disease strongly argue against the preferential use of ACE inhibitors over diuretics as initial antihypertensive treatment in black patients with metabolic syndrome.

F. **Treatment of hypertension in patients with diabetes.** Another recent *post hoc* analysis of ALLHAT data assessed the effect of initial antihypertensive treatment with thiazide-type diuretic (chlorthalidone), ACE inhibitor (lisinopril), or CCB (amlodipine) in subgroups of participants with diabetes (history of treatment with oral hypoglycemics or insulin or fasting blood glucose greater than 126 mg per dL) or impaired fasting glucose (IFG, fasting glucose between 110 and 125 mg per dL and no history of diabetes). There was no significant difference in RR for the primary outcome (fatal coronary heart disease or nonfatal MI) in patients with diabetes treated with amlodipine or lisinopril compared with chlorthalidone or in participants with IFG treated with lisinopril versus chlorthalidone. However, a significantly higher RR of the primary outcome was noted in patients treated with amlodipine compared with chlorthalidone (RR 1.73, 95% CI, 1.10-2.72). Heart failure was more common among diabetic patients treated with amlodipine (RR 1.39, 95% CI, 1.22-159) or lisinopril (RR 1.15, 95% CI, 1.00-1.32) compared to chlorthalidone. The ALLHAT findings suggest that thiazide-type diuretics should be strongly considered as first-step agents for treatment of hypertension in patients with diabetes mellitus or IFG. Moreover, the results provide no evidence of superiority for treatment with CCBs or ACE inhibitors in patients with diabetes or IFG.

The Appropriate Blood Pressure Control in Diabetes (ABCD) study was a randomized prospective intervention clinical trial with 5 years of follow-up that examined the role of intensive (goal DBP 75 mm Hg) versus standard (goal DBP 80 to 90 mm Hg) BP control in 950 patients with type 2 diabetes. Within each BP treatment goal group, patients were randomly assigned to treatment with a long-acting dihydropyridine CCB (nisoldipine) or an ACE inhibitor (enalapril). In hypertensive diabetic subjects enrolled in the ABCD study, a significant decrease in mortality was found in the intensive BP control group compared with the standard BP control group. In normotensive diabetic patients, intensive BP control also resulted in significant slowing of the progression of nephropathy (as assessed by urinary albumin excretion) and retinopathy, and was associated with fewer strokes. This occurred independently whether the initial BP treatment was with enalapril or nisoldipine. Importantly, after 4 years of follow-up, the ABCD Data and Safety Monitoring Committee halted the comparison between nisoldipine and enalapril in the hypertensive diabetic cohort because significantly fewer MIs occurred in patients with diabetes allocated to initial therapy with the ACE inhibitor enalapril. The ABCD results indicate that intensive BP control reduces all-cause mortality in diabetic patients and that ACE inhibitor therapy should be preferred over CCB therapy as part of the multidrug regimen often required for intensive treatment of hypertension in diabetic patients.

G. **Treatment of hypertension in patients with CKD.** Evidence is accumulating that strict control of BP is beneficial in slowing the rate of progression of both diabetic nephropathy and nondiabetic renal disease. Furthermore, animal and human studies have shown that progression of renal disease may be exacerbated by secondary hemodynamic factors such as intraglomerular hypertension. Therefore, a vital component of the treatment of hypertension in patients with CKD, especially those with proteinuria, is the administration of an ACE inhibitor as part of a multidrug regimen not only to optimally control BP but also with the goal of slowing the progressive loss of renal function. In the Benazepril trial, patients already in reasonable BP control were randomized to treatment with benazepril or placebo. Patients on benazepril had a greater reduction in BP and a 25% reduction in protein excretion. The risk of progression to a primary endpoint (doubling of serum creatinine or progression to dialysis) was reduced by 53% in the benazepril-treated patients. The benefits of ACE inhibitor therapy were seen mainly in patients with chronic glomerular diseases or diabetic nephropathy; whereas there was no benefit in patients with polycystic kidney disease or other CKD excreting less than 1 g of protein per day (two settings in which hemodynamically mediated factors may not be as important in disease progression). In the Ramipril Efficacy in Nephropathy (REIN) trial, patients with nondiabetic renal disease were randomized to ramipril or placebo plus other antihypertensive therapy as needed to achieve DBP below 90 mm Hg. The trial was terminated prematurely among patients excreting more than 3 g protein per day because of a significant benefit with ACE inhibitor treatment with regard to ameliorating the rate of decline of renal function. The African American Study of Kidney Disease and Hypertension (AASK) suggested that ACE inhibitor (ramipril) was more effective in slowing the progression of benign hypertensive nephrosclerosis in blacks than amlodipine or metoprolol [70]. Although the final results of the AASK trial showed no difference among the drug treatment groups in the rate of decline of GFR, the ramipril group had a 22% reduction in risk of the composite endpoint (reduction in GFR by more than 50% from baseline, ESRD, or death). In the REIN-2 trial, dihydropyridine calcium channel blocker (CCB) failed to provide renoprotection in patients with nondiabetic renal disease, despite further reduction of BP from that obtained with fixed doses of ACE inhibitors. The nondihydropyridine CCBs (diltiazem and verapamil) have antiproteinuric effects, whereas the dihydropyridines (amlodipine and nifedipine) have been shown to increase proteinuria in some studies. This paradox may be explained by the varied effect of the different classes of CCBs on renal autoregulation. In this regard, dihydropyridines cause preferential afferent arteriolar dilatation, which allows more of the systemic pressure to be transmitted to the glomerulus, thereby increasing glomerular pressure and limiting their antiproteinuric effect.

The National Kidney Foundation Kidney Disease Outcomes Quality Initiative (K/DOQI) work group on hypertension and antihypertensive agents in CKD recommends that either an ACE inhibitor or an ARB should be used as first-line antihypertensive therapy in proteinuric patients with both diabetic and nondiabetic renal disease. Although the available evidence is strongest for ACE inhibitors, ARBs may be substituted in patients who develop cough during treatment with ACE inhibitors. Although the issue is not as well studied in nondiabetic renal disease, ARBs appear to have similar antiproteinuric activity compared to ACE inhibitors and also significantly slow disease progression in patients with type 2 diabetes and nephropathy. Combination therapy with ACE inhibitor and ARB may also be beneficial given their additive antiproteinuric effect. The optimal goal is to reduce protein excretion to less than 500 to 1,000 mg per day if possible. A multidrug antihypertensive regimen is usually required to achieve the goal of reduction of BP below 130/80 mm Hg. If this BP goal is not achieved after initial therapy with an ACE inhibitor or an ARB, a diuretic should be added to the regimen. Addition of a diuretic is logical therapy given the central role of impaired natriuresis in the pathogenesis of hypertension in the setting of CKD. Thiazide diuretics may be effective in the early stages of CKD, whereas loop diuretics may be necessary in patients with more advanced kidney disease or diuretic resistance in the setting of nephrotic syndrome. If the BP goal is not achieved with combination ACE inhibitor and diuretic therapy, additional drugs may be added to the regimen including a β-blocker or a nondihydropyridine CCB (diltiazem or verapamil). Hydralazine or minoxidil (in combination with appropriate doses of β-blocker to control heart rate and diuretic to prevent fluid retention) may be added to the regimen in patients with resistant hypertension.

H. Treatment of the patient with resistant hypertension. Resistant hypertension is defined as a failure to reach BP less than 140/90 mm Hg in an adherent patient treated with a three-drug regimen including a diuretic. Truly resistant hypertension should prompt an investigation for underlying potentially treatable

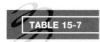

TABLE 15-7	Causes of Resistant Hypertension

Improper blood pressure (BP) measurement (use of inadequately sized BP cuff in obese patients)
Pseudohypertension in elderly individuals
White coat (office) hypertension
Volume overload or pseudotolerance
  Excess dietary sodium intake
  Fluid retention from underlying renal disease
  Inadequate diuretic therapy (failure to use loop diuretic with advanced CKD)
Noncompliance
  Patient nonadherence with therapy due to ignorance, cost, or side effects
  Physician noncompliance (inadequate drug dosage or failure to include diuretic in regimen)
Drug-induced
  Nonsteroidal anti-inflammatory agents (NSAIDs) or cyclooxygenase 2 (Cox 2) inhibitors
  Cocaine, amphetamines, or other illicit drugs
  Sympathomimetics (decongestants or anoretic agents)
  Oral contraceptives
  Adrenal steroids
  Erythropoietin
  Licorice
  Over-the-counter dietary supplements (ephedra, ma huang, bitter orange)
Excessive alcohol consumption
Identifiable secondary causes of hypertension (Table 15-3)

CKD, chronic kidney disease

forms of secondary hypertension (Table 15-3). Table 15-7 outlines other causes of resistant hypertension. Consultation with a hypertension specialist should be considered if the BP goal cannot be achieved.

VII. BENIGN VERSUS MALIGNANT HYPERTENSION. The classification of hypertension as benign or malignant is based on funduscopic examination. The finding of hypertensive neuroretinopathy (HNR) is the clinical *sine qua non* for the diagnosis of malignant hypertension (Fig. 15-3). In the absence of HNR, malignant hypertension cannot be diagnosed, regardless of the severity of the hypertension. HNR is defined by the presence of striate hemorrhages and cotton wool spots with or without papilledema (Table 15-8). The clinical importance of the finding of HNR is that it signifies the presence of a systemic hypertensive vasculopathy with fibrinoid necrosis and obliterative arteriopathy that, left untreated, will lead to ESRD or death within 1 year. Fortunately, malignant hypertension is a relatively rare disorder, occurring in less than 1% of hypertensive patients. The term *benign hypertension* is clearly a misnomer, because although the clinical course is less dramatic and precipitous than that seen in patients with malignant hypertension, the eventual cerebrovascular and cardiovascular complications are quite devastating, and they represent a major cause of morbidity and mortality in the general population. Benign hypertension is defined based on the absence of HNR. Retinal arteriosclerosis and arteriosclerotic retinopathy (Table 15-8), which are the characteristic funduscopic findings in benign hypertension, are of little clinical utility, because they may be found in elderly normotensive individuals. These findings have no predictive value with regard to the risk of cardiovascular or cerebrovascular complications.

A. Definition of hypertensive crises. The vast majority of hypertensive patients are asymptomatic for many years until complications due to atherosclerosis, cerebrovascular disease, or CHF supervene. In a minority of patients, this "benign" course is punctuated by a hypertensive crisis. A hypertensive crisis is defined as the turning point in the course of an illness at which acute management of the elevated

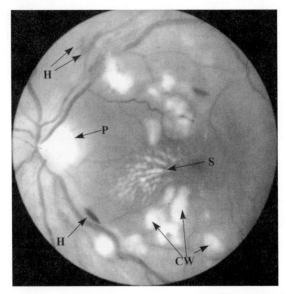

Figure 15-3. Hypertensive neuroretinopathy in malignant hypertension. Fundus photograph in a 30-year-old man with malignant hypertension demonstrates all the characteristic features of hypertensive neuroretinopathy, including striate hemorrhages (*H*), cotton wool spots (*CW*), papilledema (*P*), and a star figure at the macula (*S*).

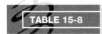

TABLE 15-8	**Classification of Hypertensive Retinopathy**

Retinal arteriosclerosis and arteriosclerotic retinopathy (characteristic of benign hypertension)
    Arteriolar narrowing (focal or diffuse)
    Arteriovenous crossing changes
    Broadening of the arteriolar light reflex
    Copper or silver wiring changes
    Perivasculitis
    Solitary round retinal hemorrhages
    Hard exudates
    Central or branch venous occlusion
Hypertensive neuroretinopathy (*sine qua non* of malignant hypertension)
    Generalized arteriolar narrowing
    Striate (flame-shaped hemorrhages)[a]
    Cotton wool spots (soft exudates)[a]
    Bilateral papilledema[a]
    Star figure at the macula

[a]These features distinguish retinal arteriosclerosis (benign hypertension) from hypertensive neuroretinopathy (malignant hypertension).
(Adapted with permission from Nolan CR. Malignant hypertension and other hypertensive crises. In: Schrier RW, ed. *Diseases of the kidney and urinary tract*, 8th ed. Boston: Lippincott Williams & Wilkins, 2007:1370–1436.)

BP plays a decisive role in the eventual outcome. The haste with which the BP must be controlled varies with the type of hypertensive crisis. However, the crucial role of hypertension in the disease process must be identified and a plan for managing the BP successfully implemented if the patient's outcome is to be optimal. The absolute level of the BP is clearly not the most important factor in determining the existence of a hypertensive crisis. For example, in children, pregnant women, and other previously normotensive individuals in whom mild to moderate hypertension develops suddenly, a hypertensive crisis can occur at a BP level that is normally well tolerated by adults with chronic hypertension. Furthermore, in adults with mild to moderate hypertension, a crisis can occur with the onset of acute end-organ dysfunction involving the heart or brain. Table 15-9 outlines the spectrum of hypertensive crises.

B. Malignant hypertension is a clinical syndrome characterized by a marked elevation of BP with widespread acute arteriolar injury (hypertensive vasculopathy). Funduscopy reveals HNR with flame-shaped hemorrhages, cotton wool spots (soft exudates), and sometimes papilledema (Fig. 15-3). Regardless of the severity of BP elevation, in the absence of HNR, malignant hypertension cannot be diagnosed. HNR is therefore an extremely important clinical finding, indicating the presence of a hypertension-induced arteriolitis that may involve the kidneys, heart, and central nervous system. With malignant hypertension, a rapid and relentless progression to ESRD occurs if effective BP control is not implemented. Mortality can

---

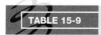 **TABLE 15-9**   **Spectrum of Hypertensive Crises**

Malignant hypertension (*hypertensive neuroretinopathy present*)
Hypertensive encephalopathy (*occurs with either malignant or severe benign hypertension*)
Nonmalignant ("benign") hypertension with acute complications (*acute end-organ dysfunction in the absence of hypertensive neuroretinopathy*)
 Acute hypertensive heart failure (pulmonary edema due to acute diastolic dysfunction)
 Acute coronary syndromes
  Acute myocardial infarction
  Unstable angina
 Acute aortic dissection
 Central nervous system catastrophe
  Hypertensive encephalopathy
  Intracerebral hemorrhage
  Subarachnoid hemorrhage
  Severe head trauma
 Catecholamine excess states
  Pheochromocytoma crisis
  Monoamine oxidase inhibitor–tyramine interactions
  Antihypertensive drug withdrawal syndromes
  Phenylpropanolamine overdose
 Preeclampsia and eclampsia
 Active bleeding (including postoperative bleeding)
 Poorly controlled hypertension in patients requiring emergency surgery
 Severe postoperative hypertension
  Postcoronary artery bypass hypertension
  Postcarotid endarterectomy hypertension
 Scleroderma renal crisis
 Autonomic hyperreflexia in quadriplegic patients

(Adapted from Nolan CR. Malignant hypertension and other hypertensive crises. In: Schrier RW, ed. *Diseases of the kidney and urinary tract,* 8th ed. Boston: Lippincott Williams & Wilkins, 2007:1370–1436.)

result from acute hypertensive heart failure, intracerebral hemorrhage, hypertensive encephalopathy, or complications of uremia. Malignant hypertension represents a hypertensive crisis; adequate control of BP clearly prevents these morbid complications.

C. **Hypertensive crises due to nonmalignant hypertension with acute complications.** Even in patients with benign hypertension, in whom HNR is absent, a hypertensive crisis may be diagnosed based on the presence of concomitant acute end-organ dysfunction (Table 15-9). Hypertensive crises due to nonmalignant hypertension with acute complications include hypertension accompanied by hypertensive encephalopathy, acute hypertensive heart failure, acute aortic dissection, intracerebral hemorrhage, subarachnoid hemorrhage, severe head trauma, acute MI or unstable angina, and active bleeding. Poorly controlled hypertension in a patient requiring surgery increases the risk of intraoperative cerebral or myocardial ischemia and postoperative acute renal failure. Severe postoperative hypertension, including post–coronary artery bypass hypertension and post–carotid endarterectomy hypertension, increases the risk of postoperative bleeding, hypertensive encephalopathy, pulmonary edema, and myocardial ischemia. The various catecholamine excess states can cause a hypertensive crisis with hypertensive encephalopathy or acute hypertensive heart failure. Preeclampsia and eclampsia represent hypertensive crises that are unique to pregnancy. Scleroderma renal crisis is a hypertensive crisis in which failure to adequately control BP with a regimen that includes an ACE inhibitor results in rapid irreversible loss of renal function. Hypertensive crises can also occur in quadriplegic patients due to autonomic hyperreflexia induced by bowel or bladder distension. The sudden onset of hypertension in this setting can lead to hypertensive encephalopathy or acute pulmonary edema.

D. **Treatment of malignant hypertension.** Malignant hypertension must be treated expeditiously to prevent complications such as hypertensive encephalopathy, acute hypertensive heart failure, and renal failure. The traditional approach to patients with malignant hypertension has been the initiation of potent parenteral agents. In general, parenteral therapy should be used in patients with evidence of acute end-organ dysfunction (hypertensive encephalopathy or pulmonary edema) or those unable to tolerate oral medications. Nitroprusside is the treatment of choice for patients requiring parenteral therapy. In general, reducing the mean arterial pressure by 20% or to a level of 160 to 170/100 to 110 mm Hg is safe. The use of a short-acting agent such as nitroprusside has obvious advantages, because BP can quickly be stabilized at a higher level if complications develop during rapid BP reduction. If no evidence of vital organ hypoperfusion is apparent during the initial reduction, the BP can gradually be lowered to less than 140/90 mm Hg over a period of 12 to 36 hours. Oral antihypertensive agents should be initiated as soon as possible to minimize the duration of parenteral therapy. The nitroprusside infusion can be weaned as the oral agents become effective. The cornerstone of initial oral therapy should be arteriolar vasodilators such as hydralazine or minoxidil. β-Blockers are required to control reflex tachycardia, and a diuretic must be initiated within a few days to prevent salt and water retention in response to vasodilatator therapy when the patient's dietary salt intake increases. Diuretics may not be necessary as a part of initial parenteral therapy, because patients with malignant hypertension often present with volume depletion due to pressure-induced natriuresis. Although many patients with malignant hypertension definitely require initial parenteral therapy, some patients may not yet have evidence of cerebral or cardiac dysfunction or rapidly deteriorating renal function and therefore do not require instantaneous control of BP. These patients can often be managed with an intensive oral regimen, often with a β-blocker and minoxidil, designed to bring the BP under control within 12 to 24 hours. After the immediate crisis has resolved and the hypertension has been controlled with initial parenteral therapy, oral therapy, or both, lifelong surveillance of BP is mandatory. If control lapses, malignant hypertension can recur even after years of successful antihypertensive therapy. Triple therapy with a diuretic, a β-blocker, and a vasodilator is often required to maintain satisfactory long-term BP control.

E. **Treatment of other hypertensive crises.** Sodium nitroprusside is the drug of choice for the management of virtually all hypertensive crises outlined in Table 15-9, including malignant hypertension, hypertensive encephalopathy, acute hypertensive heart failure, intracerebral hemorrhage, perioperative hypertension, catecholamine-related hypertensive crises, and acute aortic dissection (in combination with β-blockers). Intravenous nitroglycerin may also be useful in patients with concomitant myocardial ischemia, because it dilatates intracoronary collaterals.

Sodium nitroprusside is a potent intravenous hypotensive agent with an immediate onset and brief duration of action. The site of action is the vascular smooth muscle. It has no direct action on the myocardium, although it may indirectly affect cardiac performance through alterations in systemic hemodynamics. Nitroprusside is an iron-coordination complex with five cyanide moieties and a nitroso group. The nitroso group combines with cysteine to form nitrosocysteine, a potent activator of guanylate cyclase that causes cyclic guanosine monophosphate (cGMP) accumulation and the relaxation of vascular smooth muscle. Nitroprusside causes vasodilation of both arteriolar resistance vessels and venous capacitance vessels. Its hypotensive action is a result of decrease in SVR. The combined decrease in preload and afterload reduces myocardial wall tension and myocardial oxygen demand. The net effect of nitroprusside on cardiac output and heart rate depends on the intrinsic state of the myocardium. In patients with left ventricular systolic dysfunction and elevated left ventricular end-diastolic pressure, it causes an increase in stroke volume and cardiac output as a result of afterload reduction. Heart rate may actually decrease in response to improved cardiac performance. In contrast, in the absence of left ventricular dysfunction, venodilation and preload reduction can result in a reflex increase in sympathetic tone and heart rate. For this reason, nitroprusside must be used in conjunction with a β-blocker in acute aortic dissection.

The hypotensive action of nitroprusside appears within seconds and is immediately reversible when the infusion is stopped. The cGMP in vascular smooth muscle is rapidly degraded by cGMP-specific phosphodiesterases. Nitroprusside is rapidly metabolized, with a half-life of 3 to 4 minutes. Cyanide is formed, as a short-lived intermediate product, by direct combination with sulfhydryl groups in red blood cells and tissues. The cyanide groups are rapidly converted to thiocyanate by the liver, in a reaction in which thiosulfate acts as a sulfur donor. Thiocyanate is excreted by the kidney, with a half-life of 1 week in patients with normal renal function. Thiocyanate accumulation and toxicity can occur when a high dose or prolonged infusion is required, especially in patients with renal insufficiency. When these risk factors are present, thiocyanate levels should be monitored and the infusion stopped if the level is more than 10 mg per dL. Thiocyanate toxicity is rare in patients with normal renal function requiring less than 3 μg per kg per minute for less than 72 hours. Cyanide poisoning is a very rare complication, unless hepatic clearance of cyanide is impaired by severe liver disease, or massive doses of nitroprusside (more than 10 μg per kg per minute) are used to induce deliberate hypotension during surgery. Once the hypertensive crisis has resolved and the BP is adequately controlled, oral antihypertensive therapy should be initiated. The nitroprusside infusion is weaned as the oral antihypertensive agents become effective.

F. **Treatment of severe uncomplicated hypertension in the acute care setting.** The benefits of acute reduction in BP in the setting of true hypertensive crisis are obvious (Fig. 15-4). Fortunately, true hypertensive crises are relatively rare events that never affect the vast majority of hypertensive patients. Much more common than true hypertensive crisis is the patient who presents with markedly elevated BP (greater than 180/100 mm Hg) in the absence of HNR (malignant hypertension) or acute end-organ damage that would signify a true crisis. This entity, known as *severe uncomplicated hypertension*, is very common in the emergency department or other acute care settings. Of patients with severe uncomplicated hypertension, 60% are entirely asymptomatic and present for prescription refills or routine BP checks, or are found to have elevated pressure during routine physical examinations. The other 40% present with nonspecific findings such as headache, dizziness, or weakness in the absence of evidence of acute end-organ dysfunction.

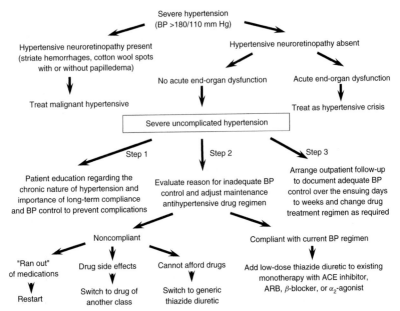

Figure 15-4. Algorithm for treatment of severe uncomplicated hypertension. (ACE, angiotensin-converting enzyme; BP, blood pressure; CCB, calcium channel blocker.) (Adapted with permission from Nolan CR. Hypertensive crises. In: Schrier RW, ed. *Atlas of diseases of the kidney*, vol. 3. Philadelphia: Current Medicine, 1999.)

In the past, this entity was referred to as *urgent hypertension*, reflecting the erroneous notion that an acute reduction of BP over a few hours before discharge from the acute care facility was essential to minimize the risk of short-term complications from severe hypertension. Commonly used treatment regimens included oral clonidine loading or sublingual nifedipine. However, the practice of acute BP reduction in severe uncomplicated hypertension is no longer considered the standard of care. The Veterans Administration Cooperative Study of patients with severe hypertension included 70 placebo-treated patients who had an average DBP of 121 mm Hg at entry. Among these untreated patients, 27 experienced morbid events at a mean of 11 (plus or minus 2) months of follow-up. However, the earliest morbid event occurred after 2 months. These data suggest that in patients with severe uncomplicated hypertension in which severe hypertension is not accompanied by evidence of malignant hypertension or acute end-organ dysfunction, eventual complications due to stroke, MI, or heart failure tend to occur over a time frame of months to years rather than hours to days. Although the long-term control of BP can clearly prevent these eventual complications, a hypertensive crisis cannot be diagnosed, because no evidence indicates that the acute reduction of BP results in an improvement in short- or long-term prognosis. Although the acute reduction of BP in patients with severe uncomplicated hypertension using sublingual nifedipine or oral clonidine loading was once the *de facto* standard of care, this practice was often an emotional response on the part of the treating physician to the dramatic elevation of BP, or it was motivated by the fear of medicolegal repercussions in the unlikely event of a hypertensive complication occurring within hours to days. Observing and documenting the dramatic fall in BP is a satisfying therapeutic maneuver, but no scientific basis for this approach exists. No literature supports the notion that some goal level of BP reduction must be achieved before the patient with severe uncomplicated hypertension leaves the acute care setting. In fact, the acute reduction of BP is often counterproductive, because it can produce untoward side effects that render the patient less likely to comply with long-term drug therapy. Instead, the acute therapeutic intervention should focus on tailoring an effective, well-tolerated maintenance antihypertensive regimen, with patient education regarding the chronic nature of the disease process and the importance of long-term compliance and medical follow-up. If the patient has simply run out of medicines, reinstitution of the previously effective drug regimen should suffice. If the patient is thought to be compliant with an existing drug regimen, a sensible change in the regimen, such as an increase in a suboptimal dosage of an existing drug or the addition of a drug of another class, is appropriate. In this regard, the addition of a low dose of a thiazide diuretic as a second-step agent to existing monotherapy with ACE inhibitor, ARB, CCB, β-blocker, or central α agonist is often remarkably effective. Another essential goal of the acute intervention should be to arrange suitable outpatient follow-up within a few days. A gradual reduction of BP to normotensive levels over a few days to a week should be accomplished in conjunction with frequent outpatient visits to modify the drug regimen and reinforce the importance of lifelong compliance with therapy. Although less dramatic than the acute reduction of BP in the acute care setting, this type of approach to the treatment of chronic hypertension is more likely to prevent long-term hypertensive complications and recurrent episodes of severe uncomplicated hypertension.

Suggested Readings

Acute Infarction Ramipril Efficacy (AIRE) Study Investigators. Effects of ramipril on mortality and morbidity of survivors of acute myocardial infarction with clinical evidence of heart failure. *Lancet* 1993;342:821–828.

Agadoa LY, Appel L, Bakris GL, et al. Effect of ramipril versus amlodipine on renal outcomes in hypertensive nephrosclerosis: a randomized controlled trail. *JAMA* 2001; 285:2719.

ALLHAT Collaborative Research Group. Major cardiovascular events in hypertensive patients randomized to doxazosin versus chlorthalidone: the antihypertensive and lipid-lowering to prevent heart attack trial (ALLHAT). *JAMA* 2000;238: 1967–1975.

ALLHAT Officers and Coordinators for the ALLHAT Collaborative Research Group. Major outcomes in high-risk hypertensive patients randomized to angiotensin-converting enzyme inhibitor, calcium channel blocker versus diuretic. *JAMA* 2002;288:2981–2997.

American Diabetes Association. Treatment of hypertension in adults with diabetes. *Diabetes Care* 2003;26(Suppl 1):S80–S82.

β-blocker Heart Attack Trial Research Group. A randomized trial of propranolol in patients with acute myocardial infarction, I: mortality results (BHAT). *JAMA* 1982; 247:1707–1714.

Black HR, Davis B, Barzhay J, et al. Metabolic and clinical outcomes in nondiabetic individuals with the metabolic syndrome assigned to chlorthalidone, amlodipine, or lisinopril as initial treatment for hypertension. A report for the Antihypertensive and Lipid-Loweriing Treatment to Prevent Heart Attack Trial (ALLHAT). *Diabetes Care* 2008;31:353–360.

Black HR, Elliott JW, Grandits G, et al. Principal results of the Controlled Onset Verapamil Investigation of Cardiovascular End Points (CONVINCE) trial. *JAMA* 2003; 289:2073–2082.

Braunwald E, Antgman EM, Beasley JW, et al. AHA 2002 guideline update for the management of patients with unstable angina and non-ST-segment elevation myocardial infarction (ACC/AHA Post MI Guideline). *J Am Coll Cardiol* 2002;40:1366–1374.

Brenner BM, Copper ME, de Zeeuq D, et al. Effects of losartan on renal and cardiovascular outcomes in patients with type 2 diabetes and nephropathy (RENAAL). *N Engl J Med* 2001;345:861–869.

Brown C, Higgins M, Donato KA, et al. Body mass index and the prevalence of hypertension and dyslipidemia. *Obes Res* 2000;8:605–619.

Capricorn Investigators. Effect of varvedilol on outcome after myocardial infarction in patients with left-ventricular dysfunction: The CAPRICORN randomized trial. *Lancet* 2001;357:1358–1390.

Chobanian AV, Bakris GL, Black HR, et al. The seventh report of the Joint National Committee on Prevention, Detection, Evaluation, and Treatment of Hypertension. The JNC 7 report. *JAMA* 2003;289:2560–2572.

CIBIS Investigators and Committees. A randomized trial of beta-blockade in heart failure: the Cardiac Insufficiency Bisprolol Study (CIBIS). *Circulation* 1994;90:1765–1773.

Cohn J, Tognoni G. A randomized trial of the angiotensin receptor blocker valsartan in chronic heart failure (ValHEFT). *N Engl J Med* 2001;345:1667–1675.

Dahlof B, Devereux RB, Kjeldsen SE, et al. Cardiovascular morbidity and mortality in the Losartan Intervention for Endpoint Reduction in Hypertension Study (LIFE). *Lancet* 2002;359:995–1003.

Estacio RO, Jeffers BW, Hiatt WH, et al. The effect of nisoldipine as compared with enalapril on cardiovascular outcomes in patients with non-insulin dependent diabetes mellitus and hypertension. *N Engl J Med* 1998;338:645–652.

Fields LE, Burt VL, Cutler JA, et al. The burden of adult hypertension in the United States 1999 to 2000: a rising tide. *Hypertension* 2004;44:398–404.

GISEN (Cruppo Italiano di Studi Epidemiologici in Nefrologia) Group. Randomized placebo-controlled trial of effect of ramipril on decline in glomerular filtration rate and risk of terminal renal failure in proteinuric, non-diabetic nephropathy (REIN). *Lancet* 1997;349:1857–1863.

Guyton AC, Manning RD, Norman RA, et al. Current concepts and perspectives of renal volume regulation in relationship to hypertension. *J Hypertens* 1986;4(Suppl 4): S49–S56.

Hager WD, Davis BR, Riba A, et al. Survival and Ventricular Enlargement (SAVE) Investigators. Absence of a deleterious effect of calcium channel blockers in patients with left ventricular dysfunction after myocardial infarction: the SAVE Study Experience. *Am Heart J* 1998;135:406–423.

Hall JE, Granger JP, Smith MJ, et al. Role of renal hemodynamics and arterial pressure in aldosterone "escape". *Hypertension* 1984;6(Suppl 1):I183–I192.

Heart Outcomes Prevention Evaluation Study Investigators. Effects of an angiotensin-converting-enzyme inhibitor, ramipril on cardiovascular events in high-risk patients (HOPE). *N Engl J Med* 2000;342:145–153.

Hunt SA, Baker DW, Chin MH, et al. ACC/AHA guidelines for the evaluation and management of chronic heart failure in the adult. *J Am Coll Cardiol* 2001;38:2101–2113.

Intersalt Cooperative Research Group. Intersalt: an international study of electrolyte excretion and blood pressure. Results for 24 hour urinary sodium and potassium excretion. *Br Med J* 1988;297:319–330.

Kober L, Torp-Pedersen C, Carlsen JE, et al. Trandolapril Cardiac Evaluation (TRACE) Study Group. A clinical trial of the angiotensin-converting enzyme inhibitor trandolapril in patients with left ventricular dysfunction after myocardial infarction. *N Engl J Med* 1995;333:1670–1676.

Lewis EJ, Hunsicker LG, Bain RP, et al. The effect of angiotensin-converting enzyme inhibitor on diabetic nephropathy: the Collaborative Study Group (Captopril Trial). *N Engl J Med* 1993;329:1456–1462.

Lewis EJ, Hunsicker LG, Clarke WR, et al. Renoprotective effect of the angiotensin-receptor antagonist irbesartan in patients with nephropathy due to type 2 diabetes (INDT). *N Engl J Med* 2001;345:851–860.

Lifton RP, Gharavi AG, Geller DS. Molecular mechanisms of human hypertension. *Cell* 2001;104:545–556.

Maschia G, Alberti D, Janin G, et al. Effect of the angiotensin-converting-enzyme inhibitor benazepril on the progression of chronic renal insufficiency. *N Engl J Med* 1996;334:939.

National Kidney Foundation. K/DOQI clinical practice guidelines for chronic kidney disease: kidney disease outcome quality initiative. *Am J Kidney Dis* 2002;39(Suppl 2): S1–S246.

National Kidney Foundation. K/DOQI clinical practice guidelines on hypertension and antihypertensive agents in chronic kidney disease. *Am J Kidney Dis* 2004, 43: (5 Suppl 1):S1.

Nolan CR. Hypertensive crises. In: RW Schrier, ed. *Atlas of diseases of the kidney*, Vol. 3. Philadelphia: Current Medicine, 1999.

Nolan CR. Malignant hypertension and other hypertensive crises. In: RW Schrier, ed. *Diseases of the kidney and urinary tract*, 7th ed. Boston: Lippincott Williams & Wilkins, 2001:1513–1592.

Nolan CR, Schrier RW. The kidney in hypertension. In: RW Schrier, ed. *Renal and electrolyte disorders*, 6th ed. Philadelphia: Lippincott Williams & Wilkins, 2003.

Packer M, Coats AJ, Fowler MB, et al. Effect of carvedolo on survival in severe chronic heart failure (COPERNICUS). *N Engl J Med* 2001;344:1651–1658.

Pitt B, Remme W, Zannad F, et al. Eplerenone, a selective aldosterone blocker, in patients with left ventricular dysfunction after myocardial infarction (EPHESUS). *N Engl J Med* 2003;348:1309–1321.

Pitt B, Zannad F, Remme WJ, et al. Randomized Aldactone Evaluation Study Investigators. The effect of spironolactone on morbidity and mortality in patients with severe heart failure (RALES). *N Engl J Med* 1999;341:709–717.

PROGRESS Collaborative Study Group. Randomised trial of perindopril-based blood pressure lowering regimen among 6105 individuals with previous stroke or transient ischaemic attack. *Lancet* 2001;358:1033–1041.

Pstay BM, Smith NL, Siscovick DS, et al. Health outcomes associated with antihypertensive therapies used as first-line agents. *JAMA* 1997;277:739–745.

Ruggenenti P, Perna A, Loriga G, et al. Blood pressure control for renoprotection in patients with non-diabetic renal disease (REIN-2): mulicentre, randomised controlled trial. *Lancet* 2005;365:939.

Schrier RW, Estacio R, Esler A, et al. Effects of aggressive blood pressure control in normotensive type 2 diabetic patients on albuminuria, retinopathy and strokes. *Kidney Int* 2002;61:1086–1097.

Schrier RW, Estacio RO, Mehler PS, et al. Appropriate blood pressue control in hypertensive and normotensive type 2 diabetes mellitus: a summary of the ABCD trial. *Nat Clin Pract Nephrol* 2007;3:428–438.

SHEP Cooperative Research Group. Prevention of stroke by antihypertensive treatment in older persons with isolated systolic hypertension. Final results of the Systolic Hypertension in the Elderly Program (SHEP). *JAMA* 1991;265:3255–3264.

SOLVD Investigators. Effect of enalapril on survival in patients with reduced left ventricular ejection fractions and congestive heart failure. *N Engl J Med* 1991;325:293–302.

Tepper D. Frontiers in congestive heart failure: effect of metoprolol CR/XL in chronic heart failure (MERIT-HF). *Congest Heart Fail* 1999;5:184–185.

UK Prospective Diabetes Study Group. Efficacy of atenolol and captopril in reducing risk of macrovascular and microvascular complications in type 2 diabetes: UKPDS 39. *Br Med J* 1998;317:713–720.

Whelton PK, Barzilay J, Cushman WC, et al. Clinical outcomes in antihypertensive treatment of type 2 diabetics, impaired fasting glucose concentration and normoglycemia. Antihypertensive and Lipid-Lowering Treatment to Prevent Heart Attack Trial (ALLHAT). *Arch Intern Med* 2005;165:1401–1409.

Wing LMH, Reid CM, Ryan P, et al. Second Australian National Blood Pressure Study Group. A comparison of outcomes with angiotensin-converting-enzyme inhibitors and diuretics for hypertension in the elderly (ANBP2). *N Engl J Med* 2003;348:583–592.

Wright JT Jr, Agadoa L, Contreras G, et al. Successful blood pressure control in African American Study of Kidney Disease and Hypertension (AASK). *Arch Intern Med* 2002;162:1636–1643.

Wright JT Jr, Harris-Haywood S, Pressel S, et al. Clinical outcomes by rate in hypertensive patients with and without the metabolic syndrome. Antihypertensive and Lipid-Lowering Treatment to Prevent Heart Attack Trail (ALLHAT). *Arch Intern Med* 2008;168:207–217.

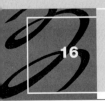

16

PRACTICAL GUIDELINES FOR DRUG DOSING IN PATIENTS WITH IMPAIRED KIDNEY FUNCTION

George R. Aronoff and Michael E. Brier

$\mathcal{U}$remia influences every organ system and every aspect of drug disposition. The physiological changes associated with renal disease have pronounced effects on the pharmacology of many drugs. The purpose of this chapter is to provide a rational schema for drug dosing in patients with decreased renal function and for those requiring renal replacement therapy.

In Figure 16-1 is outlined the approach to drug dosing in patients with renal disease. When possible, a specific diagnosis should be established before drug therapy is initiated. The use of fewer drugs and the recognition of potential drug interactions decrease adverse drug effects and the potential for drug interactions.

I. HISTORY AND PHYSICAL EXAMINATION

Clinical evaluation always begins with a careful history and physical examination. Particularly important for this purpose are the history of previous drug allergy or toxicity and the use of concurrent medications or recreational drugs. Physical assessment should include an estimate of the extracellular fluid (ECF) volume. Edema or ascites increases the distribution volume of many drugs, while dehydration contracts this volume. Measurements of body weight and height are needed to tailor the dosage regimen. For obese patients, an average of the calculated ideal body weight of the measured body weight is useful for estimating drug doses. Evidence of impaired function of other excretory organs should be sought. Stigmata of liver disease are clues that the drug dose may need to be altered.

II. MEASUREMENT OF RENAL FUNCTION

The rate of elimination of drugs excreted by the kidneys is proportional to the glomerular filtration rate (GFR). The serum creatinine or creatinine clearance is needed to determine renal function before prescribing any drug. The Cockroft-Gault equation is useful for this purpose as shown in the formula:

$$\text{Clcr} = \frac{(140 - \text{age}) \times (\text{IBW})}{72 \times \text{Scr}} \times (0.85 \text{ if female})$$

Clcr = creatinine clearance (mL per minute)
Scr = serum creatinine (mg per dL)
IBW (in kg) = Ideal body weight (men) = 50 kg + 2.3 kg per in. over 5 ft
= Ideal body weight (women) = 45.5 kg + 2.3 kg per in. over 5 ft
For obese men and women the equation should be modified:

$$\text{Clcr} = \frac{(137 - \text{age}) \times [(0.285 \times \text{wgt}) + (12.1 \times \text{hgt}^2)]}{51 \times \text{Scr}}$$
(obese men)

$$\text{Clcr} = \frac{(146 - \text{age}) \times [(0.287 \times \text{wgt}) + (9.74 \times \text{hgt}^2)]}{60 \times \text{Scr}}$$
(obese women)

wgt = patient's weight in kg
hgt = patient's height in cm

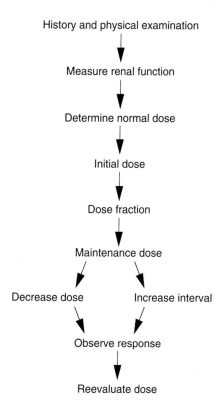

History and physical examination

Measure renal function

Determine normal dose

Initial dose

Dose fraction

Maintenance dose

Decrease dose   Increase interval

Observe response

Reevaluate dose

Figure 16-1. A schema for drug dosing in patients with impaired renal function.

In adults, the Modification of Diet in Renal Disease (MDRD) Study equation, is also frequently used to estimate the glomerular filtration rate (eGFR) for the purpose of drug dosing, where:

$$\text{eGFR (mL/min/1.73 m}^2) = 175 \times (\text{Scr})^{-1.154} \times (\text{age})^{-0.203} \times (0.742 \text{ if female})$$
$$\times (1.210 \text{ if African-American})$$

eGFR = estimated glomerular filtration rate (mL per minute)
Scr = serum creatinine (mg per dL)

The MDRD equation does not require body mass in the calculation because the results are normalized to 1.73 m² body surface area. Many commercial laboratories automatically calculate the MDRD eGFR from blood chemistries and will report the results.

In cases of changing renal function, the serum creatinine will no longer reflect the true clearance rate. In these cases, a timed urine collection is needed to estimate renal function. The midpoint serum creatinine is useful to calculate the creatinine clearance for the collection period. If the patient is oliguric, the creatinine clearance is less than 5 mL per minute.

The serum creatinine reflects muscle mass as well as GFR. Serum creatinine measurements within the "normal" range are frequently used to establish "normal" renal function. This erroneous assumption may cause serious overdose and resultant toxic drug accumulation in elderly or debilitated patients with decreased muscle mass.

III. CALCULATION OF THE INITIAL DOSE

The purpose of the initial dose is to achieve therapeutic drug concentrations rapidly. A loading dose should be considered when the half-life of a drug is particularly long in patients with impaired renal function and the clinical situation requires rapidly achieved therapeutic levels. When the physical examination suggests that the ECF is normal, the loading dose of a drug given to a patient with renal insufficiency is the same as the initial dose given to a patient with normal renal function. Initial doses for most drugs requiring loading are already known. However, the loading dose may be calculated using the following formula:

$$\text{Loading dose} = Vd(L/kg) \times Wt(kg) \times Cp(mg/L)$$

where:
  Vd = volume of distribution of the drug
  Wt = patient's ideal body weight
  Cp = desired plasma drug level
If the patient has edema or ascites a larger loading dose may be required. Conversely, dehydrated or debilitated patients should receive smaller initial drug doses.

IV. CALCULATION OF THE MAINTENANCE DOSE

Several methods can be used to decide subsequent doses. The following relationship is useful for calculating the fraction of the normal dose recommended for a patient with renal insufficiency:

$$\text{Dose fraction} = F[((Clcr/120) - 1)] + 1$$

where:
  F = fraction of the drug excreted unchanged in the urine
  $Clcr$ = creatinine clearance
When F is not known, the ratio of the drug's half-life in patients with normal renal function ($T_{1/2}$ normal) to that measure in patients with renal failure ($T_{1/2}$ renal failure) may be substituted as below:

$$\text{Dose fraction} = \frac{T_{1/2} \text{ normal}}{T_{1/2} \text{ renal failure}}[(Clcr/120) - 1] + 1$$

In Table 16-1 are listed commonly used drugs that require substantial dose alteration when used in patients with renal failure and suggestions for dose adjustment and for dialysis.

A. Use of the table

Prolonging the dose interval is often a convenient and cost-effective method for altering the drug dose in patients with renal impairment. This recommendation is indicated in the table by "I" in the method column. This method is particularly useful for drugs with wide therapeutic ranges and long plasma half-lives. Extended parenteral therapy can be completed without prolonged hospitalization when the dose interval can safely be lengthened to allow for home therapy. If the range between the therapeutic and toxic levels is too narrow, either potentially toxic or subtherapeutic plasma concentrations may result.

To maintain the same dose interval as for patients with normal renal function, one may decrease the amount of each individual dose given to renal impaired patients. This recommendation is indicated in the table by "D" in the method column. This method is effective for drugs with narrow therapeutic ranges and short plasma half-lives in patients with renal insufficiency.

In practice, a combination of the methods is often effective and convenient. The combination method uses modification of both the dose and dose interval. For drugs with particularly long half-lives in patients with impaired renal function, give the total daily dose as a single dose each day. Similarly, divide the total daily dose in half and give twice daily.

The decision to extend the dosing interval beyond a 24-hour period should be based on the necessity to maintain therapeutic peak or trough drug levels. When the peak level is most important, prolong the dose interval. However, when

TABLE 16-1 Drug Dosing Recommendations for Patients with Decreased Kidney Function and on Dialysis

Drug	Adjustment method	GFR <50 mL/min	GFR 10–50 mL/min	GFR <10 mL/min	Hemodialysis	Peritoneal dialysis	Continuous renal replacement
Abacavir	—	No change	No change	No change	None	None	—
Abacavir/lamivudine	—	1 tablet daily	Use individual drugs	Use individual drugs	Avoid	Avoid	Avoid
Abacavir/lamivudine/ zidovudine	—	100%	Avoid	Avoid	Avoid	Avoid	—
Acarbose	D	50%–100%	Avoid	Avoid	No data	No data	Avoid
Acebutolol	D	100%	50%	25%	Dose after dialysis	None	Dose for GFR 10–50
Acetaminophen	—	q4h	q6h	q8h	None	None	Dose for GFR 10–50
Acetazolamide	—	q6h	q12h	Avoid	No data	No data	Avoid
Acetohexamide	—	Avoid	Avoid	Avoid	No data	None	Avoid
Acetohydroxamic acid	D	100%	100%	Avoid	No data	No data	No data
Acetylsalicylic acid	—	q4h	q4–6h	Avoid	Dose after dialysis	None	Dose for GFR 10–50
Acrivastine	—	q.i.d.	b.i.d.–t.i.d.	b.i.d.–q24h	Dose after dialysis	Dose for GFR 10–50	Dose for GFR 10–50
Acyclovir	D, I	100% q8h	100% q12–24h	50% q24h	Dose after dialysis	Dose for GFR <10	3.5 mg/kg d
Adefovir	—	100%	10 mg q48h (q72h for <20 mL/min)	10 mg q72 hr	10 mg weekly, after dialysis	No data	—
Adenosine	D	100%	100%	100%	None	None	Dose for GFR 10–50
Albuterol (inhaled)	—	100%	100%	100%	None	None	None
Albuterol (oral)	—	100%	100%	100%	None	None	None
Alcuronium	D	Avoid	Avoid	Avoid	No data	No data	Avoid
Alfentanil	D	100%	100%	100%	Not applicable	Not applicable	Dose for GFR 10–50
Alfentanil	D	100%	100%	100%	No data	No data	Dose for GFR 10–50
Allopurinol	D, I	75%	50%	25%	1/2 dose	No data	No data

(continued)

TABLE 16-1 *(Continued)*

Drug	Adjustment method	GFR <50 mL/min	GFR 10–50 mL/min	GFR <10 mL/min	Hemodialysis	Peritoneal dialysis	Continuous renal replacement
Alprazolam	D	100%	100%	100%	None	No data	Not applicable
Alteplase [tissue-type plasminogen activator (tPa)]	D	100%	100%	100%	No data	No data	Dose for GFR 10–50
Altretamine	D	100%	100%	100%	No data	No data	Not applicable
Amantadine	I	q12h	q24–48h	q7 d	None	None	Dose for GFR 10–50
Amikacin	I	100% q12 or 24h	100% q24–72 h by levels	100% q48–72h by levels	1/2 full dose after dialysis	15–20 mg/L d	Dose for GFR 10–50 and measure levels
Amiloride	D	100%	50%	Avoid	Avoid	Avoid	Avoid
Amiodarone	D	100%	100%	100%	None	None	Dose for GFR 10–50
Amitriptyline	D	100%	100%	100%	None	None	Not applicable
Amlodipine	I	100%	100%	100%	None	None	Dose for GFR 10–50
Amoxapine	D	100%	100%	100%	None	None	Not applicable
Amoxicillin	I	q8h	q8–12h	q24h	Dose after dialysis	250 mg q12h	Dose for GFR 10–50
Amphotericin B	I	q24h	q24h	q24h	None	Dose for GFR <10	Dose for GFR 10–50
Amphotericin B colloidal dispersion	I	q24h	q24h	q24h	None	None	None
Amphotericin B lipid complex	I	q24h	q24h	q24h	None	None	None
Ampicillin	I	q6h	q6–12h	q12–24h	Dose after dialysis	250 mg q12h	Dose for GFR 10–50
Aminrone	D	100%	100%	50%–75%	No data	No data	Dose for GFR 10–50
Anistreplase	D	100%	100%	100%	Avoid	Avoid	Not applicable
Atazanavir	I	No data	No data	No data	No data	No data	No data
Atenolol	D	50–100 mg q24h	25–50 mg q24h	25 mg q24h	25–50 mg after dialysis	Dose for GFR <10	Dose for GFR 10–50

Drug							
Atovaquone	—	No data: 100%	No data: 100%	No data: 100%	No data: none	No data: none	No data: dose for GFR 10–50
Atracurium	D	100%	100%	100%	Not applicable	Not applicable	Not applicable
Auranofin	D	50%	Avoid	Avoid	None	None	None
Azatadine	—	q12h	q12h	q12–24h	Dose for GFR <10	Dose for GFR <10	Dose for GFR <10
Azathioprine	D	100%	75%	50%	Supplement 0.25 mg/kg	No data	Dose for GFR 10–50
Azithromycin	D	100%	100%	100%	None	None	None
Aztreonam	D	100%	50%	25%	0.5 g after dialysis	Dose for GFR <10	Dose for GFR 10–50
Benazepril	D	100%	50%–75%	25%–50%	None	None	Dose for GFR 10–50
Bepridil	—	No data	No data	No data	None	None	No data
Betamethasone	D	100%	100%	100%	No data	Dose for GFR <10	Not applicable
Betaxolol	D	100%	100%	50%	None	None	Dose for GFR 10–50
Bezafibrate	D	50%–100%	25%–50%	Avoid	Avoid	Avoid	Not applicable
Bisoprolol	D	100%	75%	50%	Dose after dialysis	None	Dose for GFR 10–50
Bleomycin	D	100%	75%	50%	None	No data	Dose for GFR 10–50
Bopindolol	D	100%	100%	100%	None	None	Dose for GFR 10–50
Bretylium	D	100%	25%–50%	25%	None	None	Dose for GFR 10–50
Brompheniramine	D	100%	100%	100%	Dose for normal GFR — no supplement required	Dose for normal GFR — no supplement required	Dose for normal GFR — no supplement required
Budesonide	D	100%	100%	100%	No data	No data	Dose for GFR 10–50
Bumetanide	D	100%	100%	100%	None	None	Not applicable
Bupropion	D	100%	100%	100%	No data	Dose for GFR <10	Not applicable
Buspirone	D	100%	100%	100%	Dose for GFR <10	Dose for GFR <10	Not applicable
Busulfan	D	100%	100%	100%	Dose for GFR <10	Dose for GFR <10	Not applicable
Butorphanol	D	75%	75%	50%	No data	No data	Dose for GFR 10–50
Candesartan	—	100%	100%	100%	No dose adjustment	No dose adjustment	No dose adjustment

(continued)

TABLE 16-1 *(Continued)*

Drug	Adjustment method	GFR <50 mL/min	GFR 10–50 mL/min	GFR <10 mL/min	Hemodialysis	Peritoneal dialysis	Continuous renal replacement
Capreomycin	I	q24h	q24h	q48h	Give dose after HD only	None	Dose for GFR 10–50
Captopril	D, I	100% q8–12h	75% q12–18h	50% q24h	Dose after dialysis	Dose for GFR 10–50	Dose for GFR 10–50
Carbamazepine	D	100%	100%	75%	Dose for GFR <10; give after dialysis	Dose for GFR <10	Dose for GFR 10–50
Carbidopa	D	100%	100%	100%	No data	No data	No data
Carboplatin	D	100%	50%	25%	1/2 dose	Dose for GFR <10	Dose for GFR 10–50
Carmustine	D	No data	No data	Avoid	Avoid	Avoid	Avoid
Carteolol	D	100%	50%	25%	No data	None	Dose for GFR 10–50
Carvedilol	I	100%	100%	100%	None	None	Dose for GFR 10–50
Caspofungin	I	No change	No change	No change	No adjustment necessary	No adjustment necessary	—
Cefaclor	I	100%	100%	100%	250–500 mg after dialysis	250–500 mg q8h	Not applicable
Cefadroxil	I	q12h	q12–24h	q36h	0.5–1.0 g after dialysis	0.5 g/d	Not applicable
Cefamandole	I	q6h	q6–8h	q8–12h	0.5–1.0 g after dialysis	0.5–1.0 g q12h	Dose for GFR 10–50
Cefazolin	I	100% q8h	100% q12h	50% q24–48h	15–20 mg/kg after dialysis	0.5 g q12h	Dose for GFR 10–50
Cefdinir	I	100	300 mg daily for creatinine clearance < 30 mL/min	300 mg every other day	Dose after dialysis	Dose for GFR <10	—

Cefditoren	D, I	100%	200 mg b.i.d. (q.d. for creatinine clearance <30 mL/min)	200 mg q.d.	Dose for GFR <10	No data	—
Cefepime	D, I	100%	50%–100% q24h	25%–50% dose q24h	Dose for GFR <10	Dose for GFR <10	Not recommended
Cefoperazone	D	100%	100%	100%	1.0 g after dialysis	None	None
Cefotaxime	I	q6h	q6–12h	q24h or 1/2 dose	0.5–2 g after dialysis	1.0 g/d	1.0 g q12h
Cefotetan	—	100%	1–2 g q24h	1–2 g q48h	1.0 g after dialysis	1.0 g/d	750 mg q12h
Cefoxitin	—	q6–8h	q8–12h	q24–48h	1.0 g after dialysis	1.0 g/d	Dose for GFR 10–50
Cefpodoxime	—	q12h	q24h	q24h	Dose after dialysis	Dose for GFR <10	Not applicable
Cefprozil	D, I	100% q12h	50% q12h	50% q12h	250 mg after dialysis	Dose for GFR <10	Dose for GFR <10
Ceftazidime	—	q8–12h	q12–24h	q24–48h	1.0 g after dialysis	0.5 g/d	Dose for GFR 10–50
Ceftibuten	D	100%	25%–50%	25%–50%	400 mg after dialysis only	No data: dose for GFR <10	Dose for GFR 10–50
Ceftizoxime	—	q8–12h	q12–24h	q24h	1.0 g after dialysis	0.5–1.0 g/d	Dose for GFR 10–50
Ceftriaxone	D	100%	100%	100%	None	1 g q12h	None
Cefuroxime axetil	D	100%	100%	100%	Dose after dialysis	None	Not applicable
Cefuroxime sodium	—	q8h	q8–12h	q12h	Dose after dialysis	Dose for GFR <10	1.0 g q12h
Celiprolol	D	100%	100%	75%	No data	None	Dose for GFR 10–50
Cephalexin	—	q6–8h	q8–12h	q12–24h	Dose after dialysis	Dose for GFR <10	Not applicable
Cephradine	D	100%	50%	25%	Dose after dialysis	Dose for GFR <10	Not applicable
Cetirizine	D	5–10 mg q.d.	5 mg q.d.	5 mg q.d.	Dose for GFR <10	Dose for GFR <10	Dose for GFR <10
Chlorambucil	D	100 %	75%	50%	None	Dose for GFR <10	Dose for GFR <10
Chloramphenicol	D	100%	100%	100%	None	None	None
Chlorazepate	D	100%	100%	100%	None	Dose for GFR <10	Not applicable
Chlordiazepoxide	D	100%	100%	50%	None	Dose for GFR <10	Dose for GFR <10

(continued)

TABLE 16-1 (Continued)

Drug	Adjustment method	GFR <50 mL/min	GFR 10–50 mL/min	GFR <10 mL/min	Hemodialysis	Peritoneal dialysis	Continuous renal replacement
Chloroquine	D	100%	100%	50%	Dose for GFR <10	Dose for GFR <10	None
Chlorothiazide	—	100%	100%	Ineffective	Not applicable	Not applicable	Not applicable
Chlorpheniramine	D	100%	100%	100%	None	None	None
Chlorpromazine	D	100%	100%	100%	None	Dose for GFR <10	Dose for GFR 10–50
Chlorpropamide	D	50%	Avoid	Avoid	Avoid	Avoid	Avoid
Chlorthalidone	—	q24h	q24h	Avoid	Not applicable	Not applicable	Not applicable
Cholestyramine	D	100%	100%	100%	None	None	Dose for GFR 10–50
Cibenzoline	D, I	100% q12h	100% q12h	66% q24h	None	None	Dose for GFR 10–50
Cidofovir	D	100% > 55	Avoid	Avoid	Avoid	Avoid	Avoid
Cilazapril	D, I	75% q24h	50% q24–48h	10%–25% q72h	None	None	Dose for GFR 10–50
Cimetidine	D, I	100%	50%	300 mg q8–12h	Dose after dialysis	Dose for GFR <10	Dose for GFR 10–50
Ciprofloxacin	D	100%	50%–75%	50%	250 mg q12h (200 mg if i.v.)	250 mg q8h (200 mg if i.v.)	200 mg i.v. q12h
Cisapride	D	Avoid	Avoid	Avoid	Avoid	Avoid	50%–100%
Cisplatin	D	100%	75%	50%	Yes	Dose for GFR <10	Dose for GFR 10–50
Cladribine	D	100%	75%	50%	No data	Dose for GFR <10	Not applicable
Clarithromycin	D	100%	50%–100%	50%	No data: dose after dialysis	None	None
Clemastine	D	100%	100%	50%	Dose for GFR <10	Dose for GFR <10	Dose for GFR <10
Clindamycin	D	100%	100%	100%	None	None	None
Clodronate	D	100%	25%–50%	Avoid	Not applicable	Dose for GFR <10	Not applicable
Clofazimine	—	100%	100%	100%	No data: none	No data: none	No data
Clofibrate	—	q6–12h	q12–18h	Avoid	None	Avoid	Avoid
Clomipramine	D	100%	100%	100%	None	Dose for GFR <10	Not applicable

Clonazepam	—	100%	100%	100%	None	No data	Not applicable
Clonidine	I	q12h	q12–24h	q24h	Dose after dialysis	Dose for GFR <10	Dose for GFR 10–50
Codeine	D	100%	75%	50%	No data	No data	Dose for GFR 10–50
Colchicine	D	100%	50%–100%	25%	None	Dose for GFR <10	Dose for GFR 10–50
Colestipol	D	100%	100%	100%	None	None	Not applicable
Cortisone	D	100%	100%	100%	None	None	Not applicable
Cyclophosphamide	D	100%	100%	75%	1/2 dose	Dose for GFR <10	Dose for GFR 10–50
Cycloserine	D	q12h	q24h	q36–48h	None	None	Dose for GFR 10–50
Cyclosporine	D	100%	100%	100%	None	None	100%
Cyproheptadine	I	100%	100%	50%–100%	Dose for GFR <10	Dose for GFR <10	Dose for GFR <10
Cytarabine	D	100%	100%	100%	No data	No data	Dose for GFR 10–50
Dapsone	I	No data: 100%	No data	No data	No data: none	No data: dose for GFR <10	No data
Daptomycin	—	100%	100% q24–48h	100% q48h	Dose for GFR <10	Dose for GFR <10	—
Daunorubicin	D	100%	100%	100%	None	Dose for GFR <10	Not applicable
Delavirdine	I	No data: 100%	No data: 100%	No data: 100%	No data: none	No data	No data: dose for GFR 10–50
Desferoxamine	D	100%	25%–50%	Avoid	Avoid	Avoid	Not applicable
Desipramine	D	100%	100%	100%	None	None	Not applicable
Dexamethasone	D	100%	100%	100%	None	None	Not applicable
Diazepam	D	100%	100%	100%	None	None	None
Diazoxide	I	100%	100%	100%	None	None	Dose for GFR 10–50
Diclofenac	D	50%–100%	25%–50%	25%	None	None	Dose for GFR 10–50
Dicloxacillin	D	100%	100%	100%	None	None	Not applicable
Didanosine	D	q12h	q24h	50% q24h	Dose after dialysis	Dose for GFR <10	Dose for GFR <10
Diflunisal	D	100%	50%	50%	None	None	Dose for GFR 10–50
Digitoxin	D	100%	100%	50%–75%	None	None	Dose for GFR 10–50
Digoxin	D, I	100% q24h	25%–75% q36h	10%–25% q48h	None	None	Dose for GFR 10–50
Dilevalol	D	100%	100%	100%	None	None	Dose for GFR 10–50
Diltiazem	I	100%	100%	100%	None	None	None

(continued)

TABLE 16-1 (Continued)

Drug	Adjustment method	GFR <50 mL/min	GFR 10–50 mL/min	GFR <10 mL/min	Hemodialysis	Peritoneal dialysis	Continuous renal replacement
Dimenhydrinate	I	q4–6h	q6–8h	q8h	Dose for GFR <10	Dose for GFR <10	Dose for GFR <10
Diphenhydramine	D	100%	100%	100%	None	None	None
Dipyridamole	D	100%	100%	100%	None	Dose for GFR <10	Not applicable
Dirithromycin	I	100%	100%	100%	None	No data: none	Dose for GFR 10–50
Disopyramide	I	q8h	q12–24h	q24–48h	No data	None	Dose for GFR 10–50
Dobutamine	D	100%	100%	100%	Not applicable	No data	Dose for GFR 10–50
Doxacurium	D	100%	50%	50%	Not applicable	Dose for GFR <10	Dose for GFR 10–50
Doxazosin	I	100%	100%	100%	None	None	Dose for GFR 10–50
Doxepin	D	100%	100%	100%	None	None	Dose for GFR 10–50
Doxorubicin	D	100%	100%	100%	None	None	Dose for GFR 10–50
Doxycycline	D	100%	100%	100%	None	None	Not applicable
Doxylamine	D	100%	100%	50%	Not applicable	Dose for GFR <10	Dose for GFR 10–50
Dyphylline	D	75%	50%	25%	Dose after dialysis	None	Dose for GFR <10
Efavirenz	I	100%	100%	100%	No dose adjustment	No dose adjustment	—
Emtricitabine	I	100%	100% q48–96h	100% q96h	Dose after dialysis	No data	No data
Emtricitabine/tenofovir	I	1 tablet q24h	1 tablet q48h	Avoid	Avoid	—	—
Enalapril	D	100%	50%–100%	25%	Dose after dialysis	Dose for GFR <10	Dose for GFR 10–50
Enalaprilat	D	100%	50%–100 %	25%–50 %	Dose after dialysis	Dose for GFR <10	Dose for GFR 10–50
Enfuvirtide	I	100%	100%	100%	No data	No data	—
Epirubicin	D	100%	100%	100%	None	None	Not applicable
Epoprostenol	I	100%	100%	100%	None	None	None
Eprosartan	I	100%	100%	100%	None	None	None
Ertapenem	D	100%	100% (see below)	50%	See comment below	Dose for GFR <10	—
Erythromycin	I	100%	100%	100%	None	None	None

Esmolol	D	100%	100%	100%	None	Dose for GFR 10–50
Estazolam	D	100%	100%	100%	None	Not applicable
Ethacrynic acid	—	q8–12h	q8–12h	Avoid	None	Not applicable
Ethambutol	—	q24h	q24–36h	q48h	Dose after dialysis	Dose for GFR 10–50
Ethchlorvynol	D	100%	Avoid	Avoid	Avoid	Not applicable
Ethionamide	D	100%	100%	50%	None	None
Ethosuximide	D	100%	100%	75%	Dose for normal renal function after dialysis	Increase dose by 25% and measure levels
Etodolac	D	100%	100%	100%	None	Dose for GFR 10–50
Etomidate	D	100%	100%	100%	Not applicable	Not applicable
Etoposide	D	100%	75%	50%	None	Not applicable
Famciclovir	D	100%	q12–24h	50% q24h	Dose after dialysis	No data: dose for GFR 10–50
Famotidine	D	50%–75%	10%–50%	10%	Dose after dialysis	Dose for GFR 10–50
Fazadinium	D	100%	100%	100%	None	Not applicable
Felbamate	D	75%–100%	50%–75%	50%	Dose after dialysis	Dose for GFR 10–50
Felodipine	—	100%	100%	100%	None	None
Fenoldopam	—	100%	100%	100%	None	None
Fenoprofen	D	100%	100%	50%	None	Not applicable
Fentanyl	D	75%	75%	50%	Not applicable	Not applicable
Fentanyl	D	100%	100%	100%	None	None
Fexofenadine	—	q12h	q12–24h	q24h	Dose for GFR <10	Dose for GFR <10
Flecainide	D	100%	50%	50%	None	Dose for GFR 10–50
Fluconazole	D	50%	50%	50%	Dose for GFR <10	Dose for GFR 10–50
Flucytosine	—	q12h	q12–24h	q24–48h	100% after dialysis	Dose for GFR <10
Fludarabine	D	100%	75%	50%	Dose after dialysis	Dose for GFR 10–50
Flumazenil	D	100%	100%	100%	None	Not applicable
Flunarizine	D	100%	100%	100%	None	Not applicable
Fluorouracil	D	100%	100%	100%	Give 1/2 dose	None
Fluoxetine	D	100%	100%	100%	None	Not applicable

(continued)

TABLE 16-1 *(Continued)*

Drug	Adjustment method	GFR <50 mL/min	GFR 10–50 mL/min	GFR <10 mL/min	Hemodialysis	Peritoneal dialysis	Continuous renal replacement
Flurazepam	D	100%	100%	100%	None	No data	Not applicable
Flurbiprofen	D	100%	100%	100%	None	None	Dose for GFR 10–50
Flutamide	D	100%	100%	100%	None	None	Not applicable
Fluvastatin	D	100%	100%	100%	None	None	Not applicable
Fluvoxamine	D	100%	100%	100%	None	None	Not applicable
Formoterol	—	100%	100%	100%	None	None	None
Fosamprenavir	—	No change	No change	No change	—	—	—
Fosamprenavir	—	700–1,400 mg q12	—	—	Not applicable	Not applicable	—
Foscarnet	D	28 mg/kg	15 mg/kg	6 mg/kg	Dose after dialysis	Dose for GFR <10	Dose for GFR 10–50
Fosinopril	D	100%	100%	75%–100%	None	None	Dose for GFR 10–50
Fosphenytoin	—	100%	100%	100%	None	None	None
Furosemide	—	100%	100%	100%	None	None	None
Gabapentin	D, I	400 mg t.i.d.	300 mg q12–24h	300 mg q.o.d.	300 mg load, then 200–300 post HD	300 mg q.o.d.	Dose for GFR 10–50
Gallamine	D	75%	Avoid	Avoid	Not applicable	Not applicable	Not applicable
Ganciclovir	I	50% q12–24h	25%–50% q24h	25% 3 × week	25% 3 × week	Dose for GFR <10	2.5 mg/kg q.d.
Ganciclovir-oral	D, I	1,500 mg q24h	500–1,000 mg q24h	500 mg q48–96h	500 mg 3 × weekly post HD	No data: dose for GFR <10	Not applicable
Gatifloxacin	D	100%	400 mg initially, then 200 mg daily	400 mg initially, then 200 mg daily	Dose as for GFR <10	Dose for GFR <10	—
Gemfibrozil	D	100%	75%	50%	None	Dose for GFR <10	Dose for GFR 10–50
Gemifloxacin	—	320 mg q.d.	160–320 mg q.d.	160 mg q.d.	Dose after dialysis	Dose for GFR <10	—

Drug	D/I	100% q8–24h	100% q12–48h by levels	100% q48–72h by levels	1/2 full dose after dialysis	3–4 mg/L d	Dose for GFR 10–50 and measure levels
Gentamicin	I						
Glibornuride	D	No data	No data	No data	No data	No data	Avoid
Gliclazide	D	50%–100%	Avoid	Avoid	No data	No data	Avoid
Glipizide	D	100%	50%	50%	None	Dose for GFR <10	Avoid
Glyburide	D	No data	Avoid	Avoid	None	None	Avoid
Gold sodium thiomalate	D	50%	Avoid	Avoid	None	None	Avoid
Griseofulvin	D	100%	100%	100%	None	None	None
Guanabenz	I	100%	100%	100%	None	None	Not applicable
Guanadrel	—	q12h	q12–24h	q24–48h	None	None	Not applicable
Guanethidine	—	q24h	q24h	q24–36h	No data	No data	Avoid
Guanfacine	—	100%	100%	100%	None	None	Dose for GFR 10–50
Haloperidol	D	100%	100%	100%	None	None	Not applicable
Heparin	D	100%	100%	100%	None	None	Dose for GFR 10–50
Hydralazine	—	q8h	q8h	q8–16h	Dose after dialysis	Dose for GFR <10	Dose for GFR 10–50
Hydrochlorothiazide	—	100%	100%	Ineffective	Not applicable	Not applicable	Not applicable
Hydrocortisone	D	100%	100%	100%	No data	None	No data: dose for GFR 10–50
Hydroflumethiazide	—	100%	100%	Ineffective	Not applicable	Not applicable	Not applicable
Hydroxyurea	D	100%	50%	20%	Dose after dialysis	None	Dose for GFR 10–50
Hydroxyzine	D	100%	50%	50%	Dose for GFR <10	Dose for GFR <10	Dose for GFR <10
Ibuprofen	D	100%	100%	100%	None	None	Dose for GFR 10–50
Idarubicin	—	100%	75%	50%	None	None	Avoid
Ifosfamide	D	100%	100%	75%	None	None	Dose for GFR 10–50
Iloprost	D	100%	100%	50%	None	None	Dose for GFR 10–50
Imipenem	D	100%	50%	25%	Dose after dialysis	Dose for GFR <10	Dose for GFR 10–50
Imipramine	D	100%	100%	100%	None	None	Not applicable
Indapamide	D	100%	100%	Ineffective	Ineffective	Ineffective	Ineffective

(continued)

TABLE 16-1 *(Continued)*

Drug	Adjustment method	GFR <50 mL/min	GFR 10–50 mL/min	GFR <10 mL/min	Hemodialysis	Peritoneal dialysis	Continuous renal replacement
Indinavir	—	No data: 100%	No data: 100%	No data: 100%	No adjustment necessary	No data: dose for GFR <10	No data
Indobufen	D	100%	50%	25%	No data	No data	Not applicable
Indomethacin	D	100%	100%	100%	None	None	Dose for GFR 10–50
Insulin	D	100%	75%	50%	None	None	Dose for GFR 10–50
Ipratropium	—	100%	100%	100%	None	None	None
Irbesartan	—	100%	100%	100%	No dose adjustment	No dose adjustment	No dose adjustment
Isoniazid	D	100%	100%	100%	Dose after dialysis	Dose for GFR <10	Dose for GFR <10
Isosorbide dinitrate	—	100%	100%	100%	None	None	None
Isosorbide mononitrate	—	100%	100%	100%	Dose after dialysis	None	Dose may need to be increased
Isradipine	—	100%	100%	100%	None	None	Dose for GFR 10–50
Itraconazole	D	100%	100%	50% (i.v. contraindicated)	100 mg q12–24h (oral only)	100 mg q12–24h (oral only)	Avoid
Kanamycin	—	100% q12–24h	100% q24–72h by levels	100% q48–72h by levels	1/2 fulldose after dialysis	15–20 mg/L·d	Dose for GFR 10–50 and measure levels
Ketamine	D	100%	100%	100%	Not applicable	Not applicable	Not applicable
Ketanserin	D	100%	100%	100%	None	None	Dose for GFR 10–50
Ketoconazole	D	100%	100%	100%	None	None	None
Ketoprofen	D	100%	75%	50%	None	None	Dose for GFR 10–50
Ketorolac	D	100%	50%	25%–50%	None	None	Dose for GFR 10–50
Labetalol	—	100%	100%	100%	None	None	Dose for GFR 10–50
Lamivudine	D, I	100%	50–150 mg q24h (full first dose)	25–50 mg q24h (50 mg first dose)	Dose after dialysis	No data: dose for GFR <10	Dose for GFR 10–50

Drug							
Lamivudine/zidovudine	—	100%	Avoid	Avoid	Avoid	Avoid	—
Lamotrigine	D	100%	75%	100 mg q.o.d.	100 mg after dialysis	Dose for GFR <10	Dose for GFR 10–50
Lansoprazole	D	100%	100%	100%	None	None	Not applicable
Levalbuterol	—	100%	100%	100%	None	None	None
Levetiracetam	D, I	500–1,000 mg q12h	250–750 mg q12h	500–1,000 mg q24h	250–500 mg after dialysis	Dose for GFR <10	Dose for GFR 10–50
Levodopa	D	100%	50%–100%	50%–100%	Dose after dialysis	Dose for GFR <10	Dose for GFR 10–50
Levofloxacin	D	100%	250–750 mg q24–48h (500–750 mg initial dose)	250–500 mg q48h (500 mg initial dose)	Dose for GFR <10	Dose for GFR <10	Dose for GFR 10–50
Lidocaine	D	100%	100%	100%	None	None	Dose for GFR 10–50
Lincomycin	—	q6h	q6–12h	q12–24h	None	None	Not applicable
Linezolid	—	100%	100%	100%	No dose adjustment	No dose adjustment	—
Lisinopril	D	100%	50%–75%	25%–50%	None	None	Dose for GFR 10–50
Lispro insulin	D	100%	75%	50%	None	None	None
Lithium carbonate	D	100%	50%–75%	25%–50%	Dose after dialysis	None	Dose for GFR 10–50
Lomefloxacin	D	100%	200–400 mg q24h	200 mg q24h	Dose for GFR <10	Dose for GFR <10	Not applicable
Lopinavir/ritonavir	—	400 mg q12h	400 mg q12h	400 mg q12h	No dose adjustment	No data	—
Loracarbef	—	q12h	q24h	q3–5 d	Dose after dialysis	No data: dose for GFR <10	Dose for GFR 10–50
Loratadine	—	q24h	q24–48h	q48h	Dose for GFR <10	Dose for GFR <10	Dose for GFR <10
Lorazepam	D	100%	100%	100%	None	None	Dose for GFR 10–50
Losartan	—	100%	100%	100%	None	None	None
Lovastatin	D	100%	100%	100%	Not applicable	Not applicable	Dose for GFR 10–50
Low molecular weight heparin	D	100%	100%	50%	Not applicable	Dose for GFR <10	Dose for GFR 10–50

(continued)

TABLE 16-1 *(Continued)*

Drug	Adjustment method	GFR <50 mL/min	GFR 10–50 mL/min	GFR <10 mL/min	Hemodialysis	Peritoneal dialysis	Continuous renal replacement
Mecamylamine	D	Avoid	Avoid	Avoid	Avoid	Avoid	Avoid
Meclofenamic acid	D	100%	100%	100%	None	None	Dose for GFR 10–50
Mefenamic acid	D	100%	100%	100%	None	None	Dose for GFR 10–50
Mefloquine	—	100%	No data: 100%	No data: 100%	None	No data: none	No data: dose for GFR 10–50
Melphalan	D	100%	75%	50%	Dose after dialysis	Dose for GFR <10	Dose for GFR 10–50
Meperidine	D	100%	75%	50%	Avoid	Avoid	Avoid
Meprobamate	—	q6h	q9–12h	q12–18h	None	Dose for GFR <10	Not applicable
Meropenem	D, I	100%	100% q12h	100% q24h	Dose after dialysis	Dose for GFR <10	Dose for GFR 10–50
Metaproterenol	—	100%	100%	100%	None	None	None
Metformin	D	50%	25%	Avoid	Not applicable	Avoid	Avoid
Methadone	D	100%	100%	50%–75%	None	None	Dose for GFR 10–50
Methenamine mandelate	D	100%	Avoid	Avoid	Not applicable	Not applicable	Not applicable
Methimazole	D	100%	100%	100%	None	None	Dose for GFR 10–50
Methotrexate	D	100%	50%	Avoid	Give 1/2 dose	None	Dose for GFR 10–50
Methsuximide	—	Avoid	Avoid	Avoid	No data	No data	No data: dose for GFR 10–50
Methyldopa	—	q8h	q8–12h	q12–24h	Dose after dialysis	Dose for GFR <10	Dose for GFR <10
Methylprednisolone	D	100%	100%	100%	Yes	None	Dose for GFR 10–50
Metoclopramide	D	100%	75%	50%	None	None	50%–75%
Metocurine	D	75%	50%	50%	Not applicable	Not applicable	Dose for GFR 10–50
Metolazone	D	100%	100%	100%	None	None	None
Metoprolol	D	100%	100%	100%	None	None	Dose for GFR 10–50
Metronidazole	D	100%	100%	100%	Dose after dialysis	Dose for GFR <10	Dose for GFR 10–50
Mexiletine	—	100%	100%	100%	None	None	None

Drug	Method						
Midazolam	D	100%	100%	50%	Not applicable	Not applicable	Not applicable
Midodrine	I	5–10 mg q8h	5–10 mg q8h	No data	5 mg q8h	No data	Dose for GFR 10–50
Milrinone	D	100%	100%	50%–75%	No data	No data	Dose for GFR 10–50
Minocycline	D	100%	100%	100%	None	None	None
Minoxidil	D	100%	100%	100%	Dose after dialysis	None	Dose for GFR 10–50
Mitomycin C	D	100%	100%	75%	No data	Dose for GFR <10	Not applicable
Mitoxantrone	D	100%	100%	100%	None	None	Dose for GFR 10–50
Mivacurium	D	100%	50%	50%	None	Dose for GFR <10	Not applicable
Moexipril	D	100%	50%	50%	Dose after dialysis	Dose for GFR <10	Dose for GFR 10–50
Moricizine	D	100%	100%	100%	None	None	Dose for GFR 10–50
Morphine	D	100%	75%	50%	None	No data	Dose for GFR 10–50
Moxifloxacin	I	100%	100%	100%	No data	No data	Dose for GFR 10–50
Nabumetone	D	100%	50%–100%	50%–100%	None	None	—
N-Acetylcysteine	D	100%	100%	75%	Not applicable	Dose for GFR <10	100%
N-Acetyl procainamide	D, I	100% q6–8h	50% q8–12h	25% q12–18h	None	None	Dose for GFR 10–50
Nadolol	I	q24h	q24–48h	q40–60h	Dose after dialysis	Dose for GFR <10	Dose for GFR 10–50
Nafcillin	D	100%	100%	100%	None	None	Dose for GFR 10–50
Nalidixic acid	D	Avoid	Avoid	Avoid	Avoid	Avoid	Not applicable
Naloxone	D	100%	100%	100%	Not applicable	Not applicable	Dose for GFR 10–50
Naproxen	D	100%	100%	100%	None	None	Dose for GFR 10–50
Nefazodone	D	100%	100%	100%	None	None	Not applicable
Nelfinavir	I	100%	100%	100%	None	None	No data
Neostigmine	D	100%	50%	25%	None	None	Dose for GFR 10–50
Nevirapine	I	100%	100%	100%	Dose after dialysis	No adjustment necessary	No data: dose for GFR 10–50
Nicardipine	I	100%	100%	100%	None	None	None
Nicotinic acid	D	100%	50%	25%	None	Dose for GFR <10	Dose for GFR 10–50
Nifedipine	I	100%	100%	100%	No dose adjustment	No dose adjustment	No dose adjustment
Nimodipine	D	100%	100%	100%	None	None	Dose for GFR 10–50
Nisoldipine	I	100%	100%	100%	None	None	None

(continued)

TABLE 16-1 (Continued)

Drug	Adjustment method	GFR <50 mL/min	GFR 10–50 mL/min	GFR <10 mL/min	Hemodialysis	Peritoneal dialysis	Continuous renal replacement
Nitrofurantoin	D	Avoid < 60	Avoid	Avoid	Not applicable	Not applicable	Not applicable
Nitroglycerine	D	100%	100%	100%	No data	No data	Dose for GFR 10–50
Nitroprusside	I	100%	100%	Avoid	Avoid	Avoid	Dose for GFR 10–50
Nitrosoureas	D	100%	75%	25%–50%	None	Dose for GFR <10	Not applicable
Nizatidine	D, I	75%–100%	150 mg q24–48h	150 mg q48–72h	Dose for GFR <10	Dose for GFR <10	Dose for GFR 10–50
Norfloxacin	I	q12h	q12–24h	400 mg q24h	Dose for GFR <10	Dose for GFR <10	Not applicable
Nortriptyline	D	100%	100%	100%	None	None	Not applicable
Ofloxacin	D	100%	200–400 mg q24h	200 mg q24h	100–200 mg after dialysis	Dose for GFR <10	300 mg/d
Olmesartan	D	100%	100%	50%	None	Dose for GFR <10	None
Omeprazole	D	100%	100%	100%	None	None	Not applicable
Ondansetron	D	100%	100%	100%	None	None	Not applicable
Orphenadrine	D	100%	100%	100%	Dose for GFR <10	Dose for GFR <10	Dose for GFR <10
Oseltamivir	I	100%	q.d. (treatment); q.o.d. (prophylaxis)	q.o.d.	30 mg on nondialysis days	30 mg twice weekly	100%
Ouabain	I	q12–24h	q24–36h	q36–48h	None	None	Dose for GFR 10–50
Oxaproxin	D	100%	100%	100%	None	None	Dose for GFR 10–50
Oxatomide	D	100%	100%	100%	Dose for GFR <10	Dose for GFR <10	Dose for GFR <10
Oxazepam	D	100%	100%	100%	None	None	Not applicable
Oxcarbazepine	D	100%	75%–100%	50%	Dose for GRF <10; give after dialysis	Dose for GFR <10	Dose for GFR 10–50
Paclitaxel	D	100%	100%	100%	None	None	Not applicable
Pancuronium	D	100%	50%	Avoid	Avoid	Avoid	Not applicable

Paroxetine	D	100%	50%–75%	50%	None	Dose for GFR <10	Not applicable
PAS	D	100%	50%–75%	50%	Dose after dialysis	Dose for GFR <10	Dose for GFR <10
Penbutolol	D	100%	100%	100%	None	None	Dose for GFR 10–50
Penicillamine	D	100%	Avoid	Avoid	1/3 dose	Avoid	Not applicable
Penicillin G	D	100%	75%	20%–50%	Dose after dialysis	Dose for GFR <10	Dose for GFR 10–50
Penicillin VK	D	100%	100%	100%	Dose after dialysis	Dose for GFR <10	Not applicable
Pentamidine (i.v.)	I	q24h	q24h	q24–36h	Dose for GFR <10; 0.75 g after each HD	Dose for GFR <10	None
Pentazocine	D	100%	75%	50%	None	No data	Not applicable
Pentobarbital	D	100%	100%	100%	None	None	Not applicable
Pentopril	D	100%	50%–75%	50%	No data	No data	Dose for GFR 10–50
Pentoxifylline	—	q8–12h	q12–24h	q24h	None	Dose for GFR <10	Not applicable
Perindopril	D, I	2 mg q24h	2 mg q24–48h	2 mg q48h	Dose before dialysis; 1/2 dose after dialysis	Dose for GFR <10	Dose for GFR 10–50
Phenobarbital	I	q8–12h	q8–12h	q12–16h	Dose for GFR <10	1/2 normal dose	Normal dose and measure levels
Phenoxybenzamine	—	100%	1 mg t.i.d.	Avoid	Avoid	Avoid	Avoid
Phenylbutazone	D	100%	50%	Avoid	None	None	Not applicable
Phenytoin	—	100%	100%	100%	None	None	None
Pindolol	D	100%	100%	100%	None	None	Dose for GFR 10–50
Pipecuronium	D	100%	50%	25%	None	None	Dose for GFR 10–50
Piperacillin	—	q6h	q6–12h	q12h	2 g q8h plus 1 g after HD	Dose for GFR <10	Dose for GFR 10–50
Piperacillin/tazobactam	D, I	100%	2.25 g q6h (q8h if <20)	2.25 g q8h	Dose for GFR <10; 1.125 g after HD	4.5 g q12h	4.5 g q8h
Pirbuterol	—	100%	100%	100%	None	None	None
Piretanide	D	100%	100%	100%	None	None	Not applicable
Piroxicam	D	100%	100%	100%	None	None	Dose for GFR 10–50
Plicamycin	D	100%	75%	50%	None	Dose for GFR <10	Not applicable

(continued)

TABLE 16-1 (Continued)

Drug	Adjustment method	GFR <50 mL/min	GFR 10–50 mL/min	GFR <10 mL/min	Hemodialysis	Peritoneal dialysis	Continuous renal replacement
Polythiazide	D	100%	100%	Ineffective	Ineffective	Ineffective	Ineffective
Pravastatin	D	100%	100%	100%	None	None	Not applicable
Prazosin	I	100%	100%	100%	None	None	Not applicable
Prednisolone	D	100%	100%	100%	Yes	None	Not applicable
Prednisone	D	100%	100%	100%	None	None	Not applicable
Primaquine	I	No data: 100%	No data: 100%	No data: 100%	No data: none	No data: none	No data: dose for GFR 10–50
Primidone	I	q12h	q12–24h	q24h	Dose after dialysis	No data	No data
Probenecid	D	100%	Avoid	Avoid	Avoid	None	Avoid
Probucol	D	100%	100%	100%	None	None	Not applicable
Procainamide	I	q4h	q6–12h	q8–24h	Follow levels	None	Dose for GFR 10–50
Promethazine	D	100%	100%	100%	Dose for GFR <10	Dose for GFR <10	Dose for GFR <10
Promethazine	D	100%	100%	100%	None	None	Not applicable
Propafenone	I	100%	100%	100%	None	None	None
Propofol	D	100%	100%	100%	None	None	Not applicable
Propoxyphene	D	100%	100%	Avoid	Avoid	Avoid	Avoid
Propranolol	I	100%	100%	100%	None	None	Dose for GFR 10–50
Propylthiouracil	D	100%	100%	100%	None	None	Not applicable
Protriptyline	D	100%	100%	100%	None	None	Not applicable
Pyrazinimide	D	100%	100%	50%–100%	40 mg/kg 24h before each 3 times/wk dialysis	100%	No data
Pyridostigmine	D	50%	35%	20%	None	None	Dose for GFR 10–50
Pyrimethamine	I	100%	100%	100%	None	None	None
Quazepam	D	100%	100%	100%	None	None	Not applicable

Drug							
Quinapril	D	100%	2.5–5 mg q24h	2.5 mg	Dose for GFR <10	Dose for GFR <10	Dose for GFR 10–50
Quinidine	D	100%	100%	75%	Dose after dialysis	None	None
Quinine	—	q8h	q8–12h	q24h	Dose after dialysis	Dose for GFR <10	Dose for GFR 10–50
Quinupristin/ dalfopristin	—	100%	100%	100%	No dose adjustment	No dose adjustment	—
Ramipril	D	100%	25%–50%	25%	Dose after dialysis	Dose for GFR <10	Dose for GFR 10–50
Ranitidine	D, I	75%	150 mg q12–24h	75–150 mg q24h	Dose after dialysis	Dose for GFR <10	Dose for GFR 10–50
Reserpine	D	100%	100%	Avoid	None	None	Not applicable
Ribavirin	D	100%	Avoid	Avoid	Avoid	Avoid	Avoid
Rifabutin	—	100%	100%	100%	None	None	No data: dose for GFR 10–50
Rifampin	D	100%	50%–100%	50%–100%	None	Dose for GFR <10	Dose for GFR <10
Rifaximin	—	200 mg p.o. t.i.d.	100%	100%	—	—	—
Ritonavir	—	100%	100%	100%	None	None	No data: dose for GFR 10–50
Salmeterol	—	100%	100%	100%	None	None	None
Saquinavir	—	100%	100%	100%	None	No data: dose for GFR <10	No data: dose for GFR 10–50
Secobarbital	D	100%	100%	100%	None	None	Not applicable
SEE COMMENT							
Sertraline	D	100%	100%	100%	None	None	Not applicable
Simvastatin	D	100%	100%	100%	None	None	Not applicable
Sotalol	—	q12h	q24–48h	q48–72h	Dose after dialysis	None	Dose for GFR <10
Spectinomycin	D	100%	100%	100%	None	None	None
Spironolactone	—	q6–12h	q12–24h	Avoid	None	None	Avoid
Stavudine	D, I	100%	50% q12–24h	50% q24h	Dose for GFR <10 (after dialysis)	No data	No data: dose for GFR 10–50
Streptokinase	D	100%	100%	100%	Not applicable	Not applicable	Not applicable

(continued)

TABLE 16-1 *(Continued)*

Drug	Adjustment method	GFR <50 mL/min	GFR 10–50 mL/min	GFR <10 mL/min	Hemodialysis	Peritoneal dialysis	Continuous renal replacement
Streptomycin	D, I	q24h	q24–72h	q72–96h	1/2 normal dose after dialysis	20–40 mg/L d	Dose for GFR 10–50 and measure levels
Streptozocin	D	100%	75%	50%	Not applicable	Not applicable	Not applicable
Succinylcholine	D	100%	100%	100%	Not applicable	Dose for GFR <10	Not applicable
Sufentanil	D	100%	100%	100%	No data	No data	Dose for GFR 10–50
Sufentanil	D	100%	100%	100%	Not applicable	Not applicable	Dose for GFR 10–50
Sulfamethoxazole	—	q12h	q18h	q24h	1.0 g after dialysis	1.0 g/d	Dose for GFR 10–50
Sulfinpyrazone	D	100%	50%	Avoid	None	None	Dose for GFR 10–50
Sulfisoxazole	—	q6h	q8–12h	q12–24h	2.0 g after dialysis	3.0 g/d	Not applicable
Sulindac	D	100%	100%	100%	None	None	Not applicable
Sulotroban	D	50%	30%	10%	No data	No data	No data
Tamoxifen	D	100%	100%	100%	None	None	Not applicable
Telithromycin	—	100%	100%	100%	No data	No data	No data
Telmisartan	—	100%	100%	100%	None	None	None
Temazepam	D	100%	100%	100%	None	None	Not applicable
Teniposide	D	100%	100%	100%	None	None	Not applicable
Tenofovir	—	100%	Avoid	Avoid	Avoid	Avoid	—
Terazosin	—	100%	100%	100%	None	None	Dose for GFR 10–50
Terbutaline	—	100%	50%	50%	Dose after dialysis	None	None
Tetracycline	D	q8–12h	q12–24h	q24h	None	None	Dose for GFR 10–50
Theophylline	— D	100%	100%	100%	125% during dialysis	None	125% during CRRT and measure levels
Thiazides	D	100%	100%	Avoid	Not applicable	Not applicable	Not applicable
Thiopental	D	100%	100%	75%	Not applicable	Not applicable	Not applicable

Drug	Method						
Tiagabine	—	100%	100%	100%	None	None	Dose for GFR 10–50
Ticarcillin/clavulanate	D, I	100%	3.1 g q8–12h	2 g q12h	Dose for GFR <10 and 3.1 g after dialysis	3.1 g q12h	Dose for GFR 10–50
Ticlopidine	D	100%	100%	100%	None	None	Not applicable
Timolol	—	100%	100%	100%	No dose adjustment	No dose adjustment	Dose for GFR 10–50
Tobramycin	I	100% q8–24h	100% q24–48h by levels	100% q48–72h by levels	1/2 full dose after dialysis	3–4 mg/L d	Dose for GFR 10–50 and measure levels
Tocainide	D	100%	100%	50%	Dose after dialysis	None	Dose for GFR 10–50
Tolazamide	D	100%	100%	100%	None	None	Avoid
Tolbutamide	D	100%	100%	100%	None	None	Avoid
Tolmetin	D	100%	100%	100%	None	None	Not applicable
Topiramate	D	100%	50%	25%	Dose for normal renal function after dialysis	Dose for GFR 10–50	Dose for normal renal function during CRRT
Topotecan	D	75%	50%	25%	Avoid	Avoid	Not applicable
Torsemide	—	100%	100%	100%	None	None	None
Trandolapril	—	100%	50%–100 %	50%	None	None	Dose for GFR 10–50
Tranexamic acid	D	50%	25%	10%	Avoid	Avoid	Not applicable
Trazodone	D	100%	100%	100%	None	None	Not applicable
Triamcinolone	D	100%	100%	100%	None	None	Not applicable
Triamterene	—	q12h	Avoid	Avoid	Not applicable	Not applicable	Not applicable
Triazolam	D	100%	100%	100%	None	None	Not applicable
Trimethoprim	—	q12h	q12h above 30 mL/min, q18h for 10–30 mL/min	q24h	Dose after dialysis	Dose for GFR <10	q18h

(continued)

TABLE 16-1 *(Continued)*

Drug	Adjustment method	GFR <50 mL/min	GFR 10–50 mL/min	GFR <10 mL/min	Hemodialysis	Peritoneal dialysis	Continuous renal replacement
Trimetrexate	D	100%	No data: 50%–100%; avoid for serum creatinine >2.5 mg/dL	Avoid	No data	No data	No data
Trimipramine	D	100%	100%	100%	None	None	Not applicable
Tripelennamine	–	No data	No data	No data	No data	No data	No data
Triprolidine	–	No data	No data	No data	No data	No data	Not applicable
Tubocurarine	D	75%	50%	Avoid	Not applicable	Not applicable	Not applicable
Urokinase	D	100%	100%	100%	None	None	Not applicable
Valacyclovir	D, I	100%	Full dose q12–24h	0.5 g q24h	Dose after dialysis	Dose for GFR <10	No data: dose for GFR 10–50
Valganciclovir	D, I	GFR 40–59; induction 450 mg b.i.d.; maintenance 450 mg q.d.	GFR 25–39; induction 450 mg q.d.; maintenance 450 mg q2 d	GFR 10–24; induction 450 mg q2 d; maintenance 450 mg twice weekly	Dose after dialysis	Dose for GFR <10	–
Valproic acid	D	100%	100%	100%	Dose after dialysis	Dose for GFR <10	None
Valsartan	–	100%	100%	100%	None	None	None
Vancomycin	D, I	1.0 g q12–24h	1.0 g q24–96h	1.0 g q4–7 d	Dose for GFR <10	Dose for GFR <10	Dose for GFR 10–50
Vecuronium	D	100%	100%	100%	Not applicable	Not applicable	Not applicable
Venlafaxine	D	75%	50%	50%	None	None	None
Verapamil	–	100%	100%	100%	None	None	None
Vigabatrin	I	q24h	q48h	q48–72h	Dose after dialysis	Dose for GFR <10	q24h during CRRT

	Method	100% (>50)	(10–50)	(<10)			
Vinblastine	D	100%	100%	100%	None	None	Not applicable
Vincristine	D	100%	100%	100%	None	None	Not applicable
Vinorelbine	D	100%	100%	100%	None	None	Not applicable
Voriconazole	—	100%	100% (i.v. not recommended)	100% (i.v. not recommended)	No adjustment necessary (oral only)	No adjustment necessary (oral only)	—
Warfarin	D	100%	100%	100%	None	None	None
Zafirlukast	D	100%	100%	100%	None	None	Not applicable
Zalcitabine	I, D	100%	q12h	q24h	No data: dose after dialysis	No data	No data: dose for GFR 10–50
Zanamivir	D	100%	100%	100%	No dose adjustment	No dose adjustment	—
Zidovudine	D, I	100%	100%	100 mg q8h	Dose for GFR <10	Dose for GFR <10	100 mg q8h
Zileuton	—	100%	100%	100%	None	None	Not applicable
Zonisamide	D	75%–100%	50%–75%	50%	Dose for GFR <10	Dose for GFR <10	Dose for GFR 10–50

GFR, glomerular filtration rate; HD, hemodialysis.

the minimum trough level must be maintained, modification of the individual dose or a combination of the dose and interval methods may be preferred.

V. DRUG DOSING IN PATIENTS ON DIALYSIS

Drug removal by hemodialysis (HD) is most effective for drugs that weigh less than 500 Da, are less than 90% protein bound, and those that have small volumes of distribution. In Table 16-1 are also listed commonly used drugs removed by HD or peritoneal dialysis. For many drugs, alter the dosage schedule such that the dose can be given at the end of the HD treatment, thereby eliminating the need for a reloading dose. For example, give aminoglycosides to patients on chronic HD as a postdialysis dose.

Continuous renal replacement therapies (CRRTs), such as continuous venovenous hemofiltration (CVVH) and sustained low-efficiency dialysis (SLED) are frequently used to maintain fluid and electrolyte homeostasis and remove waste products in critically ill patients. The rate and extent of drug removal by CRRT depends less on the molecular weight of the drug and more on the degree of drug protein binding, volume of distribution, membrane characteristics, blood flow rate, the amount of hemofiltration by convection, and the addition of dialysate to the extracorporeal circuit. During continuous therapies, substantial drug removal may occur. Following drug levels during prolonged continuous or frequent intermittent renal replacement therapies will be the best guide to drug dosing. The serum creatinine, as an estimate of creatinine clearance, can be used as an estimate of drug clearance during CRRT for drugs that are not highly protein bound and have relatively small volumes of distribution. Underestimating drug removal in these circumstances risks ineffective therapy.

VI. ADVERSE DRUG REACTIONS

Adverse drug reactions occur more frequently in patients with impaired renal function. Untoward effects may be the result of direct toxicity or additive effects of the drug or its metabolites. The lack of efficacy of the drug in patients with compromised renal function, or increased drug-induced metabolic load also causes adverse drug effects. The acute onset of any unexplained symptoms should alert clinicians of a possible adverse drug effect.

VII. THERAPEUTIC DRUG MONITORING

Measurement of plasma drug concentrations may be helpful in assessing a particular drug-dosing regimen when efficacy or toxicity corresponds to drug levels. These measurements are most important for drugs with a narrow therapeutic range or for drugs whose pharmacologic effects are not easily measured.

Measure serum levels following administration of an appropriate loading dose. If no loading dose is administered, give three or four doses of the drug before measuring serum levels to ensure that steady-state serum concentrations have been established. For some drugs, both maximum and minimum concentrations are relevant. Peak levels are most meaningful when measured after rapid drug distribution has occurred. For example, measure aminoglycoside peak concentrations 30 minutes after the end of the infusion; minimum concentrations are usually measured just before administration of the next scheduled dose. Included in Table 16-1 are recommendations for drug level monitoring. Appropriate pharmacokinetic application of drug level measurements can improve patient care and decrease cost.

Patients with renal disease are heterogeneous and their responses to drug therapy are variable. Dosage nomograms, drug tables, and computer-assisted dosing recommendations should not be taken as a fixed approach to therapy in patients with decreased renal function. They are initial attempts to arrive at an effective dose regimen. Physicians using sound clinical judgment in caring for patients with renal disease evaluate each situation, choose a drug regimen based on all factors, and continually reevaluate the response to therapy.

Suggested Readings

Aronoff GR. Drugs and the kidney. *Curr Opin Nephrol Hypertens* 1993;2(2):187–191.
Aronoff GR, Bennett WM, Berns JS, et al. *Drug prescribing in renal failure. Dosing guidelines for adults and children.* Philadelphia: American College of Physicians, 2007.

Note: Page numbers followed by *f* indicate figures; those followed by *t* indicate tables.